Patrick Kenis, Bernd Marin (Eds.)

Managing AIDS

Organizational Responses in Six European Countries

Ashgate

Aldershot · Brookfield USA · Singapore · Sydney

Published by

Ashgate Publishing Limited
Gower House
Croft Road
Aldershot
Hants GU11 3HR
England

Ashgate Publishing Company
Old Post Road
Brookfield
Vermont 05036
USA

Composition: Michael Eigner
European Centre for Social Welfare Policy and Research
Berggasse 17
1090 Vienna
Austria

British Library Cataloguing-in-Publication Data. A catalogue record for this book is available from the British Library.

ISBN 1-85972-126-5

Printed by Druck Partner Rübelmann, Germany.

Contents

List of Figures and Tables

A) List of Figures

B)   List of Tables

Preface

Studying the "organizational response" to a phenomenon such as HIV/AIDS, which is having a profound and personal effect on so many individuals, might at first sight be seen as yet another detached scientific interpretation of a grave situation by researchers addressing a problem by applying traditional disciplines and approaches. Although most researchers who have contributed to the present Volume are indeed organizational researchers, their *Erkenntnisinteresse* for turning their attention to HIV/AIDS was quite a different one. After a first period, in which many scientists focused on the medical aspects of HIV/AIDS, a number of significant social aspects and consequences which arose from the phenomenon and this approach to it became apparent. One of them was that organizations seemed to react in decidedly different ways to this new disease and to those affected by it. Some reactions were uneducated, even hostile, or helpless at best; some organizations, however, developed conspicuously constructive, open-minded and innovative initiatives. It was particularly this manifest difference in human effectiveness between different organizations in dealing with the issue, and the fact that this distinction has a significant influence on the prevention of HIV transmissions and the personal and social consequences of HIV/AIDS, which motivated us to look into the reasons for these differences in organizational responses in greater detail.

The *Managing AIDS* project, of which some results are published in the present Volume, began in 1989 as a WHO Collaborative Study. Its design was developed in close collaboration with the World Health Organization (WHO) and the European Council of Aids Service Organizations (EuroCASO). One of the main initial challenges of the project was to find country teams who were able to mobilize the resources necessary to carry out this quite unconventional type of research – compared to the great number of medical or behavioural studies which have been initiated and undertaken in this area. We are fortunate that six of the initially started nine countries made it to this Volume (one country is only presented by one of its regions however, i.e. Belgium). The data for the study were collected in the period between 1992 and 1995.

The Volume presents the results of these country studies. All chapters are comparable since all countries used the same research design, however, they at the same time also pointed out and reflected on the specifics of the particular country under analysis. In Chapter One we summarize the motivation for and the logic of the research design. Since this research design has undergone a number of changes (as natural consequence of a project's life-cycle), we also include the original research design for documentary reasons (Annex II). For methodological reasons, the two main research instruments used by the different countries, i.e. the "European AIDS Service Organizations Inventory Sheet" (Annex III) and the "*Managing AIDS* Questionnaire" (Annex IV) are also included. Although the findings reported in the country chapters primarily rely on data gathered from the first research instrument, the second research instrument elucidates the chosen approach more comprehensively. Furthermore, a number of other publications produced in the context of the *Managing AIDS* project, which are cited throughout the different country chapters, also primarily rely on data from the *Managing AIDS* Questionnaire.

This volume would never have come about without the help of many organizations and dedicated persons. First of all we would like to thank the literally thousands of organizations active in the field of HIV/AIDS who shared their time, insights, and information with us – without whom this study simply could not have been undertaken. We would also like to thank those who were decisive in the initial phase of this project and who helped get the study off the ground: Jan Branckaerts, Svein-Erik Ekeid, Brigitte Gredler, Henning Mikkelsen, and Gorm Kirsch of WHO/Euro and Kurt Krickler and Arne Husdal of EuroCASO. We are also indebted to the home institutions of the different country teams who provided the necessary financial support. We would also like to thank not just those country teams presented in this volume but also those who invested quite some time and energy in contributing to the research design and lively exchanges over country experiences but who could not hold with the project to the end due to the lack of research resources: Pat Warren and Andrew Bebbington from the U.K., Mauro Guillén and Charles Perrow from the USA, Alain Anciaux and Françoise Weil from the French part of Belgium, Hugues Lagrange and Sebastian Roché from France, Endre Sik, Éva István and Agnes Czako from Hungary, Fausto Amaro and Vitoria Mourão from Portugal, and Michel Perreault from Canada.

Finally, our thanks go out to the staff at the European Centre for their dedicated and continuous help in the revisions and finalization of this Volume. Klarissa Guzei and Christiana Nöstlinger had an essential role in the project in helping to manage, systematize, classify and make sense of the enormous amount of data produced in this project. Michael Eigner, Vanessa Proudman and Willem Stamatiou have given key inputs to the legibility of the text, tables and graphs.

We would like to dedicate this book to all those people whom we met in the course of this project and who personally managed to live dignified lives with HIV/AIDS. They taught us what it means to live up to one's own life – which, according to Karl Kraus one doesn't even live once – under great uncertainties, and what one can do to fight AIDS. Their courage and wisdom acquired under adverse circumstances of painful human deficiencies helps us also to come alive to the fact that this study is only a very small contribution to what can and should be done, and it is intended to learn from and assist to upgrade what *is* being done.

October 1997 Patrick Kenis (Constance) / Bernd Marin (Vienna)

CHAPTER 1

Managing AIDS: Analysing the Organizational Responses to HIV/AIDS in European Countries

Patrick Kenis
Bernd Marin

1   HIV/AIDS: Analysing Organizational Responses

1.1   Introduction

The sudden emergence of HIV/AIDS in the 1980s turned out to be a disaster for the communities most grievously affected, and indeed for society as a whole. HIV/AIDS is publicly much less dramatically discussed nowadays compared to the mid-1980s when the problem was perceived as a national crisis in most European countries, even though the number of persons affected by HIV/AIDS is still steadily increasing worldwide. In most European countries it is not only the number of persons living with HIV/AIDS which is on the increase, but also the number of newly diagnosed AIDS cases (see Figure A2 in Annex 1).

Given the reality of this crisis which affects many individuals, social groups and societies, and given the fact that we have learned that modern societies can and will be confronted with new, destructive and lasting diseases such as HIV/AIDS, the crucial question is who and how should they intervene in such a situation?

The present volume sets out to empirically describe and analyse one specific and admittedly limited – although highly under-investigated – type of intervention, namely the organizational response to HIV/AIDS. In contrast to most of the existing social science contributions within the field of HIV/AIDS, which analyse the response either on the micro-level of individual behaviour or on the national macro-level, this study's focus of attention will be on the meso-level of organiza-tions. Analysing the organizational response to HIV/AIDS implies studying the degree of organizational representation as well as the conditions which explain the difference in the frequency, type and distribution of organizations which develop activities for reducing HIV transmissions and for improving the personal and social impact of HIV/AIDS. Consequently, the study is less to be seen as a public policy analysis of national HIV/AIDS policies, but rather as a study of the response by a wide variety of sources of collective action, such as public organizations, private organizations, non-profit organizations, community-based organizations, etc., which provide a wide variety of activities, such as prevention, care, policy coordination, interest intermediation, fund-raising, etc.

Before turning to a detailed description of what is meant by the organizational response, and how it has been analysed in the present study, our approach will be compared to a number of more commonly studied forms of interventions or insti-tutional responses which have been developed in the last 15 years to cope with HIV/AIDS.

1.2   The Institutional Response to HIV/AIDS

Apart from the "non-response" to or the "repression" of the HIV/AIDS problem, four other types of responses can be distinguished: the medical, the behavioural, the administrative and the organizational. These different types of responses should clearly be seen as ideal-typical or paradigmatic constructions. The pure form of response exists very seldom in reality. However, they correlate with and therefore point to specific phenomena such as the types of solutions chosen in practice, specific types of actors assigned to the problem, the areas to which resources are allocated, the specific norms, values and belief systems on which policies are based, etc. The best way to imagine what is meant here is to ask oneself the question what would I do were I to have to decide how to solve the problem of HIV/AIDS. One tends to think in a paradigmatic way and either the virus, the individual behaviour of persons, laws and regulations or social contexts (such as communities or or-ganizations) comes to one's mind.

The order in which the responses will be presented below coincides by and large with the order in which they have appeared on the policy scene.

After a period of *non-response*[1] (Perrow/Guillén, 1991), medical research suc-cessfully defined the new disease as AIDS,[2] identified its cause, i.e. the Human Immune Deficiency Virus,[3] identified the modes of transmission of the HIV[4] and developed a test[5] to identify carriers of the virus. It is consequently the virus and its symptoms which are at the centre of attention of the *medical response*. The medical knowledge about HIV and AIDS has increased considerably in the last ten years. Medicines to directly combat the virus (e.g. AZT, ddI, ddC, etc.) have turned out to be marginally effective in increasing the life chances of persons infected. They also help lengthen the a-symptomatic period[6] of HIV infection. In general, medicine has indeed contributed a lot to the increase of the average life expectancy of people with AIDS. The fact remains, however, that at this moment in time neither a totally effective treatment nor a vaccine exists; it is also widely recognized that such a treatment or vaccine will neither be available in the near future.

Having realized that due to the complexity of HIV and the AIDS disease, a medical solution to the problem would take a long and too long a time to develop, a response appeared which considered *behavioural change* as the solution to the problem of the transmission of HIV. This solution is based on the supply of "information" on the risks of certain behaviour with respect to the transmission of the HIV. The idea is that people should change their behaviour as a result of fear of a possible risk situation. Consequently, a great deal of information is being supplied, much of it especially directed towards the general public. It is, however, questionable and many studies have indeed shown that it is unlikely that people will only change their behaviour on the basis of information on the expected risks of particular choices. On the basis of an argument made by Hirschman (1982), one can assume that people in such situations rather change their behaviour on the basis of the "experiences of risk" instead of on the basis of the "expectations of risk". However, experience of risk is contingent on many more factors than the supply of information as will be shown later.

Parallel to the development of the behavioural response and in some cases as a consequence of the fact that it turned out that people do not simply change their behaviour on the basis of information, *regulative responses* have developed in some countries, inducing mandatory behavioural rules. Whereas in the previous approach, the idea is to leave the problem to the individual, here, the idea is to have rules for behaviour specified by a third party, i.e. usually the state. Examples of political and administrative regulations that deal with the problem of HIV/AIDS are: compulsory testing (e.g. pre-employment HIV screening), bringing HIV/AIDS into the sphere of criminal law (by prosecuting those who infect others) or isolating HIV-positive persons or people with AIDS. The state is confronted with a fundamental problem when it comes to such administrative regulation (de Vroom, 1991): on the one hand, it must protect the individual freedom of its citizens and ensure that there is no discrimination, but on the other hand, health is seen as a public good which must also be assured by that very same state. Therefore, the state faces the dilemma of having to choose between protecting individual freedom at the expense of public well-being – or vice versa, protecting public health and welfare at the expense of personal freedom. Aside from this dilemma, another problem arises with regard to political and administrative regulation (especially when it comes to prevention): it is almost impossible for the state to regulate social phenomena which are so closely linked to the private sphere. Aside from the many normative problems, state intervention would at the same time imply a "larger bureaucracy than anyone has yet conceived and methods of surveillance bigger than Big Brother" (Wildavsky cited in Bayer, 1989: 82).

A whole spectrum of *organizational responses* have developed which have run in parallel to all of the above responses and which started very early on in the crisis. However, their potentiality as an effective response to alleviating the problem of HIV/AIDS remained remarkably unnoticed by scientists and policy-makers for considerable time. Although many would agree with Perrow and Guillén's statement that "... it is inconceivable that a serious social problem such as an epidemic could have any other solution or mitigation than an organizational one ..." (Perrow/ Guillén, 1990: 150), it took researchers and policy-makers a while to recognize that the degree of HIV transmissions as well as that of the personal and social impact of HIV/AIDS was in fact greatly dependent on the development and responsiveness of organizations.

A graphical overview of the different institutional responses described above is presented in Figure 1.1.

Figure 1.1:   Institutional Responses to the Problem of HIV/AIDS

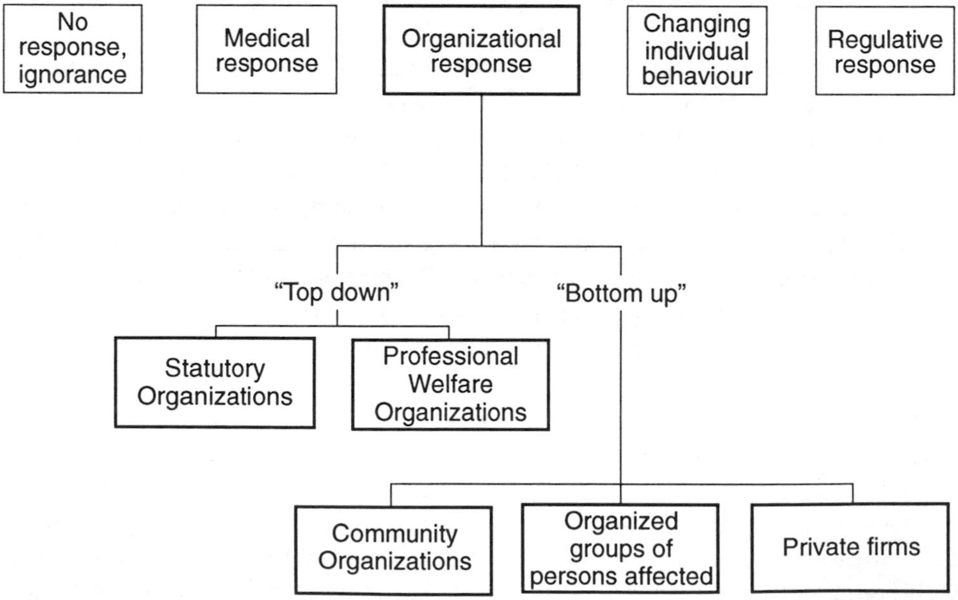

Source: Kenis/de Vroom, 1996.

Whereas there is an enormous amount of research in the area of the medical and behavioural response and a considerable amount of research on the regulatory response, the study of the organizational response to HIV/AIDS has been neglected. Only a handful of studies exist which look at the contribution organizations have made to alleviating the problem of HIV/AIDS in a specific and systematic way.[7] A double bias, either *micro* or *macro*, seems to exist in the literature on HIV/AIDS (the *micro* level being the level of behaviour, and the *macro* level being the level of political discourse, policy and planning). The present study is on the other hand located on the *meso* level or the intermediate level, i.e. the level on which organizations are located. The significance of considering this level as an independent level of analysis will become especially apparent in the different country studies. It will be illustrated that the organizational response is only weakly determined by micro-level phenomena, i.e. the needs of people, epidemiological case-loads, etc. Second, it will also become clear that although the macro-level, i.e. the level of planning and policy, to a certain extent influences the organizational level, it does not do so in a deterministic way. One can observe, however, that existing general health and welfare policies and AIDS policies – often countervailing organizational activities – have nevertheless been developed from the bottom-up which are only loosely coupled to the macro level of policy-making.[8] This phenomenon is clearly illustrated by one of the questions Bennet and Ferlie pose in their study on the National Health Service in Britain: "how is it possible to develop drug service organizations in a community where there is a strong value system that operates to condemn any form of drug use?" (Bennet/Ferlie, 1994: 53). Concentrating exclusively on either the micro or macro level does in fact hide much of what is really going on in a country, region or social group.

As will be seen later, there are many different ways of portraying types and forms of organizational responses. One example is provided in Figure 1.1 where the organizational response is classified by whether it is "top-down" or "bottom-up". It is the contribution that these type of organizations make to solving the problem of HIV/AIDS as well as organizations classified by other criteria which are matters at the centre of attention in the "Managing AIDS" project and the present volume in which some of its findings are presented.

It should be mentioned that the term "organizational response", as one type of institutional response, is far from ideal, since even within the other mentioned institutional responses (especially the medical and administrative ones) organizations are often the main actors (research labs, ministries, parliaments, etc.). Using the label "organizational response" does, however, seem nevertheless useful for the type of phenomena our study is primarily interested in. First, the label specifically directs one's attention to the importance of the organizational dimension in the existence and availability of HIV/AIDS-specific activities, e.g. Why do some organizations become active in the context of HIV/AIDS and why do others not?

Secondly, in social policy literature there is no concept which more effectively conceptualizes what is meant here by organizational response given its specificity as presented in Figure 1.1.[9] The usefulness of applying an organizational response framework will become more clear below, especially on the basis of the type of empirical results presented.

1.3 The Significance of Studying Organizational Responses to HIV/AIDS

Apart from the fact that only little research has been done on the organizational response to HIV/AIDS so far, there are a number of other reasons why studying this type of response should be done in a specific and systematic way. First, the response by organizations is an empirically important phenomenon. Secondly, the organizational level is often the more appropriate level of analysis. Thirdly, the organizational response is often the more effective one.

From an empirical point of view, it is obvious that organizations which provide HIV/AIDS activities have an extremely significant and positive influence on the problem. Most countries had both new and already established organizations in the field of health and welfare which have developed activities for preventing HIV transmissions and reducing the negative personal and social impact of HIV/AIDS. The variety of these activities covers an entire spectrum. For example, buddy programmes were developed to give persons with AIDS a special friend to help him or her in daily matters, such as buying groceries or picking up prescriptions as well as giving emotional support. AIDS hotlines were set up to give specific information concerning HIV/AIDS. Legal services were developed to help people receive benefits. AIDS nutritional training programmes were established. The distribution of AIDS educational information was organized. Initiatives were set up to reach out to intravenous drug users, etc. The development of organizations which provide HIV/AIDS programmes and activities varies greatly across countries, however. Indeed, one of the main purposes of the present volume is to both describe and explain this variation in number of such organizations.

Secondly, analysing the organizational response implies a different, but often a more appropriate, level of analysis than the level of analysis HIV/AIDS research has commonly concentrated on. In the study of the organizational response the unit of analysis is the organizations and not the HI-Virus or persons. The approach assumes that a person's risk of becoming infected as well as the type and degree of personal and social consequences he or she has to cope with are primarily determined by the social (organizational) context in which the person lives rather than on his or her behavioural choices. Clearly, it is indeed the person itself who acts (i.e. puts on a condom), and not the environment nor the social context. The fact that action is located at the level of the person does not, however, imply that this response has to be explained at the level of the person itself (e.g. by personal characteristics such as his or her willingness, readiness, degree of compliance, intelligence, information received and stored, etc.). Instead, options for action are conditioned by the social context in which a person lives and therefore should, at least partially, be explained by contextual factors. There are different types of social factors which are relevant here, such as for example the communication structure (e.g. between sexual partners or needle-sharing drug users), the existing legal measures (e.g. regarding sexual behaviour), societal norms, or the type and number of organizations concerned with HIV/AIDS in the person's environment. The present study considers this last type of social context, often being the appropriate level of analysis for studying the given options a person has when trying to avoid HIV transmissions or when dealing with the personal and social impact of HIV/AIDS.[10]

Thirdly, the organizational response is often the more effective response to deal with the problem of HIV/AIDS. For example, in the area of prevention, it has been illustrated that through the intermediation of organizations, situations might develop through which specific groups can learn of the risks involved, and even experience them. Through the development of a certain type of organization in certain situations, a *solidarity culture* can develop which could help to create a *culture of responsibility* between infected and non-infected members of the group. Such solidarity can then strengthen the development of group activities, besides producing regulating effects regarding behaviour. Strengthening solidarity is often done through bringing about *solidaristic goods* – such as organizing discussion groups, parties and recreation activities, or providing meeting places for social contacts, producing newsletters and badges, etc.

It is also in the area of care where it is obvious that the presence of a differentiated set of organizations can have a significant influence, e.g. on the length of stay in hospital for people with AIDS. It is even in the field of testing where the presence of organizations which provide HIV/AIDS activities seems to make a considerable difference. For example, the mass HIV screening in Viennese hospitals, being a regulative measure, has been much less effective in identifying HIV cases than voluntary testing done through a specialized organization, e.g. the *Österreichische AIDS-Hilfe*, which at the time of data collection provided such HIV testing as one of its many HIV/AIDS-related activities. Through routine HIV screening in Viennese hospitals, there was a ratio of 26 cases to every 100,000 tests performed in 1990; but with the *Österreichische AIDS-Hilfe*, the ratio was 1,600 cases per 100,000 tests.

This is, of course, not an extensive list of the advantages of studying the organizational response to HIV/AIDS. Ultimately, it is the successive country chapters that will have to illustrate the advantages of this approach. In section 3 of this chapter some of the benefits of this approach will be summarized as they result from these country chapters.

1.4 Defining the Organizational Response

Generally speaking, the degree of organizational response (being the dependent variable in this study) is defined as the degree to which an organization or a group of organizations responds to HIV/AIDS, i.e. where they develop specific activities which are directed to deal with the problems of reducing the number of HIV transmissions and/or to reducing the negative personal and social consequences of HIV/AIDS.

Any type of organization which offers any type of activity which contributes to dealing with the above-mentioned problems is defined here as having an organizational response to HIV/AIDS, as long as these activities are provided in a specific and specialized way.[11] Organizations can be statutory organizations, non-profit organizations, private organizations, exclusive organizations, inclusive organizations, professional organizations, local or national organizations, small or large ones, membership organizations, old or new ones, etc.

Organizations are considered in the present study as having an organizational response as long as they provide at least one activity in the area of HIV/AIDS.

The type of activity provided by these organizations can also be of any type as long as it contributes to one of either problems mentioned above. They can be prevention activities, education and information, health care and social services, policy coordination, interest representation, fund-raising, care activities, interest intermediation, monitoring activities, etc.

Finally, it should be mentioned that – as will be seen in the country chapters – the degree of organizational response can be analysed on different levels. It can be analysed on the level of the single organization, i.e. it can be assessed how far a single organization develops as a reaction to HIV/AIDS-specific responses (organizational level). Moreover, a specific group of organizations, such as public organizations or community-based organizations can be assessed on their organizational response (the sectoral level). Or, finally, organizations in a specific region, such as a province or country, can be assessed on their organizational response (on a regional level).

1.5 Countries Covered and Research Methods Used in Analysing Organizational Responses

The data presented here are the results of a cross-national comparative study in six European countries, which first developed, and then applied a common research design.

The selection of countries included in the study resulted from practical considerations rather than from theoretical ones. The initial idea was to limit the study for comparative reasons to European and North-American countries and to include, for both practical and comparative reasons, not too many nor too few countries in the study. Initially, all countries from the above-mentioned region were invited to participate in the WHO-Collaborative Project "Managing AIDS". There are a number of reasons why some countries were unable to participate in the end: first, difficulties in identifying organizational researchers who were committed to studying the field of HIV/AIDS (e.g. Spain and Denmark); secondly, the impossibility of mobilizing funding sources for the project in some countries[12] (e.g. France and the UK); thirdly, the opposition of some powerful AIDS service organizations in some countries to have the organizational response in their country evaluated (e.g. Germany and Canada); and fourth, the fact that the research design is rather heavy to carry out for large countries (e.g. USA and France; the fact that Italy is the only large country which could be included in the studied is due to the fact that almost a complete database of relevant organizations was already in existence at the beginning of the study). Despite this heavy and difficult process in identifying participating countries, eight countries fully participated in the "Managing AIDS" project: Austria, Belgium (with two research teams, one from the Flemish Region and one from the Walloon Region), Hungary, Italy, the Netherlands, Portugal, Sweden and Switzerland. Due to a lack of resources and changes in the working positions of some research team members the country reports for Hungary, Portugal and the Walloon Region could not be completed and are therefore not included in this volume. The data for these three cases are, however, available and will be included in some of the tables which follow.

The first step of the research project was to agree on a common and comparative research design for mapping the dependent variable, being the organizational response to HIV/AIDS.

In a second step, the organizations were identified which provided HIV/AIDS activities in the different countries. The procedure for identifying such relevant organizations took place in different stages. Firstly, all generally known organizations in the field were addressed. Secondly, information was requested from all organizations of a specific type, e.g. hospitals, prisons, counselling centres – which are theoretically able to provide the kind of services dealt with in this project. Thirdly, experts in the field, e.g. as care providers, doctors, experts, etc. were asked to name any organizations they knew of which provided HIV/AIDS activities. Fourth, we used the so-called "reputational method": this means asking previously-identified organizations whether they knew of any other organizations within their geographical area which also provide HIV/AIDS activities.

In a third research step, all identified organizations received a Standardized Inventory Sheet from which the following information was gathered: first, basic information (name, address); second, information on the organizations' HIV/AIDS activities; and third, information on the organizational context in which the activities are provided (legal status, age, size, geographical scope, general type of organization, etc.).

In a fourth research step, the resulting data from the Inventory Sheet were entered into a database (called "AIDSINST").[13]

In addition, the research design foresaw the collection of a limited number of independent variables such as the case-load and the institutional structure of the health and welfare system. In general, however, a considerable leeway was given to the different country teams in explaining the organizational response identified, accommodating for, on the one hand, the specificities of the different countries involved, and on the other hand, for the different research backgrounds and interests of the researchers involved in the project. This approach resulted in the end in a rich and thick description and enumeration of a large number of factors throughout the different country studies – accounting for the development of the organizational response to a crisis such as HIV/AIDS.

2   Some Dimensions in the Organizational Responses to HIV/AIDS

2.1   The Overall Organizational Response to HIV/AIDS in the Countries Studied

As specified above, the main research question in the present study is to analyse and explain the organizational response to HIV/AIDS in various European countries. Almost 2,400 organizations were active in this area of interest in 1993 in the eight countries studied; this is represented in Table 1.1.

Table 1.1 clearly indicates that the number of organizations varies considerably between countries. On the one end of the scale we find countries like Hungary and Portugal with only a few organizations active in this area, respectively 7 and 16, and on the other, we find small countries such as Switzerland and the Netherlands with respectively about 300 and 700 organizations, and Italy with over 1,100 organizations. Between these extremes, we find Austria and Belgium with several dozen organizations.

The numbers do not seem to indicate a direct relationship between the number of organizations in the field of HIV/AIDS and the AIDS-epidemic. This is illustrated by the indicators for *Organizational Density I* in Table 1.1: the number of organizations per 100 AIDS cases varies between less than 1 and 28. The relationship to the population size is neither very strong and varies between 1 and 47 (Table 1.1: *Organizational Density-II*). This finding confirms one of the most important assumptions the present research is based on, i.e. that the organizational response can neither be explained by the case-load (i.e. epidemiological size) nor by the size of the country. How else can the organizational response to HIV/AIDS in a particular country be explained? To answer this question, one should take a number of alternative explanatory factors into consideration, e.g. the existing intermediary structures in health and welfare, the associative tradition in a country, public policies in the health and welfare sector as well as its institutional characteristics in a given country, types of legal regulations regarding HIV/AIDS, the political structure of a given country (e.g. federal versus unitary states), the role of opinion-makers, the

Table 1.1:   The AIDS Epidemic and the Organizational Response and Organizational Density in Eight European Countries

Country	Number of Organizations	Number of AIDS Cases (cumulative)	Number of Inhabitants (Millions)	OD I[c]	OD II[d]
Netherlands	711	2,567	15.2	28	47
Switzerland	306	3,240	6.8	9	45
Belgium[a]	50	1,114	5.8	4	9
Austria	104	921	7.9	11	13
Sweden[b]	63	797	8.6	n.a.	n.a.
Italy	1,135	20,282	57.5	0.06	20
Portugal	16	1,352	9.8	1	2
Hungary	7	115	10.4	6	1

[a]   only Flanders.
[b]   The Swedish study did not, in contrast to the other country studies, include all organizations; all non-profit organizations and a sample of public organizations are included in this figure; n.a. = not applicable.
[c]   OD I (Organizational Density I): Organizations per 100 AIDS cases.
[d]   OD II (Organizational Density II): Organizations per million inhabitants.

Sources: "Managing AIDS" (European Centre/WHO Collaborative Study) (1993); European Centre for the Epidemiological Monitoring of AIDS (1993); Eurostat – Statistische Grundzahlen der Gemeinschaft 1993, Luxembourg.

existence of platforms, committees, etc. These factors, as well as their significance will be presented in greater detail in the following country chapters.

Whereas the overall organizational response in a country may give a general indication of its extent, it is more important to analyse the functional and structural differentiation of the organizational response in a country. Analysing the functional and structural differentiation is not only important for portraying the degree of the distribution of organizational responses across social groups or geographical areas but it can also give indications as to the structural causes leading to organizational response other than the case-load motive.

Three functional and structural dimensions were identified in the course of the empirical research; they significantly contribute to effectively describing and analysing the organizational response in a country. The first functional dimension relates to the types of activities provided. As will be shown below, the overall organizational response can be broken down by types of activities and we find a difference in the type of structure in the distribution of such activities in the various countries. Secondly, the overall organizational responses do also differ significantly when it comes to the types of organizations involved in the organizational response. A detailed analysis of this structural dimension is believed to be a key to a better explanation and understanding of the causes leading to organizational responses. Thirdly, organizational response can also be analysed in terms of how it is distributed across social groups and geographical areas. As will be seen in the country studies, the organizational response is neither equally distributed across social groups nor across geographical areas within any one country. Analysing the form of distribution of these activities also contributes to a better understanding of the degree of organizational response. It is these three dimensions, types of activities, types of organizations and forms of distribution, which have been found to constitute a useful common and minimal framework for identifying and making explicit important independent variables for explaining differences in the organizational response to HIV/AIDS. These dimensions will be presented in somewhat more detail, presenting the first general findings of this study.

It should be mentioned that although these dimensions constitute a minimal comparative framework and were found to be relevant in each of the country studies presented, they do not constitute a complete list of relevant and discriminating dimensions. Additional dimensions have been identified for the respective countries which help to explain the degree of organizational response in the particular country studied.

2.2 Types of Activities Provided

Important factors for understanding the organizational response to HIV/AIDS can be derived by mapping out in more detail and comparing the different types of activities which are provided in a specific country. Certain types of activities have been found to be more common in some countries than in others, thus pointing towards the importance of certain types of factors which seem to be at stake in these countries.

In the present study, all kinds of activities have been identified which contribute to reducing HIV transmissions or reducing the personal and social impact of HIV/AIDS. The approximately 100 different, specific types of activities which were initially identified were grouped into 25 specific types of activities which, in turn, have been grouped into six different groups of activities (see Table 1.2).

The analysis has shown that the prevalence of the different types of activities differs significantly both across and within the different countries studied (see Table 1.3).

Analysing the data along this dimension reveals the importance of factors such as the existence of legal regulations regarding HIV/AIDS, the importance of the non-profit sector in health and welfare in general, the political/administrative tradition, etc. in explaining the organizational response to HIV/AIDS.

Table 1.2:   Types of Activities Analysed in the "Managing AIDS" Project

Prevention
   Hotline
   Production of information material
   AIDS information campaigns
   Educational and information work
   Drug-related prevention
   Training of volunteers and health care professionals

Care
   Primary health care/medical services
   Care/psychological support of people with HIV/AIDS
   Face-to-face counselling
   Home care services
   Hospices, shelters, housing facilities
   Voluntary HIV-testing and counselling
   Buddy system
   Referral services
   Food bank

Research

Control and Monitoring
   AIDS policy coordination and implementation
   Control of blood/plasma product safety
   HIV-screening, testing, identification

Interest Representation
   Self-help groups of people with HIV/AIDS
   Counselling for insurance/welfare entitlements
   Civil and human rights/protection against discrimination
   Political lobbying
   Legal advice

Fund-raising for HIV/AIDS programmes

Table 1.3:   Percentage of Organizations Providing Specific Types of Activities

Country	Prevention	Care	Research	Control, Monito-ring	Interest Represen-tation	Fund-raising
Netherlands						
Switzerland[a]	34	44	n.a.	12	4	6
Belgium[b]	86.2	62.7	27.5	33.3	1.9	19.6
Austria	78.1	77.1	21.9	21.0	37.1	10.5
Sweden	90.5	47.6	41.3	27.0	15.9	14.3
Italy[c]	44.2	43.2	n.a.	10.7	1.8	0.1

[a] in Switzerland organizations were asked to name only their main area of activity; "research" was not considered as a category in its own right so that multiple answers were excluded and the distribution could not exceed 100%.

[b] only Flanders.

[c] in Italy it is not the distribution of organizations across the different areas of activities which is indicated but the distribution of all activities so that multiple answers were excluded and the distribution could not exceed 100%; "research" was not considered a category in its own right.

Source: "Managing AIDS" (European Centre/WHO Collaborative Study), 1993.

Not only the prevalence of the six types of activities has been analysed but also the presence or absence of single types of activities in the different countries. Apart from the fact that the identification of the absence of single activities (such as buddy systems or hospices) reveals important deficits in the provisions for people affected by HIV/AIDS, at the same time, it again hints at specific factors which are relevant for understanding the development of the organizational response.

2.3   Types of Organizations Involved

Another important dimension which pictures, as well as enables one to reveal further factors behind the organizational response to HIV/AIDS, is to analyse the organizational response by the type of organization involved. It can be clearly shown that different types of organizations respond to different extents to the problem of HIV/AIDS for a number of reasons. These responses once again do not directly relate to the case-loads they are confronted with.

There are many different ways to differentiate organizational types. In the present study two typologies have been developed which seem particularly relevant in differentiating organizations according to their degrees of organizational response:

legal status and orientation of the organization. Both types will be expanded upon below. There are of course many other possibilities of how to classify organizations and some of them are certainly also relevant when it comes to identifying the organizations' degree of responsiveness to HIV/AIDS. A number of these are presented in the different country chapters. Only the above-named types will be presented in this introductory chapter since they play an important role in all of the countries studied.

2.3.1 Public and Non-profit Organizations

The legal status of organizations (public, private non-profit, private for-profit organizations which provide HIV/AIDS activities) was found to be an important dimension for various reasons. For example, it is an indication for the degree to which different societal sectors (the market, the state, civil society) take their responsibility in a crisis such as HIV/AIDS as well as the degree to which they collaborate in such a crisis ("welfare mix"). It also reveals important causes for the over- or under-representation of certain types of activities.

Classifying the different organizations according to their legal status is interesting as there is a difference both in the organizational response between organizations of *different* legal status as well as between organizations of the *same* legal status between different countries (see Table 1.4).

Table 1.4: Legal Status of Organizations

Country	Public organizations		Private non-profit organizations		Private for-profit organizations		Total	
	N	%	N	%	N	%	N	%
Netherlands	168	24	526	75	3	1	697[*]	100
Switzerland	149	50	141	46	12	4	307	100
Belgium[a]	6	12	42	84	2	4	50	100
Austria	40	38	63	60	2	2	105	100
Sweden	18[**]	n.a	45	n.a	0	n.a.	63	n.a.
Italy	549	41	779	58	5	1	1,335[***]	100

[a] Only the Flemish region.
[*] 14 organizations could not be classified.
[**] only a sample of public organizations.
[***] 2 organizations could not be classified.

Source: "Managing AIDS" (European Centre/WHO Collaborative Study), 1993.

As will become clear in the different country chapters (also on the basis of the structural differentiation of the organizational response) a number of factors can be identified which explain the degree of organizational response to HIV/AIDS. It is obvious that in countries where state organizations play a more important role than non-profit organizations different types of organizational response are evident. It is important to point out that the extent to which certain types of organizations respond to HIV/AIDS when compared to other types does indeed have an important effect on the overall organizational response identified in a country.

2.3.2 Exclusive versus Inclusive Organizations

Another distinction which can be made is the one between *inclusive* and *exclusive* HIV/AIDS organizations. So-called "Exclusives" are HIV/AIDS organizations which are only active in the field of HIV/AIDS. Those organizations are by definition new organizations, explicitly founded as a response to the epidemic. Inclusive HIV/AIDS organizations, on the other hand, have a broader problem orientation. Here, activities in the field of HIV/AIDS are perceived as merely a new task in addition to a whole range of already existing activities. Inclusives are predominantly organizations which already existed when the epidemic broke out. The project has found that differentiating the organizational response along this dimension to be a better way of understanding the dynamics on which the development of the organizational response is based in a particular country. Table 1.5 presents the number of exclusives and inclusives in the different countries studied.

Table 1.5:   Orientation of Organizations

Country	Inclusive organizations		Exclusive organizations		Total	
	N	%	N	%	N	%
Netherlands	652	89	80	11	732	100
Switzerland	239	78	67	22	306	100
Belgium	54	73	20	27	74	100
Austria	47	73	17	27	64	100
Sweden	34	58	25	42	59	100
Italy	15	94	1	6	16	100
Total	1,043	83	215	17	1,258	100

[a]   Only the Flemish region.

Source: "Managing AIDS" (European Centre/WHO Collaborative Study), 1993.

In Table 1.5 the organizational response in the six countries is compared according to the distinction "inclusive" versus "exclusive" HIV/AIDS organizations. The countries differ both in the absolute and the relative numbers of these organizations. It is in general the inclusive organizations that dominate the organizational response. However, the number of exclusive organizations is – at least in some countries – remarkable. As will become clear in the different country reports, it is especially the development of the number of these exclusive organizations which gives rise to a significant amount of insights into the organizational response in a particular country. Do they develop because of the particularity of the problem they have to deal with? Do they develop because traditional (inclusive) health and welfare organizations fail to respond? Do they develop because groups are affected which were previously not organized, or just the other way around? etc.

2.4 How Organizational Responses Are Distributed

Another way to analyse or break down the overall organizational response in order to better understand its underlying structures or determinants is to consider the way the overall organizational response is distributed across social groups or geographical areas or, in other words, to enquire into the political economy of the organizational response.

2.4.1 Distribution of the Organizational Response across Social Groups

The involvement of particular organized communities and communities at risk is illustrated in Table 1.5. From these figures it becomes clear that when combining them with the epidemiological figures (see Annex 1), they hardly correlate with one another. Whether social groups are organizationally covered or not is more dependent on such factors as whether these groups were already organized before the HIV/AIDS problem, dependent on the size of the group at risk and on the level of social cohesion of the group at risk. These and other explanatory variables will be explained in greater detail in the different country studies.

2.4.2 Distribution of the Organizational Response by Geographical Areas

Another important dimension which provides important indicators for the structure of the organizational response is the degree to which this organizational response is distributed geographically. It is not possible to summarize these findings in a summary table since the type and number of regions differ considerable across countries. Be that as it may, what becomes clear from the data presented in the different country studies is that highly variable regional distributions exist, and this does not necessarily correlate with the problem-load or size of the region (as is also the case with the countries). Consequently, regional specificities regarding policy-making, organizational culture, etc. also seem to play a more important role in explaining the availability of organizational response to HIV/AIDS.

Table 1.6: National Patterns of Organized Communities and Organized Groups at Risk in Six European Countries

	NL	CH	A	S	P	H	Total
Organized communities	*191*	*27*	*17*	*23*	*1*	*1*	*260*
Gay community	37	7	9	3		1	57
(IV-) drug users	4	4	2				10
Haemophiliacs	2	1	1	2	1		7
Women	1						1
Prostitutes	1	2					3
Migrants	1			8			9
Parents	2			1			3
Religious org., etc.	7	7					14
Red cross, etc.	67			5			72
Others	69	6	5	4			84
Organized groups at risk	*18*	*11*	*6*	*5*	*2*	*1*	*43*
People with AIDS/HIV	9	8	4	4	2	1	28
Gay community	1	1					2
Women	1	1					2
(IV-) drug users				1			1
Buddies	7		1				8
Others		1	1				2
Total	*209*	*38*	*23*	*28*	*3*	*2*	*307*

The above-mentioned dimensions are only a selection of the important issues which could be used to describe and analyse the organizational response in a particular country. They have been mentioned here in some detail since they are common to all studies and are believed to give a first indication of the type of data collected in the "Managing AIDS" project. Examples of other fruitful ways of looking at the data collected are by considering the cooperative structures which underlie the organizational response (particularly pronounced in the chapters on the Netherlands and Switzerland) or by looking at the organizational response in terms of the welfare mix (Cattacin/Panchaud, 1995).

3   Preliminary Conclusions and Future Research

In this final part the benefits of analysing the organizational response to a problem such as HIV/AIDS will be addressed once again. This time it will be on the basis of findings in the different country studies and it will be shown that the organizational response approach does indeed produce relevant, interesting and surprising results. In a second part it will be argued that this approach has a much greater potential as far as future research possibilities are concerned than what could be accomplished in the "Managing AIDS" project up to now. A number of such possibilities regarding the study of the organizational response to HIV/AIDS will therefore be outlined below.

3.1   Types of Findings Produced by the Organizational Response Approach

The approach presented above, and which has been applied in the following country chapters, produces a range of different insights into different levels of analysis. Studying the organizational response produces knowledge regarding HIV/AIDS on the societal, the sectoral, the organizational, and the personal levels.

Concerning how *societies* as a whole have dealt with the problem of HIV/AIDS, a number of important findings resulted from the organizational response approach. For example, it became clear that almost no society applied the existing epidemic laws to deal with this problem, but rather mobilized (to a larger or lesser extent) societal actors to deal with the problem. Not only has this specific societal mode of coping with a modern problem been identified, but it has been possible to distinguish societies or provide a typology of countries regarding their societal response to HIV/AIDS on the basis of organizational response data (for such a typology see Cattacin/Panchaud 1996, for example).

The applied organizational response approach also gives important insights into the *sectoral level,* i.e. the level of health and welfare systems. On the basis of organizational response data, it can be analysed whether these sectors are flexible and respond to a new challenge such as HIV/AIDS (as has been the case in Switzerland) or whether these traditional sectors are more or less "immune deficient" to such a new problem and hardly properly react to it in a substantive way (as is the case for Austria for example). Moreover, the organizational response data can show in greater detail what the often cited "new division of labour" which took place in these sectors in some countries as a result of HIV/AIDS is based on (see e.g. Rosenbrock, 1991). Is it more based on the existence of new types of organizations within these sectors or on the re-orientation of existing organizations? Will this new division of labour be limited to the problem of HIV/AIDS or are there indications that it will spill off to other problems?, etc. Addressing these questions, the approach is moreover consistent with and can greatly contribute to recent trends in social policy analysis. This has developed from an approach which focuses on the social policy as state policy to an approach which focuses on the welfare state as a whole and concentrates on the analysis of the so-called "welfare-mix" (e.g. the original research outline, Marin/Kenis, 1989 [see Annex II]; Evers, 1993; Kenis/ de Vroom, 1996).

It is obvious that the organizational response approach can clearly in part answer the question as to how single *organizations* deal with the problem of HIV/ AIDS. On the basis of the data in the "Managing AIDS" project, systematic findings are presented for the first time on the so-called "responsiveness" of single organizations and of types of organizations which dealt with the problem of HIV/ AIDS. Questions regarding the degree of responsiveness, types of activities provided, conditions for organizational development, conditions for organizational effectiveness, etc. can and will be answered in the following chapters.

Finally, the organizational responsiveness approach also substantially contributes to the knowledge regarding the existing possibilities of coping with HIV/AIDS on a *personal level*. By mapping out and analysing the organizational response to HIV/ AIDS a lot of information is produced regarding the life chances and social and personal consequences of people living with HIV/AIDS. For example, psycho-neuroimmunological research suggests that social support and attitudes contribute to the survival chances for people with a life-threatening illness (Kiecolt-Glaser/ Glaser, 1988). Such social support is also (but of course not exclusively) provided through community-based organizations, offering buddies to people with AIDS to provide practical and emotional support, etc. Seen from such a perspective, analysing the organizational response means at the same time, to a certain extent, providing information on how people living with HIV/AIDS manage illness.

The above are only a few examples of the many different questions, levels and areas an organizational response approach can contribute to the analysis of coping mechanisms for the problem of HIV/AIDS, be it on the societal, sectoral, organizational or personal level. Many more applications and examples will be found in the country studies. The country studies do not, however, only illustrate the actual power and efficiency of this approach for analysing different areas and questions, but also point out further important areas and questions for follow-up research.

3.2   Follow-up Research

Instead of mainly studying the organizational response as an aggregate phenomenon, a more important task for follow-up research would be to concentrate more on the interaction between the different organizations when dealing with the problem of HIV/AIDS. As will be seen in many instances in the country chapters, the importance of the role of communication between organizations rather than strategies carried out by single organizations has been indicated regarding the provision of HIV/AIDS related activities. The importance of such phenomena as welfare mixes (Evers/Olk, 1996), micro-solidarities (Evers, 1990), inter-organizational networks (Marin, 1990a and b; Kenis, 1996), policy networks (Marin/Mayntz, 1991; Kenis/Schneider, 1991), etc. become apparent. Future research should enquire in greater detail into the role, structure and sustainability of such cooperative structures in the provision of HIV/AIDS related activities.

A second line of follow-up research could be to treat the organizational response as an independent variable. Since the present volume has successfully illustrated the relevance of studying the organizational response as a dependent variable, follow-up research could start using this variable for explaining phenomena such as the quality or content of programmes such as prevention campaigns, public policies towards HIV/AIDS, etc.

A third possibility for follow-up research would be to analyse the data of the "Managing AIDS" project in a more cross-national perspective in order to arrive at typologies or national models of HIV/AIDS policy. These conflicting models could consequently be assessed on their effectiveness (for the first of such studies see Cattacin/Panchaud, 1996; Kenis/de Vroom, 1996).

A fourth possibility for follow-up would be to concentrate on the explanation of the organizational response less by means of contextual factors and more by those of organizational ones. It can be assumed that the organizational response of a single organization also and often depends on intra-organizational factors such as conflicts, decision structures, types of professionals and staff, financing structures, etc. The importance of these variables for explaining the responsiveness of single organizations should be analysed in greater detail (for such a study which mainly concentrates on organizational failure see Perrow/Guillén, 1990).

A fifth task for follow-up research could be to study the development of the organizational response in the different countries. Since the "Managing AIDS" project is an asynchronic study it is difficult to assess how the organizational response will change over time. The question is, for example, whether the societal "normalization" of HIV/AIDS (which is something desirable) also leads to a normalization of the organizational response to HIV/AIDS (which is less desirable). Or the question whether the momentum which the organizational response gained during the 1980s will upsurge in the 1990s when new groups (such as women) are increasingly affected by the risks of infection.

A sixth fruitful type of follow-up research would be to compare the findings of the "Managing AIDS" project with those in other sectors, using a similar organizational responsiveness approach. Such a strategy could not only help to introduce additional explanatory variables but could also help to answer the question as to whether the specific findings of the "Managing AIDS" project are linked to the specificity of the HIV/AIDS problem or whether they are rather linked to the type of research design applied (first such cross-sectoral studies have been done for alcohol [Bütschi/Cattacin, 1994] and drugs [Cattacin et al., 1996]).

Finally, a more theoretically-oriented follow-up could be to assess how issues that have emerged are related to HIV, and how the study of HIV could improve our understanding of social science and the social-scientific approach to the study of a social problem. The analysis of HIV/AIDS has turned out to be more than another problem that can be treated as an interesting case-study of more fundamental processes (Albrecht/Zimmerman, 1993). HIV/AIDS has rather pointed towards the limits, new possibilities and challenges when applying existing paradigms and theories. These limits have been recognized right from the beginning in the "Managing AIDS" project (also because of EuroCASO's involvement in the specification of the research design) and has consequently led to the formulation of a less theory-driven and mainly descriptively-oriented research design. On the basis of this approach and its subsequent findings, it now becomes possible, however, to re-evaluate theories and models (especially in the field of organization theory and research, the study of public policy and social policy, and political science) to sharpen theories, improve our methods, and lay better groundwork for informed social policy.

Notes

1 In the initial period it was especially the gay community which developed strategies and activities regarding the HIV/AIDS issue (which probably results from the fact that AIDS first affected homosexual persons, and was consequently called the "Gay Men's Disease"). Generally, it took some time before "established" science and policy circles considered the problem of public importance. This "non-response" period existed in most countries and still exists in some. It is also especially still prevalent regarding specific social groups. For example, in many Western European countries, of those newly HIV-infected persons the majority is now women. However, this fact is only rarely reflected in the development of specific responses for this social group.
2 The definition of AIDS has been changed several times, however, and is often considered to be matter of controversy.
3 It has generally been accepted that the HI-virus causes AIDS. There are, however, some immunologists who pertain that HIV does not cause AIDS and that the HIV-virus is merely a co-factor (e.g. Duesberg, 1991).
4 Its possible modes of transmission are unprotected anal intercourse, intravenous drug injection, via blood transfusion and blood products, perinatal transmission from mother to child and unprotected heterosexual intercourse.
5 The HIV antibody test shows whether the body has started to build antibodies to HIV. It is consequently indirectly shown whether an HIV infection has taken place or not.
6 The a-symptomatic infection is characterized by the absence of symptoms in the case of an HIV infection. The length of this period varies extremely from person to person and can be ten years or even much more.
7 Exceptions being Perrow/Guillén (1991); Bennet/Ferlie (1994); Panem (1988); the Special Issue "The Response of the Voluntary Sector to the AIDS Pandemic" of the *Non-profit and Voluntary Sector Quarterly* (1991).

8   The most extreme cases in this respect are those where organizations develop activities which are forbidden by law but which nevertheless exist and often contribute significantly to dealing with the problem of HIV/AIDS. For example, some forms of homosexual community organizations are still formally forbidden by law in Austria – though tolerated – and are some of the most effective organizations for HIV prevention.

9   The literature distinguishes such aggregates as "third" sector, non-profit sector, private sector, "civil society", "welfare mix", etc. The "organizational response" distinct construct is somewhat inverted to the above concepts, and is, as such, at the same time more limited and more comprehensive.

10   Concentrating on this level of analysis has additional normative implications. Whereas concentrating on the level of the individual person can lead to strategies such as "identify and isolate the carrier" approach (as suggested by some variants of the regulative approach) or the "change your behaviour or die" approach, which is the sad message of the behavioural approach, the organizational approach would suggest strategies for improving the responsiveness of organizations rather than that of persons.

11   This means that organizations which do not explicitly deal with HIV/AIDS in a different or differentiated way have been excluded from this study. An example of such an organization would be one providing housing facilities for people in crisis situations: such an organization might also do this for seropositive persons or those with AIDS, perhaps even without knowledge of their particular medical condition or even disregarding it. Another example would be a family planning centre which offers information on AIDS as one sexually-transmitted disease among many without offering any AIDS-specific educational activities.

12   An important constraint in this respect was that one of the conditions the general assembly of EuroCASO (The European Council of AIDS Service Organizations) posed prior to the implementation of the project was that it would not use any national AIDS-specific funding sources, but would only apply to general research funding agencies. It should be noted that WHO agreed to the implementation of the *Managing AIDS* project as a WHO-Collaborative Study under the condition that EuroCASO would be regularly informed and have its say in some of the practical matters.

13   These data are also publicly available, sometimes in the form of handbooks (Nöstlinger/Kenis, 1993; Pestoff/Walden-Laing, 1991) and in all cases as computer readable files.

References

Bayer, Ronald (1989) 'Aids, Privacy, and Responsibility', *Daedalus*, Journal of the American Academy of Arts and Sciences: 118-123.

Bennet, Chris/Ferlie, Ewan (1991) *Managing Crisis and Change in Health Care – The Organizational Response to HIV/AIDS*. Buckingham, Philadelphia: Open University Press.

Bütschi, Danielle/Cattacin, Sandro (1994) *Le modèle suisse du bien-être. Cooperation conflictuelle entre État et société civile: le as de l'alcoolisme et du vih/sida*. Lausanne: Éditions Réalités sociales.

Cattacin, S. et al. (1996) *Drogenpolitische Modelle – Eine vergleichende Analyse sechs europäischer Realitäten*. Zürich: Seismo Verlag.

Cattacin, Sandro/Panchaud, Christine (1994) La maîtrise du sida. Une analyse comparative des réactions organisationnelles au vih/sida en Europe de l'Ouest. Paper presented at the Conference on "Droit et sociéte", Toulouse: Université de Toulouse.

Cattacin, Sandro/Panchaud, Christine (1995) 'La maîtrise du sida. Une analyse comparative des réactions organisationelles au vih/sida en europe de l'Ouest', *Revue politiques et management public* 13 (2): 47-95.

Duesberg, Peter H. (1991) 'AIDS Epidemiology: Inconsistencies with Human Immunodeficiency Virus and with Infectious Disease', *Proceedings of the National Academy of Science of the USA* 88: 1575-1579.

European Centre for the Epidemiological Monitoring of AIDS, *HIV/AIDS Surveillance in Europe: Quarterly Reports*.

European Centre (1993) *Welfare in a Civil Society*. Vienna: European Centre for Social Welfare Policy and Research.

Evers, Adalbert (1990) 'Im intermediären Bereich – Soziale Träger und Projekte zwischen Haushalt, Staat und Markt', in *Journal für Sozialforschung* 35 (2): 189-210.

Evers, Adalbert (1993) 'The Welfare Mix Approach. Understanding the Pluralism of Welfare Systems', pp. 3-31 in: Adalbert Evers/Ivan Svetlik (eds.), *Balancing Pluralism – New Welfare Mixes in Care for the Elderly*. Aldershot: Avebury.

Evers, Adalbert/Olk, Thomas (eds.) (1996) *Wohlfahrtspluralismus – Vom Wohlfahrtsstaat zur Wohlfahrtsgesellschaft*. Opladen: Westdeutscher Verlag.

Hirschman, Albert O. (1982) *Shifting Involvements. Private Interest and Public Action*. Princeton: Princeton University Press.

Kenis, Patrick/Nöstlinger, Christiane (1993) *Handbuch AIDS – Informationen, Organisationen und Anlaufstellen für alle, die in Österreich mit HIV/AIDS zu tun haben*. Wien: Falter Verlag (in der Reihe "Die kleinen Schlauen").

Kenis, Patrick/Schneider, Volker (1991) 'Policy Networks and Policy Analysis: Scrutinizing a New Analytical Toolbox', S. 25-59 in: Bernd Marin/Renate Mayntz (eds.) *Policy Networks – Empirical Evidence and Theoretical Considerations*. Frankfurt/Main and Boulder, Colorado: Campus/Westview.

Kenis, Patrick/Schneider, Volker (1996) (eds.) *Organisation und Netzwerk*. Frankfurt/Main: Campus.

Kenis, Patrick/de Vroom, Bert (1996) 'Neue Organisationen und alte Sektoren – Eine Analyse der Organisationen im Bereich HIV/AIDS in einigen europäischen Ländern', pp. 323-346 in: A. Evers/Th. Olk (eds.), *Wohlfahrtspluralismus – Vom Wohlfahrtsstaat zur Wohlfahrtsgesellschaft*. Opladen: Westdeutscher Verlag.

Kiecolt-Glaser, Janice/Glaser, Ronald (1988) 'Psychological Influences on Immunity', *American Psychologist* 43: 892-898.

Marin, Bernd (ed.) (1990a) *Generalized Political Exchange. Antagonistic Cooperation and Integrated Policy Circuits.* Frankfurt/Main and Boulder, Colorado: Campus/Westview.

Marin, Bernd (ed.) (1990b) *Governance and Generalized Exchange. Self-Organizing Policy Networks in Action.* Frankfurt/Main and Boulder, Colorado: Campus/Westview.

Marin, Bernd/Kenis, Patrick (1989) Managing AIDS. The Role of Nonprofit Institutions in Public Health and Welfare Policy, Research Design. Vienna: European Centre for Social Welfare Policy and Research.

Marin, Bernd/Mayntz, Renate (eds.) (1991) *Policy Networks – Empirical Evidence and Theoretical Considerations.* Frankfurt/Main and Boulder, Colorado: Campus/Westview.

Panem, S (1988) *The AIDS Bureaucracy.* Cambridge, Mass.: Harvard University Press.

Perrow, Charles/Guillén, Mauro F. (1990) *The AIDS Disaster. The Failure of Organizations in New York and the Nation.* New Haven/London: Yale University Press.

Pestoff, Victor A./von Walden-Laing, Dagmar (1991) *Handbok/Directory. Organisationer och aktiviteter/Organizations and Activities.* Stockholm: Stockholms Universitet.

Rosenbrock, Rolf (1991) 'Strategien gegen AIDS', *Psychosozial* 14: IV (48): 23-32.

Shilts, R. (1987) *And the Band Played On.* London et al.: Penguin Books.

Vroom, Bert de (1991) AIDS en gedragsregulering. Dilemma's en mogelijkheden van overheidsingrijpen en categorale zelfregulering. Working Paper 34. Leyden Institute of Law and Public Policy.

CHAPTER 2

Managing AIDS: The Swiss Case (1983-1992)[1]

Danielle Bütschi
Sandro Cattacin
Christine Panchaud

Studying the organizational responses to HIV/AIDS in Switzerland cannot be done without bearing in mind the specific political organization of this country. The 26 cantons and semi-cantons that make up Switzerland have large competencies in many domains, especially regarding the social, educational and health policies, because of the federal structure of the Swiss political system. Consequently, we will analyse the management of HIV/AIDS on a national level as well as in five cantons (Bern, Geneva, Lucerne, Vaud and Zurich), which we selected as representative examples of how the Swiss welfare system is organized. With such a variety, we can analyse the effects of federalism on the organizational responses to HIV/AIDS.

After having presented the institutional, policy and epidemiological context in Switzerland, we will present an aggregate view of the management of HIV/AIDS. This second section will mainly be based on data selected from the inventory of the Swiss organizations active in managing AIDS. In a third section, we will summarize in short the development and functioning of the organizational responses to HIV/AIDS on a national level and in the five selected cantons and present a synthesis of the organizational response to HIV/AIDS in Switzerland.

1 Introduction to the Institutional, Policy and Epidemiological Context

1.1 The Epidemic

The first cases of AIDS were reported in Switzerland in 1982. However, it was later established that HIV/AIDS had been present since 1980. Considering the statistics, the epidemic has progressed since 1988, when physicians were obliged to announce the cases of seropositivity and of AIDS for the first time.[2] By the end of 1992, 2,879 AIDS cases (of which 1,916 have died) and 17,112 seropositive HIV cases had been reported. Switzerland[3] is therefore one of the European countries most affected by the epidemic. Since its appearance, we can estimate that there have been 43 AIDS cases for every 100,000 inhabitants.[4] As for the direct costs incurred by HIV/AIDS, about SFr 100 million ($ 70 million) was spent in 1991 – 0.5% of the total spending of the Swiss health system.[5]

The majority of persons affected with HIV/AIDS are intravenous drug users (IV-drug users) and homo- and bisexual men.[6] These two groups represented nearly three-quarters of the AIDS cases in Switzerland in 1992. However, in 1992 AIDS mainly progressed amongst heterosexuals. Table 2.1 elucidates the development of the epidemic in the different target groups. In general, one can observe a minor reduction in the growth rate of new AIDS cases.

AIDS is mainly a problem in large agglomerations and its prevalence varies from canton to canton. Bern, the second-largest Swiss canton in size and population, is little concerned with HIV/AIDS. Geneva, however, is the canton most affected[7] and is therefore more concerned with the problem. In the canton of Lucerne – which is at the centre of a rural region – the spread of HIV/AIDS stays minimal in comparison with other urban cantons. Even including other cantons of central Switzerland, like Unterwald, Uri, Schwyz, which benefit from some of the HIV/AIDS services available in Lucerne, AIDS prevalence remains stable (16 cases for every 100,000 inhabitants) and HIV prevalence is particularly low (18 cases for every

**Table 2.1: AIDS Cases by Target Group and Reported Year
(as at 31 December 1992)**

Group	Reported Year										Total
	1983	1984	1985	1986	1987	1988	1989	1990	1991	1992	
1. Homo-/bisexual Men	8	15	40	65	88	152	180	181	221	251	1,201
2. IV-Drug Users	-	1	7	11	48	139	179	184	255	253	1,077
3. Risks 1 and 2*	1	1	1	4	2	8	13	1	7	4	42
4. Haemophiliacs	-	-	-	2	-	2	3	6	3	2	18
5. Blood Donors	-	-	-	1	2	8	5	7	8	3	34
6. Heterosexuals	8	3	6	5	19	34	61	58	105	119	418
7. Children <15 Years of Age	-	-	2	4	1	7	4	10	5	8	41
8. Unknown/Others	1	1	1	1	4	8	10	10	11	11	58
Total	18	21	57	93	164	358	455	457	615	651	2,879

*   Homo- and bisexual IV-drug users.

Source: Federal Office for Public Health (Office fédéral de la santé publique, OFSP), 1993.

100,000 inhabitants). The canton of Vaud is moderately affected by HIV/AIDS and remains close to the Swiss average. Finally, Zurich is the canton most affected by HIV/AIDS in absolute terms (it is also the most populated canton). This high prevalence of HIV/AIDS is certainly due to the metropolitan character of Zurich, which contains more than one million inhabitants.

1.2   First Overall Reaction

The first political reaction to HIV/AIDS goes back to 1983. That year, the Federal Government decided to establish a committee of experts on HIV/AIDS. The task of this new committee was to advise the Federal Office for Public Health (Office fédéral de la santé publique, OFSP), which started an information programme on HIV/AIDS for physicians.[8]

In 1985, the Federal Government assigned an initial budget of SFr 3.5 m. ($ 2.5 m.) for HIV/AIDS research. In the following year, the Federal Office for Public Health distributed a general information booklet to every household and started a prevention campaign (the STOP-AIDS campaign) in 1987, which addressed the whole population and periodically, specific target groups. It was also in this year when the Federal Office for Public Health created the Central Office for questions related to HIV/AIDS, after having realized the increasing importance of HIV/AIDS.

1.3   Influence of the Swiss Political System

The federal structure of Switzerland has a significant impact on the organizational responses to HIV/AIDS. Cantons and municipalities have a large autonomy in domains central to the management of HIV/AIDS, namely, health and education. More precisely, cantons are able to provide the following services and activities in the field of HIV/AIDS: general support to patients and medical care; information and sex education for young people and prevention for IV-drug users. Though the federal authorities have no competencies in medical or social care, they play a crucial role in the prevention and the control of HIV/AIDS. As a matter of fact, from a legal point of view, HIV/AIDS is considered an epidemic, which means that the Federal Law against Epidemics can be applied. This law enables the federal authorities to organize activities related to HIV/AIDS: epidemiological surveillance, training of medical and social personnel, information and prevention and research incentives. Moreover, the Federal Office for Public Health is in charge of the coordination of the different measures taken at the national level by various committees and working groups. It also elaborates on and launches various programmes and projects related to HIV/AIDS.

As a consequence of this division of activities, few organizations are present at the national level. The large majority (i.e. 73%) are active on the local and cantonal levels. Among the 27% present on the national level, 7% have an international scope beside their national activities.

2   Mapping the Services and Development of the Overall and Subsectoral Responses to HIV/AIDS

2.1   *Mapping the Development of Organizational Responses to HIV/AIDS*

2.1.1 Number of Organizations and Activities

At the end of 1990, there were 317 organizations with HIV/AIDS-related programmes in total. All these organizations offer an array of activities relevant for
the management of HIV/AIDS. Table 2.2 presents the percentage of organizations
carrying out each of these activities. The seven activities which are most under-

**Table 2.2:   Percentage of Organizations which Offer HIV/AIDS-related
               Activities**

Rank/Activities	%[*] (n=317)
1. Face-to-face counselling	43
2. Psychosocial support	42
3. Education or information	39
4. Training of health personnel, volunteers, etc.	31
5. Drug-related HIV/AIDS prevention	27
6. Hotline (information, emergency)	27
7. Referral service	26
8. Production of information material	25
9. Information campaigns	24
10. Primary health care and medical care	22
11. Voluntary HIV-testing and counselling	20
12. AIDS policy coordination and implementation	18
13. Counselling in insurance and welfare entitlements	17
14. Epidemiological and social research	13
15. Civil and human rights/protection against discrimination	12
16. Contact-tracing	12
17. Self-help groups of people with HIV/AIDS	10
18. Legal advice	9
19. Political lobbying	8
20. Home care services	8
21. Fund-raising	8
22. Shelter, housing facilities	6
23. Blood product screening	5
24. Foodbank	5
25. Buddy system	4

* More than one answer was possible.

taken by HIV/AIDS organizations come under the category of Care and Social Services. Moreover, prevention also seems to be an important dimension in the management of HIV/AIDS in Switzerland.

2.1.2 Organizational Development

These 317 organizations emerged progressively. Their modification in number can be divided into two phases, as shown in Figure 2.1. After a first and rapid phase of development which lasted until 1987, with a 60% increase in the number of organizations, a declining phase started in 1988 with the growth rate of the organizations' number going down from 42% in 1988, to 7% in 1990.

Comparing this trend and the variation in AIDS cases cannot alone explain the two phases just described. Such a comparison might be valuable for the first phase when it is clear that the rapid growth of the number of organizations is the result of a reaction to the emergence of HIV/AIDS. However, in the second phase, whereas

Figure 2.1:   The Development of HIV/AIDS Organizations and Progression of AIDS Cases

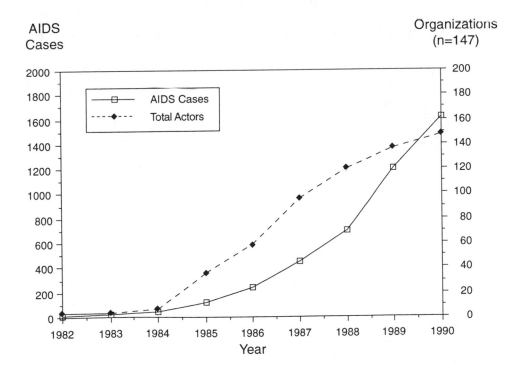

(missing data = 170)

there has been a constant and rapid increase in AIDS cases, the number of HIV/ AIDS organizations diminishes and it then seems that the AIDS field enters into a consolidating phase. Several factors can be considered to explain this change:

- the organizations created during the first phase cover the whole HIV/AIDS field relatively well;
- public financial support is stagnant;
- the organizations created during the first phase diversify their tasks and activities and focus more on their work and on a better coordination between organizations than on the creation of new organizations;
- the field of HIV/AIDS is still developing internally (i.e. organizations are getting bigger).

Explanations for these facts are explored in more detail in the third part of this chapter.

2.1.3 The Simultaneous Development of Public and Non-Profit Organizations

The organizational responses to HIV/AIDS are apparent just as much in public organizations as in non-profit organizations – the latter constituting about half of the Swiss HIV/AIDS organizations. At the end of 1990 there were 149 public

Figure 2.2: Development of Public Services and Non-profit Organizations

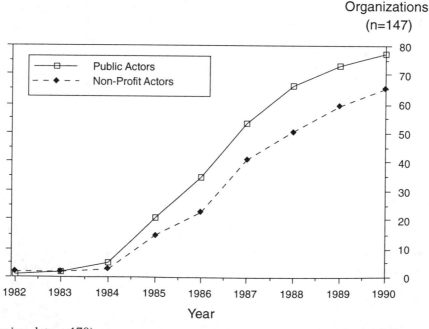

(missing data = 170)

services[9] and 168 private organizations with HIV/AIDS programmes. Among the 168 private organizations, 158 were non-profit and 10 were for-profit organizations (private societies close to the HIV/AIDS organizations which sell condoms, pharmaceutical industries and private laboratories). The for-profit organizations will not be considered in the following analysis as there are so very few of them.

Public as well as non-profit organizations have concerned themselves to an equal extent with HIV/AIDS since the very beginning. On observing the development of the number of public and non-profit organizations, the aggregate analysis shows no difference between these two types of organizations.[10] Figure 2.2 illustrates the simultaneous development of public services and non-profit organizations fighting against HIV/AIDS.

This result does not mean that there is no difference between public and non-profit organizations. Differences do exist, especially regarding the activities offered by public organizations and exclusive non-profit organizations. Table 2.3 presents these differences, showing the percentage of public, inclusive and exclu-

Table 2.3: **Distribution of Organizations by Legal Status and Organizational Orientation**

Main Activity	Type of Organization	Public Organizations %	Non-Profit Organizations		Total %
			Exclusive %	Inclusive %	
Prevention		36	19	36	34
Health & Psychosocial Care		47 hospitals=21	28	46 IV-drug=25	44
Controlling/Research		16	5	9	12
Interest Representation		–	12	7	4
Fund-raising		1	37	1	6
Total		100 (n=146)	100 (n=43)	100 (n=109)	100 (n=298)

(missing data = 9)

sive non-profit organizations whose main tasks are in the areas of prevention, care, control and monitoring, research, interest representation or fund-raising.

This table discloses that public services and inclusive non-profit organizations centre their activities around prevention and health care. In fact, 21% of the public services with HIV/AIDS-related activities are hospitals and 25% of the inclusive non-profit organizations are consultation and treatment centres for IV-drug users. Moreover, public organizations are much more active in the areas of control and monitoring, and research than non-profit organizations. However, no public organization has interest representation as its main duty, whereas 12% of exclusives and 7% of inclusive non-profit organizations do. As a rule, exclusive organizations are the ones that involve themselves with interest representation.

The field of HIV/AIDS is thus characterized by a division of tasks between public and non-profit organizations, as well as between inclusive and exclusive non-profit organizations. When we consider all the activities one organization has on offer, the same functional differentiation appears, though less distinctly (Table 2.4).

We notice that three-quarters of all the organizations – public or non-profit – have a preventive message.[11] Health care activities also strongly characterize all organizations. Again, one notes that interest representation and fund-raising mainly

Table 2.4: Number of Activities by Legal Status and Organizational Orientation*

Main Activity	Public Organizations % (n=149)	Non-Profit Organizations		Total % (n=307)
		Exclusive % (n=43)	Inclusive % (n=115)	
Prevention	72	86	78	76
Medical & Psychosocial Care	69	88	65	69
Controlling/Research	47	28	20	35
Interest Representation	17	65	32	29
Fund-raising	5	30	4	8

*   The total in each column is more than 100% because one actor can realize several activities in each category.

exist in exclusive non-profit organizations, and that monitoring and research activities are realized by public organizations.

In summary, the development of public and non-profit organizations, as well as the division of tasks between these different types of organization, testifies that non-profit organizations do not have a promotional role in the management of HIV/AIDS in Switzerland – at least on the aggregate level of analysis. One can claim – and we will verify it in the following sections – that public organizations have established the basic structure for managing HIV/AIDS and that non-profit organizations have filled in the gap of this basic structure.

2.1.4 The Influence of Federalism on Organizational Responses

As has already been mentioned, the Swiss federal structure gives a large autonomy to cantons and municipalities. This not only gives much responsibility to cantonal and local authorities in the field of HIV/AIDS, but it also has an influence on the activities of all HIV/AIDS organizations, be they public or non-profit. Table 2.5 looks at organizations according to their scope of action (local/cantonal and national) and shows what kind of activities they supply.

This table suggests the following:

- In accordance with the federal structure of Switzerland, one notices that local and cantonal organizations supply all HIV/AIDS-related activities.
- Local and cantonal organizations, because they are close to their clients, are naturally well represented within the domain of personal social services (personal counselling, psychological support, education and information, drug prevention, monitoring, health care, self-help, home care services, food banks, hotlines, buddy systems).
- National organizations offer more technical activities with no direct client contact (training, information campaigns, political coordination, professional counselling, interest representation, lobbying, fund-raising, blood screeening, plasma and blood product safety).
- Medical research and the production of prevention material are two important activities for the national organizations. In fact, the federal authorities have decided to play a central role in these fields. As they generally only have the right to support national organizations, federalism has no great influence on these two kinds of activities.

Federalism not only influences the activities, but also their territorial distribution. Thanks to the federal structure, almost every canton has at least one HIV/AIDS organization. Schwyz and Obwald – very small cantons – arc the only ones without any HIV/AIDS organization, but their inhabitants can refer to organizations in neighbouring cantons with problems related to HIV/AIDS. However, differences exist in the legal status of the organizations as there are differences in the various territorial contexts. Generally speaking, if there is a division of tasks between public

Table 2.5: Number of Activities in Local/Cantonal and National Organizations*

| | Organizations | |
Activities	Local/ Cantonal %	National %
Local/Cantonal Actors		
Face-to-face counselling	50	24
Psychosocial support	47	24
Education or information	41	31
Drug-related HIV/AIDS prevention	31	18
Hotline	30	15
Referral services	30	15
Primary health care and medical care	25	13
Self-help groups of persons with HIV/AIDS	12	5
Home care services	10	4
Foodbank	7	1
Buddy system	5	1
Equal Proportion between Local/Cantonal & National Actors		
Training of health personnel and voluntaries, etc.	30	33
Information campaigns	26	19
Voluntary HIV-testing and counselling	21	15
AIDS policy coordination and implementation	19	15
Counselling in insurance and welfare entitlements	19	11
Civil & human rights/protection against discrimination	11	17
Legal advice	9	8
Political lobbying	7	12
Fund-raising	8	9
Shelter, housing facilities	5	8
Blood product screening	5	6
National Actors		
Production of information material	20	40
Epidemiological and social research	9	23
Contact-tracing	9	18
	(n=224)	(n=85)

*   The total in each column is more than 100% because one actor can realise several
    activities in each category.

and non-profit organizations, only public organizations are present in managing HIV/AIDS in peripheral cantons (this is especially the case for Appenzell, Glaris, Nidwald and Uri).

The population density also influences the number of HIV/AIDS organizations. In the five largest Swiss towns – Zurich, Basel, Geneva, Bern, and Lausanne (with about one-seventh of the Swiss population) – 104 organizations with HIV/AIDS programmes exist, i.e. about one-third of all HIV/AIDS organizations identified in Switzerland.

Federalism therefore guarantees a homogeneous territorial distribution of organizations, as well as the existence of various organizational structures, even in peripheral regions. However, this situation does not mean that responses to HIV/AIDS have been uniform in Switzerland. As cantons have a large autonomy in the field of health and education – and thus in the field of HIV/AIDS – the organizational responses to the epidemic differ considerably from canton to canton. Table 2.6 presents some of the important cantonal measures which have been adopted to fight HIV/AIDS, as well as the number of organizations in each canton.

This table clearly presents how autonomous cantons are in the management of HIV/AIDS as well as the variety of measures taken by the different cantons. Information in schools is offered in every canton, but the didactic material is only elaborated upon by a few cantons (see Imhof, 1989). The anonymous HIV test, as well as medical and psychological services, are only provided in some cantons. Regarding IV-drug users, measures vary greatly from one canton to another.[12] Moreover, whereas the majority of cantons have official committees and working groups, six of them do not possess such structures. Other differences, especially as to when the various measures were introduced, distinguish the Swiss cantons from one another.

It seems that there are neither linguistic nor cultural differentiations which might explain these variations between cantons. There seem to be more differences between the central cantons and the periphery. For instance, it is mainly in cantons with large cities – also more concerned with the epidemic – where HIV/AIDS has been politicized. Zurich, Bern and Basel-city have experienced parliamentary interventions much more than other cantons.[13] In addition to this however, urban cantons have all experienced numerous organizational responses to HIV/AIDS, as well as having taken a large number of new measures themselves. Contrary to this, the organizational responses to the new epidemic have been less important in peripheral cantons – with a low rate of urbanization and HIV/AIDS cases. Only a few HIV/AIDS measures have been promoted in the cantons of central Switzerland in particular, and the number of HIV/AIDS organizations is very low there.

2.1.5 The Role of Exclusive Organizations

HIV/AIDS specifications decisively influence what kinds of organizations have emerged in this field. Aggregate data for Switzerland show how important exclusive organizations are in the management of HIV/AIDS: 43 organizations have been

Table 2.6: **Cantonal Measures, Activities and Number of HIV/AIDS Organizations in Each Canton**

Cantons	Total of Parliamentary Interventions	Commissions/ Working Groups	Care & Prevention Structures	Psychological Services	Anonymous HIV-Testing	Liberalisation of Methadone Programmes	Disposal of Sterile Syringes	Own Didactical Material	Didactical Material OFSP	Didactical Material other Canton	Information in Schools	Subventions to AIDS-Antennas	Number of Cantonal Organizations
Zurich	11	X	X	X	X	X	X	X		X	X	X	31
Bern	13	X	X	X	X	X	X	X			X	X	23
Lucerne	5	X	X	X		X	X	X	X	BE	X	X	9
Uri	1	X									X	X	2
Schwyz		X			X	X	X		X	X	X		
Obwalden		X					X		X		X	X	
Nidwalden		X							X		X	X	3
Glarus	1			X		X			X		X	X	2
Zug		X		X	X	X	X		X	BE	X	X	5
Fribourg	1	X			X		X		X		X	X	14
Solothurn	2	X	X	X	X	X	X	X	X	BE	X	X	10
Basel-City	10	X	X	X	X		X		X		X	X	31
Basel	4		X	X	X	X	X				X	X	8
Schaffhausen	2	X					X			ZH	X	X	3
Appenzell R.		X		X			X		X		X		2
Appenzell I.								X	X	ZH	X		2
St. Gallen	2	X	X	X	X		X		X	X	X	X	10
Graubünden	2	X		X	X	X	X		X	X	X	X	6
Aargau	4	X									X		9
Thurgau	1		X		X	X	X				X	X	5
Ticino	1		X		X	X	X				X	X	5
Vaud	3	X	X	X	X	X		X		BE	X	X	19
Valais	2	X			X						X		10
Neuchâtel		X	X	X	X		X		X	BE	X		12
Geneva	2	X	X	X	X		X	X			X	X	19
Jura	3						X	X			X		7

Source: AIDS Infotek 4/91 and own data.

created to fight HIV/AIDS in particular. Although these organizations are in a minority, their weight must not be underestimated. In 1990, their total budgets were about SFr 11.5 m. ($ 8.2 m.). Moreover, 200 professionals worked in such organizations, as well as about 750 volunteers.[14]

Exclusive organizations can be distinguished from inclusive ones by their internal and external operating logic:

- Concerning the internal logic, exclusive organizations are more often than not member organizations where the decisional power is mainly in the members' hands. In fact, whereas only 57% of inclusive organizations are member organizations, 76% of exclusive organizations have a membership structure and are, therefore, more dependent on their members' decisions.

  Another difference concerns the degree of professionalism. There are more volunteers and less professionals in exclusive organizations than in inclusive ones. Exclusive organizations estimate a median rate of 23 volunteers for every 10 professionals, whereas inclusive ones 9 volunteers for every 10 professionals.

- Considering the external logic of these organizations – that is, their impact on the environment – exclusive organizations have a greater number of activities addressed to the public than inclusives (hotlines, information material production and information campaigns). Moreover, they have more political activities (coordination and participation in HIV/AIDS policies, human and civil rights protection and lobbying activities): 79% of the exclusive organizations maintain public activities and 49%, political activities; these figures for inclusives are respectively 35% and 25%.

We estimate that it is above all because of the specificity of homosexual groups (which were at the origin of a large number of exclusive organizations) that such differences exist among non-profit organizations. The pre-existing capacity for self-mobilization which the homosexual community had already had before HIV/AIDS appeared gave them the opportunity not to be only the clients or passive members of an organization, but to actively become involved in a common reality. Moreover, we think that inclusive organizations did not constitute a relevant structure for homosexuals because such structures could not respond to their specific interests and did not offer them places where they could meet and assert themselves.

2.1.6 Organizational Integration

The different organizations active in the field of HIV/AIDS are well integrated with one another. Vertically, there are many affiliations between non-profit organizations; horizontally, collaboration exists between them. Several aspects can be pointed out to illustrate this integration:

- More than half the HIV/AIDS non-profit organizations are affiliated to other HIV/AIDS organizations.
- When a non-profit organization is affiliated to another one, it is often with an organization of the same type: 90% of exclusive affiliated organizations have relations with another exclusive, and 86% of inclusive affiliated organizations have relations with another inclusive.

- Horizontal integration, i.e. collaboration, mainly occurs with two organizations: the Swiss AIDS Foundation (Aide suisse contre le sida, ASS) and the Federal Office for Public Health. Twenty-one per cent of HIV/AIDS organizations collaborate directly with the Swiss AIDS Foundation. However, this number is in reality not completely accurate as many organizations work together with the cantonal antennas[15] of the Swiss AIDS Foundation. Thus, 61% of all organizations collaborate directly or indirectly with the Swiss AIDS Foundation. There are also many organizations that work together with the Federal Office for Public Health: 18% of all organizations directly collaborate with the Federal Office for Public Health through its committees and the HIV/AIDS Central Office.

From these results, it appears that efforts have been made to integrate organizations managing the HIV/AIDS epidemic. Moreover, it seems that it is possible for central organizations to coordinate the various interventions which have taken place in the area of HIV/AIDS.

2.1.7 Intermediary Conclusions from the Aggregate Data

This statistical summary of information shows that in Switzerland, public and non-profit organizations have reacted simultaneously and rather rapidly to the emergence of HIV/AIDS.[16] However, after an initial phase, the number of newly constituted HIV/AIDS organizations seems to have become stagnant. Nevertheless, HIV/AIDS organizations are distributed rather homogeneously and are present in nearly every canton.

Considering, more specifically, the role of non-profit organizations in the management of HIV/AIDS, it is interesting to mention once more that in opposition to more traditional fields – such as alcoholism – where non-profit organizations reacted first, HIV/AIDS non-profit organizations have worked parallel to public services since the beginning of the epidemic. Nevertheless, non-profit organizations cannot be assimilated to public structures and their critical potential towards influencing political decisions must not be underestimated. Their reactions, especially public and political interventions, have been of special importance in fighting the stigmatization and risks of discrimination which threaten all persons affected with HIV/AIDS in one way or another.

2.2   The Setting Up and Operation of the Networks

2.2.1 The National Network

Taking its sources from the gay movement in 1983,[17] the national network spread little by little, with numerous newly involved actors and bound agreements with 51 groups, organizations and institutions (15 public services, 24 inclusive non-profit organizations, 9 exclusive non-profit organizations and 3 private companies) by the end of 1990. Its focal points are the Federal Office for Public Health and the

Figure 2.3: The Development of the National Network

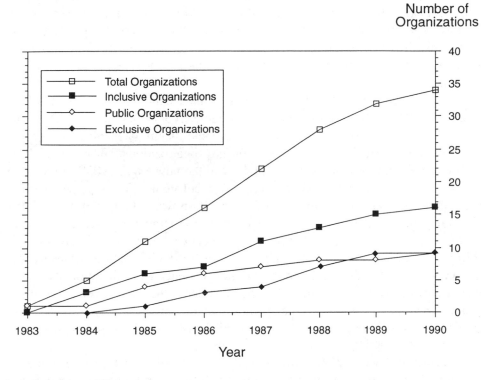

(missing data = 17)

Swiss AIDS Foundation. Figure 2.3 shows the development of the national network.

Three phases can be distinguished in this development. During the first phase (1983-1985) – which we can call "the first epidemic" – the gay organizations on the federal level organized themselves unilaterally in order to fight HIV/AIDS; at the same time, the administration set up a minimum programme. The homosexuals that arrived in the gay movement after the emergence of HIV/AIDS who thought that information and education were of priority due to the quick spread of the disease decided to create a national association specifically aimed at the fight against HIV/AIDS, namely the Swiss AIDS Foundation (ASS). Until 1985, AIDS was not actually debated on the Swiss political scene and remained a subject of discussion only within the public administrative bodies and gay organizations. Therefore, the Federal Government and Parliament only treated this new epidemic marginally, considering it a "specialist's matter" which concerns only "risk groups"[18]. The idea that HIV/AIDS had to be treated following a medical logic and technical projects, was common to all administrations which dealt with HIV/AIDS in one way or another – on both the federal and cantonal levels. At the same time, there was a debate within the gay organizational centres on the social aspects of the infection (discrimination, marginalization, stigmatization), which resulted in information and interest representation programmes (see Staub, 1988). During this phase, the extent of the diffusion of the infection was often underestimated and the structures set up were far from efficient and had remained underdeveloped for a long period of time.

During a second phase (1985-1986), which can be called the "awakening of the epidemic", the discussions on HIV/AIDS became broader, and more incisive. The Federal Administration endeavoured to overcome its purely medical conception of HIV/AIDS and tried to draw nearer to the gay organizations. The Federal Office for Public Health took up serious contact with the new Swiss AIDS Foundation in order to organize preventive measures, even before its official presentation to the public. As soon as the Swiss AIDS Foundation was established in 1985, the Federal Office for Public Health asked to become a member in order to feel closer to the people with risk behaviour (namely homosexuals) and to maintain its credibility amongst them. In fact, the Federal Office for Public Health was aware that the success of an HIV/AIDS programme was dependent on the utilization of existing social networks (see Somaini, 1989) and considered the gay movement as a decisive partner. For the homosexuals, whose movement was not very powerful in the 1980s, the collaboration with the Federal Office for Public Health gave them some means of action.

As far as the Swiss AIDS Foundation was specifically concerned, the collaboration with the Federal Administration was befitting as it legitimized it as being an expert and central agent, as well as guaranteeing its future financially. It was at this time when the first state measures were taken, i.e. particularly the HIV test. Since the establishment of the Swiss AIDS Foundation, prevention has been able to move on from the gay subculture, allowing other organizations to enter the field of HIV/AIDS and proposing services to other groups than homosexuals. Nevertheless, the reaction remained rather weak as only a few inclusive organizations integrated HIV/AIDS programmes into their agendas and only very few exclusive ones appeared. Among them, the Swiss Association of Workers Dealing with Drug Addiction (VSD/ASIT) played a promotional role in the prevention of HIV/AIDS and IV-drugs. The problem in this phase was that one had to create a consensus on the importance and urgency of taking serious measures to fight against HIV/AIDS.

It was only in 1987 that the third phase of reaction to the epidemic and reinforcement of the network started when the first consensus was found on a national level. This consensus permitted the setting-up of a programme based on information and prevention and the release of a succession of measures in the cantons as well as affirming the launch of the national STOP-AIDS campaign in 1987. The national campaign was aimed at the general population and was to be regularly repeated. Its main message was to promote the use of condoms. This campaign also reinforced and elucidated the collaboration between the Swiss AIDS Foundation and the Federal Office for Public Health. The Office ensured the scientific and professional competencies and financed the campaign, and the Swiss AIDS Foundation was in charge of carrying out the campaign – in addition to its own activities – using its experience and proximity with people at risk. This campaign is of great importance because of the impact it had on the population, but also because it sent out a political signal, being a public policy measure.

The time-lag between the awareness of the disease by the Federal Administration in 1983 and the beginning of the campaign in 1987 can be explained by the non-existence of a national structure which could administer a risk situation like HIV/AIDS. As public health matters are under the canton's responsibility, it was indeed necessary to find a political consensus, before the Federal Government could take any preventive measures. Thus, before giving a centralized response to HIV/AIDS, and to avoid cantonal idiosyncrasies, the Federal Administration had to promote a political consensus first. This was done in order to legitimize the fight against HIV/AIDS by means of a liberal interpretation of the existing federal law on epidemics and allowing the formation of a consistent policy relating to HIV/AIDS. It has not been very easy to reach a consensus because of the conflicting, different existing opinions.

Parallel to the national campaign of the Federal Office for Public Health, the federal authorities released a whole set of subventions in 1987 (for a total amount of SFr 8.3 m. [$ 6 m.]), in order to promote the management of HIV/AIDS by the non-profit organizations active in that field. In that same year, the Federal Government adopted a "Concept for the Fight against HIV/AIDS in Switzerland". It also granted a further SFr 1.5 m. ($ 1.1 m.) to encourage research into HIV/AIDS and SFr 5 m. ($ 3.6 m.) to the WHO for its special HIV/AIDS programme. That financial resources increased, allowed the different actors active in the field of HIV/AIDS to develop their activities or even to professionalize their work. This professionalization was necessary for the Swiss AIDS Foundation, not only in order to assume its new activities, but also in order to respond efficiently to its duties as an expert in the STOP-AIDS campaign. The Swiss AIDS Foundation was also restructured with the following main results:

- the "target group" concept was replaced by a "project" concept;
- the subsectors of the national foundation were organized at a cantonal level instead of at a local one (the presently existing cantonal antennas);
- the national office limited its activities to coordination and professionalized it.

Within five years, the Swiss AIDS Foundation was transformed from a completely voluntary organization into an organization with professional management.

The financial increase in resources released by the Federal Administration also allowed for the creation of new organizations specialized in the fight against HIV/

AIDS, e.g. the foundation AIDS and Child, or Sida Info Doc Suisse which is an HIV/AIDS information centre and was created on the Federal Office for Public Health's instigation in 1988. Parallel to the creation of new organizations, the existing inclusive ones and those traditionally present in the field of social welfare in Switzerland – e.g. Caritas, The Red Cross, Pro Juventute (institution defending the interests of young people) and the ASIT/VSD (Swiss Association of Workers Dealing with Drug Addiction) – became aware of the importance of HIV/AIDS and intensified their action in that field, most of the time, with financial help from the state. Some other inclusives and traditional, well-known organizations were only then starting their activities in the field of HIV/AIDS.

Thus, instead of talking about a simultaneous development of the management of HIV/AIDS between the state and the non-profit organizations as we suggested in our analysis of aggregate data, it actually appears that it was the Federal Administration which took important measures to stimulate non-profit organizations to integrate or initiate social HIV/AIDS-related programmes – sometimes even the Federal Administration independently created such an organization. The non-profit organizations which responded quickly to the HIV/AIDS problem got public funding and thus participated in the HIV/AIDS national policy. However, one must point out that the non-profit organizations actually developed their activities only once an HIV/AIDS national public policy and various programmes had been conceived.

To complete the presentation of the national network, the situation in some cantons should be described to show in what ways subsidiary governing powers and federalism give them autonomy in the field of public health. We will clarify the relationships between non-profit and public actors in each case, as well as the specific role the latter have played in this matter.

2.2.2 The Network in the Canton of Bern

The approach in the canton of Bern was to integrate the non-profit organizations into the cantonal policy from the beginning. The response towards HIV and AIDS is vast and covers medical care as much as prevention. By the end of 1990, the HIV/AIDS network in Bern consisted of 21 organizations or institutions, 12 of which were public services. Six of the non-profit organizations had already existed before the outbreak of HIV/AIDS and also had activities in other social sectors (inclusive organizations), three of them were non-profit organizations specializing in the field of HIV/AIDS. A great deal of these actors are located in the cantonal capital, Bern. The rest of the canton is mainly covered by public services. The non-profit organizations are rather concerned with the more inhabited area of the territory.

The response in this canton was rather quick and can be divided into two phases. Both phases were initiated by parliamentary interventions in the Cantonal Parliament. The first phase, which began in 1985, was essentially devoted to the elaboration and transmission of information from the political authorities of the canton to the whole population – this was even before the first national campaign was launched. Several parallel measures were taken to accompany the cantonal campaign (information passed on to health professionals, blood tests, etc.) and the Cantonal Parliament asked its administration to develop a clear concept on the fight against HIV/AIDS, which was legally realized at the end of 1986. During the second phase, which started in 1987, the political authorities tried to put this concept into practice:

- The division of work was organized as proposed by the Cantonal Chief Medical Officer[19]. Public institutions became responsible for the treatment of the infection and the non-profit organizations dealt more specifically with all the non-medical aspects of HIV/AIDS.
- An HIV/AIDS reference centre (an HIV/AIDS consultation centre) was created between 1987 and 1990 in each of the five regional hospitals of the canton. They include prevention, care and psychological help for people living with HIV/AIDS as part of their programme and constitute a part of the original cantonal network.
- A cantonal office of coordination for problems related to HIV/AIDS was created to deal with educational activities and proficiency courses for employees on a regional basis.[20]

The medical and psychosocial administration is therefore based on decentralized units of HIV/AIDS consultation, which are centrally coordinated. The Cantonal Department of Education is in charge of the general prevention (information, campaigns, etc.), which permits the large diffusion of prevention, even through schools.

The non-profit actors were not inactive. It was already in 1985 when the members of the Homosexuals' Base Groups in the Canton of Bern (HAB), created an HIV/AIDS specialized non-profit organization. Other inclusive non-profit organizations working in the field of drug addiction had been pressurized to help drug abusers as they were severely affected by the problem of HIV/AIDS. The authorities in Bern have actually been giving grants from the beginning to the Cantonal HIV/AIDS Antenna, which set up the basic services to fight against HIV/AIDS. Finally, it has been since 1987 that the cantonal HIV/AIDS concept has been giving important room to the non-profit organizations, i.e. putting them in charge of the psychosocial activities related to HIV/AIDS.

An actual policy to fight against the diffusion of HIV/AIDS throughout the IV-drug addict population was, compared to other cantons, quickly set up in Bern. The cantonal authorities gave the green light very early on for the free distribution of syringes and favoured methadone programmes. Later, the canton had a liberal attitude, authorizing syringe distribution in prisons or demanding a modification of the federal law on drugs in order to allow the distribution of heroin under medical supervision for instance.

The clear differentiation between public and non-profit actors is evident from the HIV/AIDS model in Bern. There is clearly one network with two centres: the HIV/AIDS Antenna and the Cantonal HIV/AIDS Coordination; they communicate with one another, but independently coordinate each of the two sub-networks. This division of work between a public and a private sub-network has not created competition amongst the different actors, but rather cooperation between those responsible for the HIV/AIDS Antenna and the Cantonal HIV/AIDS Coordination. The collaboration between the two sectors (public and non-profit) is selective and thus essentially concentrates on the exchange of information and client experiences. In addition, there are several exclusively financial collaborations, i.e. where the non-profit organizations ask the authorities for subventions. Therefore, the non-profit organizations are relatively independent in managing their activities, even though they heavily depend on the state for their financial support.

2.2.3 The Network in the Canton of Geneva

The rather important room given to the non-profit sector by the cantonal authorities in the management of HIV/AIDS is characteristic of the welfare mix which has existed in Geneva since 1985. The state limited its action to financing the actors active in the area of HIV/AIDS and sometimes incited them to create new structures or to organize new projects. However, the state allowed the actors to organize themselves in the network to realize these initiatives. In 1990 those with activities or programmes related to HIV/AIDS constituted a network of 12 public services, three exclusive and four inclusive non-profit organizations.

The response in the canton of Geneva can be divided into three phases. In 1985, the first reactions were to be detected in the gay movement when its association, Dialogai, decided to start activities related to HIV/AIDS and to join the very newly created Swiss AIDS Foundation. The prostitutes also reacted with the introduction of an AIDS group within their association, namely Aspasie, in order to discuss questions related to the disease and to evaluate the possibilities of getting an HIV test for prostitutes. The cantonal authorities became aware of the seriousness of HIV/AIDS and in October 1985, the head of the Cantonal Department for Public Health gave a press conference, with representatives of Dialogai and Aspasie, to outline the objectives of the cantonal HIV/AIDS policy, which were:
• to put the decrees set out by the Federal Office for Public Health into practice;
• to avoid all kinds of discrimination;
• to make sure that all means would be found in order to set up the necessary structures to fight against HIV/AIDS.
A final reaction came in the same year from the Cantonal Chief Medical Officer who rather spontaneously and informally created a Cantonal Committee for questions related to HIV/AIDS, gathering several actors (public and non-profit) concerned with HIV/AIDS, which operated as a kind of platform for discussion.

Nevertheless, the response remained purposely precarious on the side of the authorities as they wanted to avoid politicizing the debate. In addition to this, there was the difficulty in allocating greater subventions to a gay organization like Dialogai, which was at that time with Aspasie – the only non-profit organization active in the field of HIV/AIDS. With the increase in HIV/AIDS cases, this attitude was no longer possible. To get information as well as moral support, more and more people affected by HIV/AIDS could not identify themselves with a gay or prostitute interest group and expressed the need for a more neutral organization. Such an organization was also needed in order to facilitate the allocation of public funds. Therefore, other organizations already present in the field of social welfare in the canton of Geneva were asked by the Cantonal Department for Public Health to organize a kind of neutral federation, called the Geneva AIDS Group (GSG). Therefore, since the end of 1986-1987, larger subventions have been allocated to the Geneva AIDS Group which allots part of the money to Dialogai and part of it to the cantonal University Hospital – the medical reference centre.

The allocation of these subventions represented the end of political controversies and the beginning of a second period, characterized by the realization of the HIV/AIDS policy decided in 1985 and the allocation of steadily greater funds for the fight against HIV/AIDS.

New structures have been created since 1987. In fact, mainly in 1988, an HIV/AIDS Consultative Committee was set up at the cantonal University Hospital and two non-profit organizations, Sid'Aide and Sid'Accueil (housing facilities), were founded, whose objectives were to respond to the needs of primary care for the people in the last stages of the disease.

Since the second half of 1990, collaborations and projects were gathering all kinds of actors – public and non-profit – which created some problems of coordination.

Concerning drug addiction, the canton of Geneva went through an important development in 1988, i.e. from pursuing a policy exclusively oriented to a "drug-free" attitude, to a policy favouring harm reduction. The introduction of syringe exchanges in chemists was then made possible and it also brought an end to the "methadone conflict", which had been the centre of discussion for more than 10 years. However, it was only in 1990 when a real programme associating HIV/AIDS prevention and intravenous drug addiction was set up.

In Geneva, all actors, non-profit or public, have a lot of contact with one another (especially regarding the exchange of information and client experiences). On the other hand, coordination remains limited and not very intensive. It is purposely that the cantonal authorities have not implemented a strong centre of coordination – as is the case in Bern – as their aims were to make the existing organizations integrate the problems of HIV/AIDS in a larger prevention policy.

Geneva did not elaborate an official concept on HIV/AIDS and the HIV/AIDS policy remained mainly based on non-profit initiatives. Nevertheless, the solution adopted by the authorities in Geneva is not illustrative of the traditional subsidiary system present in the field of social welfare in Switzerland, because the authorities "used" the non-profit organizations in order to realize their own objectives. This way of action is new, especially in Geneva, where until the end of the 1970s, social policy was essentially the responsibility of large public institutions and the health care system was centred on the hospital structure, prevention remaining marginal. It has been only since the beginning of the 1980s that a new offer of various services outside the large, public institutions has started to develop. Since then, the state has had to learn to communicate and generate a real partnership with the non-profit sector.

To avoid any politicization of the HIV/AIDS issue, numerous actors were allowed to contribute to the HIV/AIDS policy – even those who did not exactly follow the government's lines. This was clearly a positive move. With the integration of as many professionals as possible in the discussions and field, the cantonal authorities in Geneva have favoured a pragmatic management of HIV/AIDS, in which the professionals and the administration have most of the say. Despite the intolerance which marked the first period of the fight against HIV/AIDS in Geneva, the state has managed to moderate the debate and has succeeded in promoting a policy centred on the fight against discrimination. However, this policy also has its negative sides, mainly because it can slow the whole process down. In fact, even if the administration is open to many projects, the professionals still have to convince the politicians of their ideas and these efforts of persuasion can cost a lot of time and effort which slows down the adoption of practical measures. Nevertheless, the Geneva case shows that through collaboration, these difficulties can be overcome.

2.2.4 The Network in the Canton of Lucerne

The originality of this canton is that it assumes the management of HIV/AIDS not only in Lucerne but also in some of its small bordering cantons (Uri, Unterwald and a part of Schwyz). The town of Lucerne is the only urban centre in the whole area and therefore the services which are provided there are of great importance to these bordering cantons. At the end of 1990, the HIV/AIDS network consisted of 22 organizations or institutions, of which 15 were public and 7 non-profit. The HIV/AIDS Antenna in Lucerne is the only exclusive one.

The management of HIV/AIDS started at the beginning of 1985 and has gone through two main phases. The first one, which lasted until 1987/88, is characterized by a parallel and distinct development of two realities, with little interaction between them:

• On the "official" side, a working group was created; it was promoted by the Physicians' Cantonal Foundation. Its objective was, in its initial phase, to discuss the strictly medical implications of the disease. Up until 1987/88, this group had been the main discussion partner in the field of HIV/AIDS for the cantonal and local authorities, as well as for the religious structures.

- The Homosexuals' Basis Group (HaLu) and the social workers dealing with drug addiction decided to organize minimal assistance for people affected with HIV/AIDS at the end of 1985, namely homosexuals and IV-drug addicts. In March 1986, the Cantonal HIV/AIDS Antenna was created thanks to the help of the Swiss AIDS Foundation. The Antenna quickly became the network centre of communication for all non-traditional, non-profit organizations.

The second phase started at the end of 1987 and was characterized by a better integration of the two networks, thanks to several factors which influenced them both:

- The group promoted by the physicians adopted more realistic options and had a more global view at the end of 1987. It actually acquired an information and formal consultative function for the authorities, a function which was regulated in 1987. Since then, the group has become an official state committee (Cantonal AIDS Committee). This institutionalization permitted the group to have more impact on the cantonal action against HIV/AIDS.
- However, the network of the non-profit organizations was no longer able to face up to the increasing demands made upon them. Voluntary services had to be abandoned in May 1987 and the HIV/AIDS Antenna became professionalized in order to face the global prevention of HIV/AIDS and to adapt itself to the needs of the people affected with HIV/AIDS in the canton.

Action and thought during this second phase were more all-encompassing and the division of work between the two sub-networks became more effective. The public network organized itself around the Cantonal AIDS Committee. It dealt with HIV/AIDS-related problems in hospitals and set up a new programme on HIV/AIDS prevention to be taught to all schoolchildren. The non-profit network organized its coordination around the HIV/AIDS Antenna and set up programmes dealing with psychosocial care, prevention and education of target groups.

These two networks did not work separately, unlike in the canton of Bern. Institutional connections were set up and used by the actors of the two networks. In addition to this, more informal and direct contacts, even everyday contacts, existed between the actors.

Concerning drug addiction and the HIV/AIDS policy, the canton of Lucerne has been rather tolerant: syringe distribution has been authorized and methadone programmes are available. The town of Lucerne has also planned to organize an injection room where IV-drug addicts have hygienic conditions and medical help at their disposal.

The cantonal authority and its administrative as well as political structures, are therefore partially absent from managing HIV/AIDS. This absence and the negative effects of the subsidiary set-up in the canton of Lucerne is counterbalanced by the intervention of national actors (the Swiss AIDS Foundation and the Federal Office for Public Health) in the cantonal network. The relative gap between the official position (rather conservative) and the everyday practice (pragmatic and tolerant) can be explained by the strategy adopted by the Cantonal Government. The idea was to differentiate the official political position from practical measures in order to preserve the conservative image attached to the canton in general as well as that of the political parties in the government. At the same time, they wanted to permit realistic and innovative actions in the field of practice. This strategy has also favoured the integration of the HIV/AIDS problem into the activities of existing institutions and organizations. Nevertheless, the differentiation between political and practical spheres can also slow down or even block innovations in situations where a political debate is unavoidable, e.g. when important funds are required for a project and must therefore be voted on by the Cantonal Parliament.

2.2.5 The Network in the Canton of Vaud

The HIV/AIDS model in the canton of Vaud integrates public and non-profit actors. The Cantonal Department of the Interior and Public Health and its head are of great influence on the whole policy in the canton of Vaud. Therefore, unlike in other cantons where the state intervention remains modest and mainly supports the Cantonal HIV/AIDS Antenna financially, the authorities are very active in the canton of Vaud, not only by taking charge of all the medical aspects, but also by delegating a certain number of tasks concerning psychosocial aspects of HIV/AIDS to non-profit structures. The Cantonal Department of Public Health and the Cantonal Chief Medical Officer have an important coordinative function. They are the political and organizational point of reference for the whole network. The cantonal University Hospital is also a central structure as the unique medical centre of reference – also because all other organizations need its services. Finally, unlike what happened in other cantons where many new organizations emerged to respond to HIV/AIDS, almost no structure had been specifically created for this purpose by 1989 in this canton. Furthermore, as homosexuals, drug addicts and prostitutes were not organized well enough, they were not considered valid actors for the Cantonal Government. The network essentially consists of actors who have been part of the cantonal social network for a long time. In 1990, eight public services and eleven non-profit organizations – among these, seven inclusives and four exclusives – were listed as managing HIV/AIDS.

The network was set up in three phases. Until 1986, the first reactions came from public actors and a special HIV/AIDS consultation was set up at the cantonal University Hospital in Lausanne. In addition, two existing inclusive organizations: *Point Fixe*, which is the section at the disposal of homosexuals at The Protestant Centre for Social Matters[21] and the Medical Social Centre for Family Planning were asked or encouraged by the Cantonal Department of Public Health to offer their activities in the field of HIV/AIDS to all public organizations and to increase them. These two organizations received public financial support to put these new activities into action. Since Point Fixe was the only specialized structure dealing with HIV/AIDS at that time, it quite naturally became the Cantonal HIV/AIDS Antenna as Pro Familia was in charge of all prevention in schools.

In a second period (1987-1988), the network did not develop, but remained stable and no new organizations were created. The existing actors saw their public subventions increase at the same rate as the disease became more important.

In a third period, namely since 1989, new activities and programmes have emerged to respond to some deficiencies in the system – especially concerning the care of people affected with AIDS and psychosocial help for HIV-positive people. The majority of these activities have been integrated into existing structures and have received public financing. However, new structures outside the established network were also created but with low subventions assigned to them. Nevertheless, these organizations were in a marginal position, since the main activities in the field of HIV/AIDS were already assumed by existing structures.

The drug addiction and HIV/AIDS cantonal policy also reflect the central position of the Cantonal Department of Public Health. Only the organizations which strictly follow the official policy, which is rather restrictive (that is, no large distribution or exchange of used syringes, in particular), can expect public subventions. The organizations which do not agree with the official policy must adapt if they do not want to be excluded from the network.

Nevertheless, and despite its dominant position, the state did not intervene directly nor develop a precise programme of intervention. Its objective was mainly to finance the projects and organizations within the political limits which had been enforced. In fact, the Cantonal Parliament had not formally defined an HIV/AIDS concept, nor set up an official HIV/AIDS committee, except for the School AIDS Prevention Committee. The administration, which follows the lines decided by those politically responsible, is the body really in charge of the management of HIV/AIDS.

The cantonal HIV/AIDS policy in the canton of Vaud tried to maximize the partnership between the administration and the existing non-profit actors. This policy, based on the delegation of tasks and responsibilities, is usual in the canton of Vaud. However, the cantonal authorities did not only delegate tasks and distribute mandates, they also decided on a general HIV/AIDS programme in order to define the practice of delegation and they incited certain organizations to set up special HIV/AIDS programmes. For the authorities, the organizations which asked for public funds had to respond strictly to the political programmes. Thus the cantonal policy gave great importance to the non-public sector, however, it also created a dependence on the non-public organizations or even determined their activities. In conclusion, even if this model does give great coherence to the management of HIV/AIDS, it has also brought about deficiencies which can result in a lack of innovations caused by a certain rigidity in the political decisions made.

2.2.6 The Network in the Canton of Zurich

Managing HIV/AIDS in the canton of Zurich is characterized by a parallel development of the public and non-profit organizations and by the complexity of the network. In 1990 there were more than 50 organizations or institutions in the canton which had activities related to HIV/AIDS. Among them, more than half were especially set up to face HIV/AIDS. Considering only the principal ones, there were 11 public services, 10 exclusive and 4 inclusive non-profit organizations, plus one shop specializing in condoms.

In the first period (1983-1987), the situation was a bit confused because both the public administration (schools, hospitals) and the non-profit organizations developed programmes without any coordination and thus brought about deficiencies or redundancies. However, the authorities have been making an effort to coordinate the existing services since 1987. With the nomination of a coordinator in the same year, namely the Cantonal AIDS Delegate, the state managed to reorganize the whole field of HIV/AIDS as well as to achieve a welfare mix based on a clear division of tasks between public services and non-profit organizations. The first actor dealing with HIV/AIDS was the cantonal University Hospital in Zurich (1983) – with a strictly medical approach. In 1984, the homosexual community, HAZ, also started activities; however, they were mainly related to the political and social aspects of AIDS. During this period, the authorities remained passive, despite numerous political interventions at the Cantonal Parliament, which reflected the general need for a more active attitude towards HIV/AIDS from the state.

The homosexual community was very active. The internal debate was animated and practical results were apparent, e.g. the creation of the Cantonal HIV/AIDS Antenna in 1985. The traditional, inclusive, social organizations were not conscious at that time of the seriousness of HIV/AIDS and did not do much in this area. Under these organizational conditions, and regarding the difficulty of starting up a public debate, the creation of a network was very difficult.

The launching of the national STOP AIDS campaign in 1987 gave a positive impulse to the debate, in both the political and social spheres. After years of stagnation, things started to change quickly and a new dynamic energy permitted the creation of new structures and projects:

- An AIDS committee of experts was set up to deal with the evaluation of the general situation, the counselling of the Cantonal Government, the elaboration of an HIV/AIDS concept for prevention and care and the organization of specific projects, like the prevention campaign in schools.

- The cantonal authorities modified their drug policy due to the acute aggravation of the IV-drug addiction problem because of HIV/AIDS. They abandoned a concept based on repression and started promoting a more open paradigm, including the free distribution of syringes and prevention material, vaccination campaigns against hepatitis, the facilitation of access to methadone therapies and the creation of shelter for homeless IV-drug addicts.
- The public subventions to existing or new non-profit organizations were increased in order to intensify the actions against HIV/AIDS.

All these measures were decisive for the organization of the network but did not completely solve the problems of coordination. The Cantonal AIDS Committee was not able to assume its role because of the lack of participation of the non-profit organizations and because of internal conflicts on the strategies to be adopted (information and prevention strategies were opposed to systematic tracing and control strategies). Its size (too large), its momentum (too slow) and its unilateral composition (essentially state employees) did not allow the committee to be effective. The nomination of the Cantonal Delegate was the measure which finally permitted the setting up and integration of the different initiatives and actors in the network and in 1989 the network resolved its organizational problems.

In conclusion, in 1990 the network in the canton of Zurich achieved a useful division of tasks and coordination to face the needs created by HIV/AIDS after the analysis of its global structure. Thus, after an initial delay and since the political change in 1987, the network was rapidly constituted. The only important deficiency concerned the care for people affected with the disease, who had no other choice than to stay at home or go to hospital.

Another problematic point is constituted by an eventual change in the drug policy – back to a more repressive concept – with the risk of very negative consequences on HIV/AIDS prevention among IV-drug addicts. This eventuality shows the crucial importance of political decisions on the development of the network in Zurich. The last aspect to be mentioned is a halt in the increase in expenditure by the cantonal authorities, which coincides with a policy favouring existing structures and discouraging the setting-up of new activities by new actors. This policy of stabilization seems to be convenient, but it can also block innovations if blindly applied.

2.2.7 Summary

Table 2.7 synthesizes the different phases of the management of HIV/AIDS in the five cantons chosen for our case-studies and at the national level. It shows the different general solutions adopted in the course of three phases. The first phase shows the first reactions during the period of constitution of the network; the second, the concretion of the network and the achievement of consensus. The third phase elucidates the systematization of the interventions in each canton. This table also illustrates very clearly how multifaceted the Swiss HIV/AIDS response really is.

Table 2.7:   The Facets of the Swiss Managing AIDS Model

Phase / Network	Period of Constitution	Period of Concretion	Period of Systematization
National	Parallel reactions from the Federal Administration & the homosexual movement (1983-1986)	Federal Administration (OFSP) incites public & non-profit actors to set up new services (>1987)	Autonomization of the AIDS sector with two independent centres of coordination (OFSP& ASS) (>1987)
Bern	Parallel reactions from the Cantonal Administration, homosexual & IV-drug organizations (1985-1987)	Concept created & set up by the Administration. Division of labour between non-profit (psychosocial) & public (medical) actors (1987)	Autonomization of the AIDS sector with two relatively independent centres of coordination (Coordination cantonale & AHBe) (>1988)
Geneva	Reactions among homosexual & prostitute organizations (1985-1986)	Cantonal Administration helps (up to 1989) & incites (since 1990) private & non-profit actors to set up new services	First sign of autonomization of the AIDS sector (creation of coordination centres) (>1990)
Lucerne	Reactions in the homosexual movement (with help of ASS & OFSP), IV-drug organizations & physicians foundations (1985-1986)	Administration helps public & non-profit actors to set up services (>1987)	Autonomization of two sectors with two coordination centres – relatively independent (AhLu & Commission) (>1987)
Vaud	Reaction of the cantonal University Hospital (Information-Sida) (1984-1985)	Administration organizes the AIDS sector by supporting non-profit organizations (>1986)	Autonomization of the AIDS sector with one centre of coordination (Cantonal Chief Medical Officer) (>1986)
Zurich	Reaction of the homosexual movement (1984-1987)	Creation & setting up of a cantonal policy and incitement of non-profit & public actors to set up services (1987-1988)	Autonomization of AIDS-sector with different coordinations in subsectors & with a supervisory centre (>1988)

During the first phase, in some cantons the public actors reacted first, in others, the non-public ones were the first to initiate action and in some other cases both of them reacted at the same time. However, contrary to this pattern, since the concretion period, and with very few exceptions, the administration has taken the active role in the management of HIV/AIDS. In the same way, we insist on all cantons having autonomy in the field of HIV/AIDS, although its forms are sometimes different.

3   Synthesis

3.1   First Stage: Emergence, Politicization and Development of a National Consensus

In addition to the cantonal variations, there are some common features valid for Switzerland as a whole. All the networks had been formed by 1985, but the preliminary reactions on forming a consensus were at first generally rather timid. It was only in 1987 and thereafter when a consensus on the policy to be followed was achieved, that effective measures could be taken on both a national and cantonal level. This consensus also led to efforts of coordination and systematization of the work done by the actors in the different networks.

Before becoming a public policy issue, HIV/AIDS was discussed by various administrations – mainly at the federal level and in the cantons most affected by HIV/AIDS, by homosexual organizations and by the media on a national level.

In the first discussions, HIV/AIDS was considered by the state as a problem affecting specific groups of the population which was to be treated following a purely medical logic. The representatives of the homosexual community stressed the social consequences of HIV/AIDS: discrimination and marginalization. However, in 1985, when the number of persons affected by the disease had increased, the Federal Administration decided to take measures in order to stop the diffusion of HIV/AIDS. The first measures were concerned with the control and treatment of blood products and with the reinforcement of medical research in university hospitals. These programmes can be described as "technical", in the way that they did not intervene with organizations other than medical institutions and did not define any new rules for safer behaviour. For the homosexual community, and some social workers active in the drug addiction field, the main issue was then to limit any possible discrimination which had been caused by the measures that the administration had taken at that time. Contact between the Federal Administration and those groups intensified in 1985 – especially when the Federal Office for Public Health became a member of the Swiss Aids Foundation.

In those cantons most affected by HIV/AIDS, some initiatives have been apparent since 1985, but on a national level all initiatives have remained limited, especially financially. No important, structured prevention campaign was apparent at that time. A political consensus which would have permitted the allocation of more consequent public funds was still missing and non-profit organizations dealing with HIV/AIDS also limited their activities to their own regular clients, i.e. to those homosexuals already integrated into a community as well as some IV-drug addicts.

However, these various initiatives and circumstances created a climate which finally allowed for incisive measures to be taken and a general prevention campaign to be set up. The first step was made by the Federal Office for Public Health

which managed to make the rest of the Federal Administration, cantonal administrations as well as the Federal Government aware of the seriousness of the problem. Secondly, the different Cantonal Administrations reacted quickly (even before the Cantonal Governments had made any decisions) in order to avoid as much
political interference as possible. Thirdly, homosexual organizations and public
and non-profit services dealing with problems of drug addiction approached administrations and political parties to push them to take major initiatives to fight
against HIV/AIDS. Finally, the media made the drama of HIV/AIDS public and
therefore also increased the pressure on the different political actors and institutions to act.

These crossing pressures caused the politicization of the debate before any actual
programmes had been realized. The main discussions concerned precisely the kind
of action that was to be taken and programmes that were to be initiated. The right
and the extreme right political parties, for instance, were thinking of measures of
control – even confinement of HIV-positive persons, a concept that the majority
of parties object to.

It was finally at the national level that the first programme based on information
was set up. Instead of presenting HIV/AIDS as a problem which ensued fears and
was presented in moral terms, the Swiss authorities decided that knowledge of the
means of protection against HIV/AIDS was the only valid answer.

The informative and preventive programme set up by the Federal Office for Public
Health later allowed for a clarification of the situation and got things moving again
in several cantons, which was characterized by a strong intermix of different political
forces. Nevertheless, the consensus achieved at the national level did not permit
the emergence of a clear political line or programme at the cantonal level. The
debates in the Cantonal Parliaments or Committees were still led by the political
parties, professional associations of physicians or pharmacists, or the Red Cross.
Associations, interest groups representing people affected with HIV/AIDS, and all
the professionals – public or non-profit – working in the field, were, at that time,
still excluded from the debates in the cantonal institutions responsible for the HIV/
AIDS policies. The only form of intervention they had was an indirect one, i.e.
using intermediaries to promote their views. Therefore, in this first period, the HIV/
AIDS network was not very well integrated and the symbolic political discourses
prevented the set up of an HIV/AIDS programme for a more or less long time –
although this is true to different extents depending on the canton.

This development, namely a politicization of HIV/AIDS, with the achievement
of a consensus made on the measures to be taken (but not on actual long-term
programmes), is mainly characterized by the collaboration between the homosexual
community and the public administration with the creation of the Swiss AIDS
Foundation in 1985. Their joint efforts led to a political awareness of the seriousness of the HIV/AIDS problem. Therefore, unlike the traditional mobilization

model, in which civil protests lead to political measures, here, it was the public actor, more specifically a section of the Federal Administration, which played the leading role in the politicization. In fact, the Federal Office for Public Health played a decisive part, not only at the federal level but also in the cantons, where it intervened as an expert. In this way, HIV/AIDS has revealed itself to be a specific, individual case compared to other fields under political regulation.

Therefore, the traditional Swiss procedure, namely that civil society sets up structures which are then completed by the state, does not apply to the management of HIV/AIDS. Generally speaking, at the national and at the cantonal levels, a portion of the state, i.e. the administration, decided not to wait for the reactions in civil society to start working in the field of HIV/AIDS. It was neither an "up-down" reaction, since the administration set up programmes without waiting for Government directives. HIV/AIDS was considered a medical and social emergency which needed quick, specific measures – with good reason. The administration became aware that HIV/AIDS was a risky situation which could not be controlled with the usual administrative means. The main instrument was prevention, aimed at a change in the behaviour of the whole population. That is the reason why the administration, and especially the Federal Office for Public Health, has tried to keep in contact with society by the intermediation of institutional "bridges" like the Swiss AIDS Foundation. The administration took an active part in managing HIV/AIDS, even in the cantons where reactions have been slow and weak, and a flexible social risk administration was organized in all cantons. These processes took some years and new "trial and error" processes occurred due to the lack of experience within the administrations and governments for these kinds of risk management procedures, as well as due to the slow changes in a system based on consensus.

3.2 Second Stage: Systematization through Reference Actors[22]

The dimension of "social danger", which taints HIV/AIDS and which partly determined the action of the Federal Office for Public Health and other cantonal administrations, also influenced the structure and functioning of the networks of organizations and institutions dealing with HIV/AIDS. Since forming a consensus on HIV/AIDS, one can discern two periods through which the various networks have passed. During the first period, the networks opened up to all kinds of organizations, demanding subsidies and political support and in a second period, the action became more systematized.

In the first period, networks were badly integrated and functioned on two levels – the symbolic level of committees and parliaments, and the practical level of actual services. New actors, active in the social and the political fields, asked for subventions and political support. They therefore created a stressful situation in the different political cantonal systems, which were generally overwhelmed by much non-discriminatory financial support, which was given to more or less all activities. During that period, HIV/AIDS was considered a medical and social matter of urgency, a fact which facilitated the establishment of HIV/AIDS actors in the various networks. The launching of the national STOP AIDS campaign legitimized the increase in activities and expenditure and many new projects managed to find a place in the networks. The cantonal committees, which were then made up of only politicians, medical professionals and established social actors, soon became open to new ones.

This situation of proliferation and activism in society pushed the Cantonal Governments to define strategies. Efficient administrations helped them to take strategic decisions and became central actors able to define programmes, not on a political basis but on the basis of the successful experiments which had been realized by the Federal Office for Public Health. Nevertheless, the cantonal administrations did not undertake any efforts to structure the interventions. During this stage, we can say that the network went from a period of politicization to one of concretion.

During the second period, which can be defined as one of stabilization and systematization, one observes an improvement in both the coordination between HIV/AIDS actors and a better integration of networks. This coordination was not realized by the established HIV/AIDS committees. They were often too politicized and they could not even find a political consensus for the different interests they represented. Moreover, the majority of them were characterized by their internal self-hindrance and by the externalization of their problems. Their status often limited them to merely advise their respective government. On the whole, they were not appropriated to coordinate the various actors present in the field of HIV/AIDS. Therefore, several cantons set up coordinative structures, usually formed by agencies outside the symbolic sphere of politics.

These processes of coordination had the effect of consolidating the networks: they allowed for the identification of the deficiencies and allocation of the resources in an improved way. During this period, new agents appeared outside the existing networks, but they faced difficulties in establishing their activities. Moreover, the agents that did not share the fundamental decisions of the coordinating agencies were excluded from the networks and thus lost access to public subsidies. In fact, the rationalization and sectorialization of the services and the development of a system of managing HIV/AIDS had rather important consequences on the future developments of the networks.

HIV/AIDS was then considered less and less to be an urgent social problem, which would have justified unlimited expenditure, but more and more to be a "normal" problem, as cancer for example. Expenditure therefore had to be motivated following the criteria of efficacy and efficiency to regulate the networks. This development led to a sectorialization of the field. Moreover, whereas during the whole period of the development of the networks, the state agents (the Federal Administration in particular) have played a major role, it is now mainly the actors of coordinating agencies (either public or private) who determine the operative rules of the networks and the qualitative standards of services. The welfare mix now mainly depends on the internal negotiations inside the HIV/AIDS established system, which consequently favours the existing structures. In one way, this evolution has, for the first time, the consequence of blocking innovations, but it also permits the amelioration of existing services (by professionalizing for instance certain administrative activities or using the knowledge accumulated in social work). This amelioration and stabilization is essential after all the years of turbulent development.

Finally, the control of the allocation and efficient use of resources is, with sectorialization transferred outside the traditional institutions' control (i.e. the Parliament's and the Government's), given to central actors in the network who can therefore legitimize new projects and initiatives. These actors, generally the cantonal antennas of the Swiss AIDS Foundation, have a status of official partner for the actors outside the HIV/AIDS network.

3.3   Conclusion

Managing HIV/AIDS in Switzerland is now in its second decade. The reconstruction we have made shows a successful story, crowned by international recognition and praise. Nevertheless, it is important to mention that this HIV/AIDS model is not typical of what traditionally happens in the Swiss social welfare system. Therefore, if it represents a model for other countries to follow, it is also valid for other fields of the social welfare system in Switzerland. Its strength lies in the way integration has been achieved, which respects federalism without becoming the determining factor. The incitation policy, started by the Federal Administration in 1985, introduced a prevention and care system which is the result of a conscious and determined policy. Thus, the national prevention campaign could be set up without having to take any cantonal sensitivities into consideration, but at the same time, leaving the cantons alone to conform to their own realities. The "heterarchic" network, with its national and cantonal centres, is in the end headed by the two national bodies: the Federal Office for Public Health and the Swiss AIDS Foundation. They guarantee the existence of the essential services, particularly the diffusion of preventive information, but, at the same time, allow the cantons to adapt and improve these services and information campaigns.

This development also has some dangers due to the weakness of the emerging network. The central actors in the HIV/AIDS field have only had a few years of experience and must continuously define their internal rules and sometimes even their objectives. Among the public actors, the introduction of a flexible risk administration remains problematic because the administration is not prepared for the new style of management. Neither is it politically legitimized enough for them. The flexibility in the administration is actually based on a cooperative model, this leaves an important space of action to cantonal administrative bodies. The implementation of the new model of management creates various conflicts within the Federal Administration and remains today an important issue in the different administrations. For the non-profit actors, the establishment of new services is also a source of conflict or doubt. For instance, the Swiss AIDS Foundation has experienced many conflicts throughout its history, which could have undermined its legitimacy in the eyes of the political authorities. However, they decided to keep their confidence in the Swiss AIDS Foundation, adding to the fact that there was no serious alternative. This confidence gave legitimacy to the Swiss AIDS Foundation. Similarly, the sectorialization of the field has been possible only thanks to the confidence the political actors have had towards the HIV/AIDS actors in general.

Given the still precarious consensus existing in the Cantonal Governments as well as in the Federal Government, it is quite possible to observe a change of style in the government towards a more conflicting management due to an increasing confrontation between political positions, which are also present in many political parties at the moment. Such an evolution could break the confidence existing between the different actors and destroy the kind of networks set up in Switzerland because they need large support from all factions of the political power.

Notes

1   This part of the international project has been conducted under the direction of Patrick Kenis and Bernd Marin and the Swiss country study directed by Hanspeter Kriesi. It has been financed by the Swiss National Fund for Scientific Research which, within the framework of the National Programme of Research 29 in the area of "Changes in the Ways of Life and Future of Social Security in Switzerland", made it possible to complete this project (project no. 4029-02166). The complete research also includes an analysis of the organizational response to the alcohol problem. See Bütschi/Cattacin (1994).

2   The HIV test is voluntary in Switzerland. If a person is submitted to the HIV test in hospital, anonymity is guaranteed, whereas in the doctor's consulting room it is not.

3   There were between 12,000 and 24,000 estimated cases of HIV by 1989. One can calculate from these figures that in 1995 there will be a total of 5,000 to 10,000 AIDS cases (see OFSP/Commission fédérale, 1991, *Le SIDA en Suisse – 1991. Situation actuelle, mesures prises, perspectives et recommandations jusqu'en 1993*, pp. 114-116).

4   We must however be cautious when comparing Switzerland with other countries since Switzerland has developed an efficient controlling system of the epidemic not used in other countries.

5   Figures estimated by the Commission fédérale pour les problèmes liés au SIDA (1990): 'Aspects économiques de la maladie d'immunodéficiience SIDA', *Vie économique* 3: 28.

6   This tendency must be put into perspective however, due to the long delay until the illness breaks out. The reason for the tendency towards a certain stabilization of the growth rate in the last years can also be due to the use of medicines which delay the development of the illness as well as to the prevention campaign which started in 1987 (see OFSP, 1993: 24 and next parts of this report).

7   The fact that the territory of this canton is mainly occupied by a city (the countryside is very small) can certainly be accounted for a large part of this high prevalence, but it cannot be considered as the only explanation. As a matter of fact, the semi-canton of the City of Basel that shares, with Geneva, the characteristic of being a "city-canton", is less affected by HIV/AIDS.

8   See Institut suisse de la santé publique et des hôpitaux (ISH), 1988, *Sida: vue d'ensemble sur les mesures prises par la Confédération, les cantons et les institutions privées*, p. 29.

9   Prisons are not included in this figure, although a dozen have HIV/AIDS programmes (see Harding/Manghi/Sanchez, 1990). We decided not to include them in our study because answers to the questionnaires were often missing.

10   This result contradicts the hypothesis held by Czada and Friedrich-Czada (1989) which states that public services have reacted late to the HIV/AIDS epidemic.

11   The crucial role of prevention in managing AIDS has been especially developed by Rosenbrock (1987; 1989) and by Somaini (1989) and, more generally in sexually transmitted diseases, by Widdus/Mehens/Short (1990).

12   For more details on AIDS and IV-drug use policies and their cantonal differences, see Malatesta/Joye/Spreyermann (1992).

13   Geneva seems to be an exception regarding this finding; the more detailed analysis of this canton in the next part can help us to understand why HIV/AIDS has not been as politicized as in Zurich, Bern and the canton of Basel-city.

14   From these figures, we can extrapolate that exclusive organizations' resources are as follows: in 1990 on average, SFr 274,000 ($ 195,700) with 5 professionals and 17 volunteers involved.

15   The Swiss AIDS Foundation is an umbrella association which gathers mainly collective members together. Among them are the so-called "cantonal antennas" (*antennes cantonales*), present in almost every canton. The Swiss AIDS Foundation deals at the national level with political lobbying and cooperates very closely with the Federal Office for Public Health especially in the field of prevention whereas the cantonal antennas have mainly preventive and psychosocial activities as well as political lobbying activities at the cantonal level.

16   It is not possible however – with the data collected through the inventory – to come to any conclusions concerning the quality of these first rapid reactions.

17   For a history of the homosexual movements and the emergence of HIV/AIDS in Switzerland, see Staub (1988).

18   This term has since then been abandoned and replaced by "risk behaviour". For a reflexion on the usefulness of this distinction, see Widdhus/Mehens/Short (1990), p. 183.

19   The Cantonal Chief Medical Officer is the person responsible for medical matters at the Cantonal Department of Public Health in each canton.

20   Its name being Cantonal AIDS Coordination.

21 This centre, namely *Centre Social Protestant* – founded by protestants – offers several
social services (family and marriage counselling, legal advice, launderette, etc.) and
is open to anybody, regardless of his/her religious beliefs.
22 These are private actors (federal and cantonal) recognized by the state as valid partners.

References

Bütschi, Danielle/Cattacin, Sandro (1993) 'The Third Sector in Switzerland: The
Transformation of the Subsidiary Principle', *West European Politics* 3: 362-379.
Bütschi, Danielle/Cattacin, Sandro (1994) *Le modèle suisse du bien-être*. Lausanne: Réalités
sociales.
Cattacin, Sandro/Passy, Florence (1993) 'Der Niedergang von Bewegungsorganisationen.
Zur Analyse von organisatorischen Laufbahnen', *Kölner Zeitschrift für Soziologie und
Sozialpsychologie* 3: 419-438.
Czada, Roland/Friedrich-Czada, Heidi (1989) *Aids als politisches Konfliktfeld und
Verwaltungsproblem*. Paper presented at the conference entitled "Aids und
Sozialwissenschaften", Berlin 23/24.2.1989.
Gros Dominique/Hausser, Dominique (1992) 'La lutte contre les discriminations: une
nécessité pour la prévention', in: Elena Gottraux-Biancardi (éd.), *Air pur, eau claire,
préservatif: Tuberculose, alcoolisme, sida: une histoire comparée de la prévention*.
Lausanne: Editions d'en bas.
Harding, T.-W./Manghi, R./Sanchez, G. (1990) *Le Sida en milieu carcéral. Les stratégies
de prévention dans les prisons suisses*. Berne: OFSP.
Malatesta, Dominique (1991) *Toxicomanie et prévention du sida. Etude descriptive d'une
histoire récente: Genève, 1980-1990*. Lausanne: Institut universitaire de médecine
sociale et préventive.
Malatesta, Dominique/Joye, Dominique/Spreyermann, Christine (1992) *Villes et toxicomanie. Des politiques urbaines de prévention du sida en Suisse*. Lausanne: Institut
de recherche sur l'environnement construit, Rapport de recherche No 99.
Pollack, Michael (1987) 'AIDS: Risikomanagement unter widersprüchlichen Zwängen.
Reaktionen und Verhaltensänderungen unter französischen Homosexuellen', *Journal
für Sozialforschung* 3/4.
Rosenbrock, Rolf (1987) *Soziale, medizinische une sozialwissenschaftliche Voraussetzungen
der Prävention und Bekämpfung von Aids*. Berlin: Wissenschaftszentrum für Sozial-
forschung.
Somaini, Bertino (1989) *The Basis of Prevention of AIDS and HIV*. Paper presented in the
workshop "The Social Implications of AIDS", Vienna, 17-19 October 1989.
Staub, Roger (1988) *Les homosexuels et le sida. La recherche d'une solution*. Zürich: Aide
Suisse contre le Sida.
Widdus, Roy/Mehens, André/Short, Roger (1990) 'Management of Risk in Sexually
Transmitted Diseases', *Daedalus* 199 (4): 177-191.

Documents

Aids-Infothek, 1991/4.

Commission fédérale pour les problèmes liés au SIDA (1990) 'Aspects économiques de la maladie d'immunodéficience SIDA', *Vie économique* 3: 25-29.

Imhof, Edith (1989) *Campagne anti-sida dans les écoles. Moyens utilisés, directives.* Genève: CESDOC – Centre suisse de documentation en matière d'enseignement et d'éducation.

ISH – Institut suisse de la santé publique et des hôpitaux (1988) *Sida: vue d'ensemble sur les mesures prises par la Confédération, les cantons et les institutions privées.* Aarau: ISH.

OFSP et Commission fédérale pour les problèmes liés au SIDA (1991) *Le SIDA en Suisse – 1991. Situation actuelle, mesures prises, perspectives et recommandations jusqu'en 1993*, rapport de l'Office fédéral de la santé publique et de la Commission pour les problèmes liés au SIDA.

OFSP – Office fédéral de la santé publique, Division de médecine, Section de l'épidémiologie médicale (1993) 'Aperçu général de l'épidémie de VIH et de sida en Suisse jusqu'à la fin 1992', *Bulletin de l'Office fédéral de la santé publique* 2 (25.1.1993): 18-26.

CHAPTER 3

The Netherlands:
The Strong Civil Society Response

Ineke Kester
Bert de Vroom
Armand van Wolferen

Introduction

The Dutch HIV/AIDS policy in the past decade can be characterized as having been marked by a civil society response to the problem: with a very strong involvement of private and community organizations. Compared to other countries, the Netherlands has the highest number of such organizations – with over 700. The organizational response to the HIV/AIDS epidemic in the Netherlands is not one-dimensional, but is a mixture of top-down, bottom-up and horizontal organizational structures. The overall AIDS policy and its complex organizational pattern reflects a mixture of different guiding principles of coordination and allocation: hierarchical control and coercion, organized expertise, altruism, solidarity, organized risk experience, and calculative rationality.

The size and direction of the strong civil society response cannot be explained as being merely a reflection of the size and spread of the HIV/AIDS epidemic as such. It must be explained as the result of a number of interrelated social and (partly) country- and issue-specific facts.

Firstly, the application of the existing institutional repertoire, e.g. medical technology, pharmacy, or legal coercion, in dealing with threatening public health risks have proven to be limited and inadequate in coping with the AIDS epidemic. As a result the HIV/AIDS problem has changed from a technological problem into a social or policy problem of groups at risk, so called "risk-behaviour", and has at the same time stimulated a differentiated demand for new types of services. This shift is one explanation for the increasing organizational response towards HIV/

AIDS. The number and type of organizations dealing with HIV/AIDS in the Netherlands, cannot, however, be sufficiently explained by the social structure of the epidemic since we can observe different organizational responses in other countries with almost the same type of social structure.

Secondly, the existing organizational experiences, capacities and structures are important variables, not only to explain the organizational response on the macro level, but also on the level of groups at risk (De Vroom, 1993; Kenis/De Vroom, 1996). The particular Dutch response of a huge number of organizations on the one hand, and a functional and structural differentiation and integration of the organizational pattern on the other, are the results of both organizational experience and capacity combined with a particular style of regulation.

The structure of this chapter is as follows. In section 1 we start with a general picture of the epidemiological context. The size and development of the overall HIV/AIDS epidemic in the Netherlands from 1980-1995 will be sketched out, followed by a description of the social structure and dynamics in terms of groups at risk and subepidemics. In section 2 the Dutch policy response is described and characterized as "active and liberal", indicating the explicit policy of non-intervention in individual or group behaviour. This particular national style of regulation correlates with a strong civil society response in the sense that a high number of private organizations are involved in the HIV/AIDS policy domain. The general organizational pattern and its structural differentiation is described in section 3. The functional differentiation (goals and tasks of the different organizations) is dealt with in section 4. In the concluding section (section 5) the organizational response will be analysed in policy terms, using a differentiation between top-down, bottom-up and horizontal responses. The Dutch organizational response is not only highly differentiated in structural and functional terms. It has also moved towards a mix of top-down, bottom-up and horizontal responses, which in our opinion might be a preferable model to cope with such complicated social problems like the HIV/AIDS epidemic.

1   The General Picture of the HIV/AIDS Epidemic

1.1   Size and Development of the Registered Epidemic

So far, the origin of the HIV epidemic in the Netherlands can be traced back to 1979, starting among men with homosexual contacts.[1] The first AIDS case was diagnosed at the end of 1981.[2] Between then and 1 January 1996, the cumulative number of AIDS cases had increased to 3,840. Almost 75% (approx. 2,850) of this group have died (Table 3.1).

Since there is no notification and registration system for HIV infections it is barely possible to reconstruct the size and development of the HIV epidemic in the same way as that of the AIDS epidemic. HIV infections in the Netherlands are estimated

Table 3.1:   The Development of the HIV/AIDS Epidemic in the Netherlands (1981-1995)

Year	New Diagnoses[a]	Reported Cumulative AIDS Diagnoses[b]	Cumulative Number of Persons Died[d]	Estimated HIV Infections
1981	1	1		
1982	4	5		
1983	19	24	8	
1984	31	55	24	
1985	67	122	54	
1986	136	258	117	
1987	242	500	223	10-20,000
1988	325	825	358	
1989	391	1,216	560	10-12,000
1990	416	1,632	829	
1991	446	2,078	1,123	
1992	506	2,584	1,535	
1993	459	3,043	1,962	8-12,000
1994	450	3,493	2,406	8-12,000
1995	347[c]	3,840	2,856[e]	8,000

a final year (source: Stichting Aids Fonds, *AIDS-bestrijding*, maart 1996, no. 27: 10).
b final year; adjusted for reporting delays (except 1995) (source: see footnote a).
c *not* adjusted for reporting delays.
d CBS, *Statistiek Doodsoorzaken* (1983-1994); only Dutch citizens.
e *estimation.*

on the basis of the reported AIDS cases. These estimations have been changed dramatically in recent years as a result of changing methods and assumptions. In early 1987 the number of HIV infected persons was estimated at 10,000 - 20,000 persons.[3] In early 1990 the number of HIV infections for 1989 was estimated at between 10,000 and 12,000 persons.[4] In 1995 the number of HIV infections was estimated at between 8,000 and 12,000.[5]

1.2 The Social Structure and Dynamics of the Epidemic

The particular characteristic of the HIV/AIDS epidemic is its heterogeneous pattern of different groups at risk and corresponding subepidemics which might vary between countries and which can partly explain the particular organizational responses. The following sociological variables have been used to describe the social structure of the epidemic in the Netherlands: heterogeneity, size, social cohesion and epidemic load of groups at risk.

1.2.1   Heterogeneity

For the purpose of this research we have defined heterogeneity as the extent to which the HIV/AIDS epidemic differs across subgroups concerning particular risk behaviour, risk situations and/or risk-sensitivity.[6] Heterogeneity in this context is related to policy and organizational responses in the way that a higher degree of heterogeneity is probably reflected in a more differentiated policy and organizational response.[7]

In the early years the epidemic was more or less framed as a homogeneous phenomenon concentrating on the group of men with homosexual contacts. The first AIDS case in the Netherlands got publicity at a scientific conference with the title *Fatal Diseases among Promiscuous Homosexuals* and was communicated to the general public in a national newspaper as *New 'Homosexual Disease' Takes Its First Victim*.[8] In the course of the epidemic, and as a result of epidemiological research, public debate, political mobilization and organizational response, a growing number of different groups at risk were mentioned in policy documents, the media, and in public information campaigns, e.g. intravenous drug users, heroin prostitutes, receivers of blood products, haemophiliacs, health care workers, travellers to high risk areas, sex tourists, prisoners, etc. At the same time we can observe a trend in defining broader groups at risk like: women, youngsters, and even the general public.[9]

In the course of the epidemic not only the heterogeneity between groups at risk comes to the fore but also within the groups themselves. For instance, within the group of hard drug users and with respect to risk behaviour, a distinction has been made between "domestic" users, ethnic groups and the so-called "heroin tourists". There is hardly any contact between heroin tourists and domestic users whereas Surinamese and Moroccan users look down on the Dutch injecting drug users. Drug-using prostitutes are another group isolated from both other hard drug users and other prostitutes.[10] A social gap is also reported between Dutch prostitutes and an increasing group of foreign prostitutes.[11]

Partly due to these varying views towards the epidemic on both the policy and public levels, a differentiated organizational pattern has been developed in which many, but not all of the mentioned groups at risk are organized in one way or another. This will be illustrated in section 2.

1.2.2   Size of Groups at Risk

The size of groups at risk – number of individuals in a particular population at risk – is an important variable in two respects. From an epidemiological point of view, the size is an indication of the ultimate size of the epidemic (in this group)[12] and might also be an indicator for policy priorities. From a sociological point of view, the size of a group might become an important variable for collective action by those groups (organizational response). According to literature on the subject, large (latent) groups will have more problems concerning associative action than small (privileged) groups.[13] As illustrated in Table 3.3, the estimated size of the distinguished groups varies between large (latent) groups like heterosexual men or women in the 20-45 age group and small groups like the haemophiliacs (numbering only 1,200).

1.2.3   Social Cohesion of Subgroups

Contrary to the size of the group at risk – which is more a descriptive and statistical indicator – the variable "social cohesion" gives an indication for the extent of social relationships between individual members of the group. This variable is also very important with respect to both the epidemiological and the sociological side of the HIV/AIDS epidemic. From the epidemiological point of view, a group at risk with a high level of social cohesion will probably influence the spread of HIV/AIDS within this group in a negative sense. From a sociological point of view, a high level of social cohesion might be an important condition for associative action, e.g. to change risk behaviour in this group. Social cohesion seems to create a paradoxical effect: the higher the level of social cohesion, the higher the risk of getting HIV/AIDS. However, it also offers a better possibility to change risk behaviour by associative action thus reducing the risk of getting HIV/AIDS.

Three aspects of social cohesion seem to be important in this context. *Firstly,* social cohesion indicates the extent to which members of the population are able to maintain frequent social relationships with each other instead of making diffuse or fleeting contacts. This might be the case if the group at risk is concentrated in a small geographical area instead of being spread out all over the country. In this respect, the social cohesion of the distinguished groups at risk in the Dutch context varies between two extremes. Homosexuals and intravenous drug users are concentrated in Amsterdam, whereas the other groups are more or less dispersed across the country:

> Separate attention for Amsterdam seems reasonable for a combination of reasons: the concentration of drug users (...), the differences in seroprevalence among hard drug users within and outside Amsterdam (...) and the function of Amsterdam as the international meeting place and entertainment centre for homosexual men (...). There is also a correlation between the degree of urbanization and the occurrence of prostitution and STD incidence (...)[14]

The particular pattern of the geographical spread of AIDS diagnoses seems to underline this aspect of social cohesion (see Table 3.2).

Secondly, social cohesion is influenced by the extent to which individuals of a group are able to engage in primary face-to-face contact with one another. This might be the case if there are particular public and/or underground infrastructural provisions where this is possible. Groups at risk also differ from one another here. An infrastructure of bars, meeting points, etc. for homosexuals in the Netherlands (in Amsterdam in particular) has developed in the past decades. For intravenous drug users the situation is different. Contrary to other countries, there are no "shooting galleries", but Dutch users predominantly consume "at home" or "alone".[15]

The *third* indication of social cohesion is the extent to which members of a population share a particular common culture, values and "views of the world". It is also here that the social cohesion between and within populations varies. As already mentioned, within the group of hard drug users and prostitutes there are different, more or less isolated groups with particular cultural features. There is also a frequently reported gap between domestic and ethnic groups. With respect to both the epidemiological pattern and the particular knowledge, attitude and behaviour of ethnic groups concerning sexuality and AIDS, hardly any scientific information is available in the Netherlands.[16]

Contrary to these groups, the social cohesion in terms of a shared culture is relatively high amongst the homosexual population.[17]

These features of social cohesion are also partly reflected in the organizational development and types of organizations of the different groups at risk (see the following section). It is the homosexual population in particular which has reached a relatively high level of organizational development whereas marginal groups, e.g. particular ethnic groups, are barely organized, or are reached by other organizations.

1.2.4   The Epidemiological Load of Subgroups

By epidemiological load we mean the number of cumulative AIDS cases related to the size of a particular group at risk at a certain point in time. For comparative reasons we have recalculated the cumulative number of AIDS cases of groups at risk as the number of cases per 10,000. From a sociological point of view, one might expect a correlation between the "epidemiological load" of subgroups and the type and level of organizational and policy responses. The higher the epidemic load the more one might expect either an organizational response by the population at risk and/or by other actors in the policy domain. The major different populations at risk will be described in terms of subepidemic characteristics and the respective epidemic load.

I.   THE REGIONAL POPULATIONS

As illustrated in Table 3.2 and Figure 3.1, the AIDS epidemic is not evenly spread across the country but varies very much between the 12 different provinces. We

Table 3.2: The Epidemic across Regional Populations (1993)

Region	1 Group Size by Number of Inhabitants as of 1.1.1993[a]	2 Number of Cumulative AIDS Cases		3 Epidemic Load in Number of AIDS Cases in 1993 Related to Regional Group Size in Number of AIDS Cases per Million Inhabitants	4 Epidemic Spread: Regional Number of AIDS Cases as % of the Total Number of AIDS Cases
		1 January 1993[b]	1 January 1996[c]		
Province					
URBANIZED REGIONS					
Northern Holland	2,440,200	1,404	2,066	575	54.5
Southern Holland	3,295,500	485	772	147	18.8
Utrecht	1,047,000	119	199	114	4.6
COUNTRYSIDE					
Flevoland	243,400	22	32	90	0.9
Overijssel	1,039,100	80	110	77	3.1
Limburg	1,119,900	75	101	67	2.9
Gelderland	1,839,900	120	166	65	4.7
Groningen	555,400	33	53	59	1.3
Northern-Brabant	2,243,500	105	163	47	4.1
Friesland	604,000	27	51	45	1.0
Sealand	361,200	14	22	39	0.5
Drenthe	448,300	7	10	16	0.3
unknown		11	16		0.4
Non-Dutch citizens		73	79		2.8
Total	15,239,200	2,575	3,840	169	100.0
Large cities					
Amsterdam	719,856	1,255	1,799	1,743	48.7
The Hague	444,661	160	236	360	6.2
Utrecht	234,170	54	93	231	2.1
Rotterdam	596,023	132	226	221	5.1

a   CBS, *Statistisch Jaarboek 1994*.
b   NCAB, *AIDS-bestrijding*, mei 1994, nr. 16:11; juni 1993, nr. 11:6.
c   Stichting Aids Fonds, *AIDS-bestrijding*, Maart 1996, nr. 27:10. Not adjusted for reporting delays.

Figure 3.1: The Regional Concentration of the AIDS Epidemic in the Netherlands, 1993

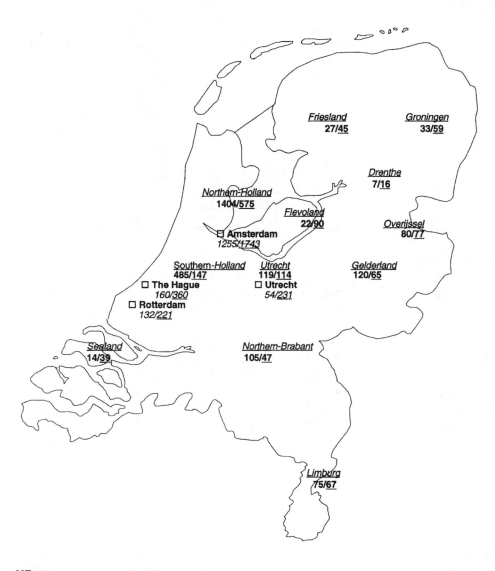

NB:

Friesland	=	province
27/45	=	cumulative number of AIDS cases per province / number of AIDS cases per million inhabitants of the province (large cities included)
☐ **Amsterdam**	=	large city

find the province of Drenthe having had only eight AIDS cases in 1994 (1 October) for example, whereas the province of Northern Holland had the very high number of 1,765 cumulative AIDS cases at the same point in time. This difference cannot be explained by the population density. In Table 2 the number of cumulative AIDS cases (1 January 1993) is related to the size of the population in the respective provinces. The urbanized regions in the western part of the country (the provinces of Northern Holland, Southern Holland and Utrecht) have by far the highest epidemic load in numbers of AIDS cases per million inhabitants (575, 147 and 114 respectively) (see also Figure 3.1). The epidemic is concentrated in the large cities of Amsterdam, The Hague, Rotterdam and Utrecht. It is particularly the city of Amsterdam which feels the intensity of the problem as it has almost 50% of all Dutch AIDS cases. This pattern corresponds with the socio-cultural fact that the most important populations at risk – homosexuals and intravenous drug users – are concentrated in the large cities of the western part of the country, therefore in Amsterdam in particular. Table 3.3 illustrates the particular social structure of the epidemic in the Netherlands.

II.   AGE GROUPS

The epidemic is more or less age-specific. Almost 60% of the AIDS diagnoses fall into the age category of 30-44. The reported AIDS diagnoses of children under the age of 15 were less than 1%. In about 56% of these cases it was a result of mother to child transmission: of 32 cumulative cases reported by 1 January 1996, 18 cases were the result of mother to child transmissions.[22] For the age group of 60 years and older, the reported AIDS diagnoses are less than 3%. Related to the group-size of the different age groups, the epidemic load in 1993 varies from 0.06/10,000 for the under 20 age group, 1.09/10,000 for the 45 age group, to 3.19/10,000 for the 20-44 age group (Table 3.3).

III.   MALES AND FEMALES

Like in most Western countries, the AIDS epidemic mainly affects the male population. In 1990, 1,344 AIDS cases (94%) were diagnosed among men (>12 years old) and 84 AIDS cases (6%) among women (>12 years old). From the 3,840 cumulative AIDS cases on 1 January 1996, 91% (3,484) were male and 9% (356), female. Since the late 1980s/early 1990s the AIDS epidemic among women has become a political issue; women's groups have emphasized the stronger increase of new diagnoses among women compared to men. Related to the group size of the respective groups, the epidemic load is 3.17 and 0.24 per 10,000 for males and females respectively (Table 3.3).

IV. THE HOMOSEXUAL POPULATION

Since the very beginning of the epidemic, men with homo-/bisexual contacts have been the largest affected group at risk. On 1 January 1996, 73.5% of all AIDS cases were men with homo-/bisexual relations (1.0% homo-/bisexual drug users are included). Their relative number has slightly decreased over the years (on 1 October 1990, 81.2%). Not only related to the overall number of AIDS cases, but also related to group-size, this group has been disproportionately attacked by the epidemic: 105/10,000 or 1 in 100 (Table 3.3).

There is no exact information about the total number of HIV infections in this population. However, the Amsterdam cohort study reveals information concerning the cumulative seroprevalence among Amsterdam males with homosexual contacts. It increased from 32% in 1984-1985 to 42% in 1989.[23] However, one should stress that this study is not representative of the whole group of men with homosexual contacts.

V. THE HETEROSEXUAL POPULATION

In 1990 the number of cumulative AIDS cases as a result of heterosexual contacts was 75 (5.2% of all AIDS cases).[18] On 1 January 1996, this number had increased to 474 (11.3%), of which 262 were men and 172, women.[19] Notwithstanding the growing number of persons infected by heterosexual contacts, it is commonly concluded that there are hardly any indications of an autonomous epidemic among the heterosexual population in the Netherlands. Even the chance of such a subepidemic taking place, judging by the initial signs, is not believed to be very realistic.[20] According to the heterosexual population, limited studies amongst pregnant women, persons with promiscuous sexual behaviour, screening by blood banks and contact tracing of persons with AIDS measured a seroprevalence of less than 1% (stg, 67).[21] If the number of AIDS cases is related to the group size, the epidemic load of this group is very low (approx. 0,2 per 10,000) (Table 3.3).

VI. INTRAVENOUS DRUG USERS

The total number of hard drug users in the Netherlands is approximately 20,000.[24] Most of them are concentrated in the western part of the country, in Amsterdam and Rotterdam in particular (approx. 7,000 and approx. 3,500 respectively).[25] Of the approximately 20,000 hard drug users, circa 8,000 are intravenous drug users. According to GG&GD Amsterdam (1992), the estimated number of 7,000 hard drug users in Amsterdam is differentiated between ±2,000 foreign users, ±3,500 Dutch users and ±1,500 ethnic users. Compared to other countries, the percentage of intravenous drug users among Dutch hard drug users is low (30%). Among ethnic addicts – Moluccan, Surinamese, Moroccan, Antillean – the percentage of intravenous drug users is low (circa 5%), whereas the percentage of intravenous drug users among heroin tourists is estimated to be as high as 70%.[26]

Table 3.3:   Populations at Risk and the Epidemic Load (1993)

Population at Risk	1 Group Size 1.1.1994	2 Number of Cumulative AIDS Cases[a] 1.1.1993	3 Number of HIV Diagnoses (Estimation)	4 Epidemic Load: AIDS Cases Related to Group Size[b] per 10,000	5 Epidemic Load: AIDS Cases as % of Total Number AIDS Cases
Total population[c]	15,341,553	2,575	8,000-12,000[d]	1.70	100.0
Age[c]:					
<20	3,751,154	24		0.06	0.9
20-44	6,169,684	1,971		3.19	76.5
≥45	5,323,028	580		1.09	22.5
Sex[c]:					
Female	7,703,914	184	630-840[e]	0.24	7.1
Male	7,535,268	2,391		3.17	92.9
Subgroup:					
Homosexual men (20-64)	192,000[f]	2,003[g]		105.00	77.8
Heterosexual men (20-64)	4,600,000[h]	115[i]		0.25	4.5
Heterosexual women (20-64)	4,500,000[h]	77[i]		0.17	3.0
Hard drug users	20,000[j]				
IV-drug users	8,000[k]	224	1,500[o]	280.00	8.7
Homo-/bisexual drug users		26			1.0
Prostitutes[l]					
- Total	17,500				
- Male	1,300				
- Drug-addicted	750				
Mother-child transmission		11			0.4
Haemophiliacs	1,200[m]	43	170[n]	342.00	1.6
Other receivers of blood products		35			1.4

a   NCAB, *AIDS-Bestrijding*, June1993; not adjusted for reporting delays.
b   in number of cumulative AIDS cases per 10,000 members of the respective subgroup.
c   CBS, *Statistisch Jaarboek 1995*.
d   NCAB, *AIDS-Bestrijding*, May1994.
e   *Bureau Vrouwen & Aids*.
f   deduced from the estimation: 4% of the population is homosexual (Van Zessen, 1990).
g   NCAB, *AIDS-Bestrijding*, June 1993: homo-/bisexual men.
h   estimation (see also f).
i   NCAB, *AIDS-Bestrijding*, June 1993.
j   estimation (GG&GD Amsterdam, 1992).
k   estimation (GG&GD Amsterdam, 1992).
l   STG 1992:58.
m   NVHP, *Hemofilie en AIDS*, September 1992:19.
n   NCAB, *AIDS-Bestrijding*, April 1993:11.
o   estimation: 1,000 in Amsterdam (GG&GD) and <10% of all intravenous drug users outside Amsterdam.

Of the 3,000 intravenous drug users in Amsterdam circa 1,000 are HIV-infected,[27] which is about 30% of the total. Outside Amsterdam the seroprevalence is estimated at lower than 10%.[28] Given these figures, the total number of HIV-infected intravenous drug users in the Netherlands is approximately 1,500. The epidemic load of this group is relatively high: 280/10,000 (Table 3.3) compared to the estimated group-size of intravenous drug users in the Netherlands.

VII. Haemophiliacs

The percentage of reported AIDS diagnoses in the group of haemophiliacs and persons who have received blood transfusions is relatively low compared to the total number of AIDS diagnoses. It has generally been assumed that the epidemic in this group has reached its limit. 13% of all haemophiliacs are infected with HIV. Compared to many other countries, this percentage is very low: in the USA the percentage of infected haemophiliacs is estimated at 70%. The relatively low epidemic load – compared to other countries – is explained by the particular Dutch institutional context and policy: no commercial blood banks, little dependence on blood from other countries and an early policy asking members of groups at risk to abstain from giving blood.[29]

If, however, the number of AIDS cases were related to the group-size, the epidemic load of this group would be by far the most severe: 342/10,000 (Table 3.3).

1.3   Summary and Conclusion

The general picture of the HIV/AIDS epidemic shows a highly differentiated pattern in the size and development of the epidemic, groups at risk and their social structure and epidemic load. While the first AIDS case was reported in 1981, in 1995 almost 3,000 AIDS-deaths had been registered. The real number of HIV infections is unclear as the result of latent infection and the Dutch voluntary testing policy. In 1995 the number of estimated HIV cases was 8,000. These estimations changed gradually as a result of changing evaluation methods and assumptions.

There is a heterogeneous pattern of social groups and a differentiation within these groups. Different social groups are labelled as HIV/AIDS risk groups. When the epidemic started it was seen as a phenomenon which exclusively concentrated on men with homosexual contacts. Later on, as a result of epidemic measures, other social groups were identified as being risk groups, i.e. intravenous drug users, haemophiliacs, etc. In time, other broader social groups will also become groups at risk, e.g. heterosexuals or health care workers. As groups at risk largely differ in numbers, they do so also in their social cohesion. For example, homosexuals, who have a relatively high social cohesion in terms of relationships, their public and/or underground infrastructures and with a shared common culture, have reached a high level of organizational development, whereas more marginal groups are reached by other organizations.

The number of AIDS cases according to the variables: region, age, sex, and social groups, demonstrate strong contrasts. By region, the epidemic is concentrated in the large cities of Amsterdam (almost 50%), Rotterdam, the Hague and Utrecht. The number of AIDS cases is largely concentrated in the relatively young age group of the 30-44 year-olds (60%). It is the male population which is largely affected, namely in 1991, 91% of the AIDS cases were diagnosed among men; this number is slightly decreasing. The number of AIDS cases as a result of heterosexual contacts is 11%; this is slowly on the increase. The epidemic load among subgroups, i.e. the number of AIDS cases related to the particular size of the subgroup, shows haemophiliacs, intravenous drug users, and homosexuals as being the most affected groups.

2   National Style of HIV/AIDS Regulation: The Active, Liberal Type

2.1   The Pre-modern Response

Medical solutions for threatening infectious epidemics like the plague, typhus, leprosy or cholera were absent in the pre-modern time of western societies. The "normal" societal response was not a struggle against the *disease* but a struggle against those individuals who were carrying the disease. As a result, those diseases were seen as the result of bad, sinful and immoral behaviour.[31] Stigmatization and exclusion of individuals – in the sense of isolation and separation from society – were not the only responses of pre-modern society. Another approach was the effort to control individual behaviour or stigmatized groups through *repression and severe preventive measures*, as was the case for cholera (De Swaan, 1988; 't Hart, 1990).

In modern welfare states, however, health policy is based on a complex and developed medical-technological and task-differentiated, professional health care system. This system has been very successful in reducing health risks and in increasing the individual's life expectancy at the same time. Contrary to the public action of pre-modern times, modern public health action is a sign of an organized attempt not to control individuals or groups but to control and reduce diseases and their symptoms. Authoritative exclusion and the coercive change in behaviour seem to have lost their meaning as "policy instruments". On the contrary, health care has increasingly become a rational choice of individuals in societies in which hazards of catching a deadly infection have been reduced to a minimum: "in those societies there is a high incentive in following an individual health care routine, since the benefit is an increasing life expectancy" (Goudsblom, 1986: 185).

However, AIDS seems to have changed this optimistic modern society model. For the first time in history, the modern welfare states are confronted by an epidemic which can neither be controlled nor terminated. At the same time, the increasing life expectancy has been brutally disturbed since it is particularly the younger part of the population which has been hit by this new disease, as is also indicated by the figures for the Netherlands (Table 3.3).

As in pre-modern societies, there is no medical solution as yet. We also know from epidemiological research that the transmission of the disease is related to particular behaviour like sexual intercourse and intravenous drug use, which could easily be connected to certain risk groups. The lack of a medical solution, combined with the knowledge about the nature of transmission, simultaneously constituted two conditions to stimulate a *pre-modern response of exclusion and coercion* towards certain risk groups.

2.2   The Modern Response

There were several reasons, however, as to why it was expected that this pre-modern response could hardly be possible in modern society. The characteristics of modern welfare state democracies and the rule of law seem to make an impregnable threshold for stigmatization, exclusion, and the extreme control and punishment of individuals and individual behaviour. The state is only in very exceptional cases allowed to intervene in the private sphere, in the intimate sphere of sexual behaviour in particular. Since the early 1960s (in most modern societies) the state has been forced to withdraw her "moral intervention" in this private sphere of sexual behaviour. Friedman has pointed out the paradoxical development of state regulation in this respect: societies which "heap rule on top of rule also deregulate sexual behaviour. Sexual life is radically free from legal control, in comparison to the past and to most historical societies" (Friedman, 1985: 144).

Others, like Bayer, have stressed the political impossibility of modern states intervening in this intimate sphere: sexual behaviours "touch on intimate decisions that only the most totalitarian society could, without great trepidation, consider the realm of appropriate direct state regulation" (Bayer, 1989: 82).

2.2.1   AIDS and the Law

The Dutch policy response more or less follows this expected logic of state intervention.

According to the Dutch jurists Kattouw and Nijboer, Dutch criminal law in principle offers possibilities to prosecute and punish behaviour that could lead to the spreading of AIDS, provided that there is evidence of "intentional or gross negligent handling of the life and health of others". The authors argue that the intentional or reckless transmission of AIDS to another person through (unprotected) intercourse can constitute a crime against life or an assault. However, in practice, few prosecutions occur as the Public Prosecutor's Office (*Openbaar Ministerie*) often decides to dismiss the charges for reasons of unlikely court conviction (*technisch sepot*) or on the basis of the court's discretion (*beleidssepot*). Often, proof of the crime is not feasible, or the physical condition of the defendant with AIDS is such that the defendant is not able to stand trial or has already died before the court decides upon the case. Kattouw and Nijboer conclude that although criminal law has a role to play in the realm of HIV/AIDS, albeit no particular one, no real contribution is to be expected from the criminal justice system here. Furthermore, the authors see little in the normative force of criminal law: moral conduct such as safe sex "belongs to the own responsibility of people to decide for themselves what risk they are willing to take". Moreover, symbolic penalizing can contribute to "criminalization" and "renewed tabooing of sexuality".

In general, Dutch governmental policy, with regard to controlling of the AIDS epidemic, has abstained from interfering in private life, nor has the government tried to juridize or criminalize the problem of AIDS by explicitly incorporating it into criminal law (apart from the arguments based on the right to private life and the prohibition of discrimination, this is due to the fact that there is no efficacious treatment for AIDS as yet). The absence of such a treatment has also played a part in deciding not to bring AIDS under the operation of the Act on the Control of Infectious Diseases and the Tracing of the Cause of Diseases (*Wet bestrijding infectieziekten en opsporing ziekte oorzaken*). The former Health Minister, Elco Brinkman, formulated it as follows: "by bringing AIDS under the operation of this act, the government purposefully participates in maintaining the illusion that this disease can be controlled by such measures".

2.2.2   Choices for State Intervention

State intervention in this respect can be related to the following different domains: (1) the detection of people with HIV (is a preventive measure), (2) the registration of people with AIDS and/or HIV positives, (3) the regulation of individual behaviour (4) the exclusion of people with AIDS or HIV positives from certain sectors within society or from society in general (like the old response). A choice can be made between regulation on a compulsory or a voluntary basis for each domain, and regulation of the public or of specific groups. The Dutch policy response can be classified as the "active liberal type" as illustrated in Table 3.4. This table also illustrates the country-specific Dutch response from a cross-national perspective. The cross-national comparison unveils that the regulative responses vary between authoritative, coercive responses on the one hand and active liberal responses the other. All countries (in Table 3.4) register people with AIDS, three of them (Sweden, Switzerland and Portugal) also register HIV positives. Five of the countries do it on a mandatory basis whereas Portugal, Belgium and the Netherlands have a voluntary system. With respect to the regulation of individual behaviour, which means measures against antisocial behaviour (wilful contagion), times combined with penal codes or based on criminal law, we again see the five countries with a mandatory system in this respect, in particular for HIV people. For example, in Sweden HIV positives are obliged to go for regular check-ups, there are strict regulations for sexual practices (formally) and ligation to inform the general practitioner and dentist of any HIV infec

	behaviour			Regulation of Exclusion/Isolation							Screening and Testing	
	HIV	Mandat.	Volunt.	No	Anti	Pro	PWA	HIV	Mandat.	Volunt.	Mandat.	Volunt.
	X[1]	X	X		X[2]	X[3]	X	X	X	X	X[4]	X
	X	X	X	X[6]	X[7]						—[8]	X
	X	X	X			X[9]					X[10]	X
	X	X	X			X		X[11]	X		X[12]	X
	X	X	X		X	X	X	X	X		X[13]	X[14]
						X[15]					X[16]	X[17]

General responses

Portugal	X	X	X				X		X	X		X
Belgium	X	X	X	X[18]		X[19]	X	X			X[20]	
Netherlands	X	X	X		X		X	X			—[21]	X[22]

Sources: WHO, *Health Legislation and Ethics in the Field of AIDS and HIV Infection*, 1988. A.Hendriks, *AIDS, HIV Prevalence and AIDS? HIV Policies in Europe: A Survey*, 1991. WHO, *Current Status of HIV/AIDS Prevention and Control Policies in the European Region*, 1990.

1   HIV-positives are bound by a range of legal restrictions, including regular medical checks, strict rules of sexual practice, and an obligation to inform their general practitioner and dentist.

2   Regulation of non-discriminatory acceptance for standard health and pension insurance; as well as legal protection against dismissals for HIV-positives showing no AIDS symptoms.

3   According to the Prevention of Infectious Diseases Act, HIV-positives and people with AIDS can be isolated after court-decision. Since 1987 there is an official isolation clinic for HIV-positives who continue to engage in risky behaviour.

4   "Anyone who suspects being infected"; "suspicious persons"; in cases of rape.

5   In 1987 this changed from voluntary to compulsory.

6   No legal protection against dismissals for HIV-positives showing no AIDS symptoms.

7   Regulation to prescribe non-discriminatory acceptance for standard health and pension insurance, however, only for *minimum coverage*.

8   The Swiss Epidemic Law would permit compulsory testing on particular patients or population groups. In the case of AIDS this is considered "disproportional".

9   In accordance with the AIDS Law, HIV-positive prostitutes' licenses are not renewed.

10 Prostitutes. For other persons no formal compulsory testing. There is, however, widespread practice in Vienna and Klagenfurt.

11 Prison inmates. Immigrants: according to the new immigration law, immigrants should not be HIV positive.

12 Immigrants.

13 Particular professions: nurses, the army, police, fire-brigade, etc.

14 Drug users.

15 Prison inmates until 1989.

16 Prison inmates.

17 Pregnant women; alternative test places.

18 Insurance companies. As an effect of non-regulation insurance, certain applicants might be excluded.

19 Asylum seekers (effect of a general health examination).

20 Asylum seekers; insurance applicants (as a result of non-regulation); foreign students (formally not enacted but there is strong evidence that Belgian universities apply tests).

21 The same situation as in Switzerland (see note 8). There is, however, in cases of collective insurance for workers, a creeping practice of insurance companies to test individual employees. This is not forbidden by law. In the case of getting oneself insured, insurance companies are allowed to oblige applicants to take an AIDS test. Hfl 200,000 and over. In the last three years there have been 95 compulsory tests (7 x: HIV-positive).

22 There are a number of "alternative test places" where people can ask for a voluntary test.

relevant question is whether modern states exclude people with AIDS or HIV positives from society or whether they only react on anti-exclusion regulation. Here we see more differentiated patterns between pro- and anti-exclusion regulations, sometimes both and in most occasions regulations for particular groups. For example, Sweden has laws against discrimination in the case of health and pension insurance, as well as legal dismissals for HIV positives. At the same time, HIV positives and PWAs can be isolated on the basis of court-decision; since 1987 Sweden has had an official isolation clinic for HIV positives who continue to engage in risky behaviour.

Can these different responses be explained by country-specific cultural, institutional or political circumstances or are these differences the result of a particular pattern of the AIDS epidemic? If we compare the structure of the AIDS epidemic in the first half of the last decade (1986) then there only seems to be a relation between Switzerland and the Netherlands. Switzerland, with a relatively high incidence rate of 25.2 in 1986, and the Netherlands with a relatively low incidence rate of 9.4 at the same point in time, respond in a coercive and liberal way to the epidemic. If we compare the other countries which are all in the group of a relatively low incidence rate, then we see that they vary between all the possibilities of coercive and liberal responses (Figure 3.1). The coercive response by those countries with a relatively low incidence rate at that time, e.g. Austria (2.8) and Italy (7.9) is explained by some authors as an example of "symbolic" response. According to the authors of the Austrian and Italian reports in this publication, the Austrian and Italian governments reacted before the first AIDS case was even reported. Apart from the question as to how to evaluate the meaning of symbolic regulation which has been disputed, we still have to explain why one country reacts in the first phase of the epidemic by coercive regulation, whereas other countries with the same epidemic problem react in another way.

Another explanation might be the way the disease has been legally *framed* in the respective countries: the way a certain problem is defined often correlates to a particular institutional response. With respect to the AIDS epidemic, there might be two possibilities of definition; either defining it as a classic *public-health crisis*, which usually means it is a temporary threat requiring special policies selected from the existing repertoire of institutions used in crisis type situations, or defining it as a *chronic problem*. In that case the crisis type response might not work and a new AIDS-specific policy health strategy might be stimulated. AIDS was defined as a public health crisis (as an *epidemic*) in all the selected countries in its first phase, but as the epidemic has not yet disappeared we can observe a creeping re-definition of the problem in the direction of a chronic problem. This is of course not just a matter of its superstructure but it simultaneously reflects the actual transformation of the epidemic. However, so far, the changing re-definition of the AIDS disease cannot explain the differences between the respective countries since one can observe a more or less similar transformation from a crisis problem to a chronic problem in all the areas studied.

On a lower level of abstraction we do, however, see some interesting differences in defining the AIDS crisis in the first phase, which partly explains why some countries use coercive regulations, while others do not. A clear-cut example is Sweden. This country is the only one of the eight countries that defined AIDS as a *venereal disease* at the very beginning of the epidemic. Consequently, it has used the whole range of procedures and regulations which have traditionally been applied to sexually-transmitted diseases. In contrast, other countries have purposefully not put AIDS into one of the existing legal frames. In the Netherlands, the government has refused to deal with AIDS within the frame of the existing Act on the Control of Infectious Diseases and the Tracing of the Causes of Diseases (*Wet bestrijding infectieziekten en opsporing ziekte oorzaken*), which would have allowed coercive government intervention.

Since a medical solution has not (yet) been reached, and a policy of changing behaviour or reducing risks by means of strictly regulating individual or group behaviour was rejected in the Dutch case, the question arises as to how civil society could effectively respond to the epidemic. In the next section this question is dealt with from an organizational sociological perspective.

2.3   Summary and Conclusion

The Dutch governmental policy is characterized by its active and liberal direction. While in pre-modern times, the common societal response was exclusion, coercion and stigmatization of the individuals as there were no medical solutions for threatening infectious diseases, the modern (public health) action is directed towards the control and reduction of the disease and its symptoms. Today's policy instruments show this. The Dutch government has abstained from interfering in private life, has not juridicized or criminalized AIDS by incorporating it into criminal law, and has not brought AIDS under the operation of the Act on the Control of Infectious Diseases and the Tracing of the Cause of Diseases (as is the case in some other countries).

State intervention is very much based on the voluntary cooperation of (groups of) individuals and private organizations. The detection of people with HIV takes place on a voluntary basis; the registration of people with HIV/AIDS is voluntary. The regulation of individual behaviour takes place on a voluntary basis and by the social groups themselves. The exclusion of people with HIV/AIDS is consequently avoided by not bringing AIDS under the existing Act on the Control of Infectious Diseases.

3   The Organizational Response: General Pattern and Structure

For this study, the organizational configuration comprises all organizations involved in the HIV/AIDS policy domain. Organizations are defined as involved in this policy domain if (1) they perform a specific HIV/AIDS task, and/or (2) they dispose of HIV/AIDS specific financial or personnel resources, and/or (3) they are mentioned[32] by other organizations in the HIV/AIDS policy domain as part of the organizational network. In the following subsectors we will deal with the organizational density and organizational structure of this overall organizational pattern.

3.1   Organizational Density

711 organizations were involved in the HIV/AIDS policy domain (for 1993). For comparative reasons we will use *organizational density* as one measure to indicate the relative importance of the organizational response in the Netherlands. We can relate the number of organizations to three different types of populations to indicate a certain organizational density: the *size of the total population* of the country under study, the size of the HIV epidemic in terms of the *number of HIV-infected people*, or the size of the AIDS epidemic by the *number of people with AIDS* (Table 3.5).

The Dutch figures have been compared with those of other countries in the European Region (Table 3.6) to illuminate the possible country-specific organizational density. As one can see, the number of HIV/AIDS organizations vastly differs from one country to another. While countries such as Hungary and Portugal have generated only a handful of HIV/AIDS organizations, the Netherlands and Switzerland form the other end of the spectrum with several hundreds of organizations.

**Table 3.5:   Organizational Density in the HIV/AIDS Policy Domain –
The Netherlands (1993)**

Number of Organizations in the HIV/AIDS policy domain	Number of Inhabitants x million	Cumulative AIDS Cases 1.1.1993 (adjusted for reporting delays)	Number of estimated HIV-positives	Organizational Density by the number of organizations per:		
				I 100 AIDS Cases	II 100 HIV- infected persons	III Million inhabitants
711	15.2	2,580	10,000[a]	28	7	47

a   average of the estimation in 1993 (see Table 3.1).

Table 3.6:   Organizational Response and Organizational Density in the Netherlands, Compared to Other Countries in the European Region (1993)

Country	Number of Organizations in the HIV/AIDS Policy Domain	Number of Inhabitants x million	Cumulative AIDS Cases[a]	Organizational Density by the number of organizations per:	
				I 100 AIDS Cases	III Million Inhabitants
Netherlands	711	15.2	2,567	28	47
Switzerland	306	6.8	3,240	9	45
Austria	104	7.9	921	11	13
Sweden	63	8.6	797	8	7
Belgium[b]	50	5.8	1,114	4	9
Portugal	16	9.8	1,352	1	2
Hungary	7	10.4	115	6	1

a   number of cumulative AIDS cases as on 31 December 1993, not adjusted for reporting delays.

b   only *Flanders*.

Sources: *Managing AIDS* (European Centre/WHO-Collaborative Study). *AIDS Surveillance in Europe*, quarterly report no. 36, 30 December 1992; European Centre for the Epidemiological Monitoring of AIDS, Paris.

Table 3.6 also indicates that there is no direct, causal relation between the size of the epidemic or the number of inhabitants and the size of the organizational response (as illustrated by the varying organizational densities). However, on closer appraisal, three groups of organizational density (related to the size of the epidemic) can be distinguished, two extremes and one in the mean. On the one end we find Portugal and Belgium with an organizational density of one and four respectively. At the other end we find the Netherlands with an organizational density of 28. The other countries are more or less in between the two extremes with an organizational density between six and eleven. If we relate the organizational density to the total population (III), the picture is almost the same, with the exception of Switzerland and Hungary. Switzerland now almost has the same figure as the Netherlands whereas Hungary ends up at the lower end of the low density group.

3.2   Interorganizational Differentiation

The number of organizations as such does not explain that much. A high number might even indicate a high level of overlap between organizations. From an organizational development point of view, the relevant question is in fact whether the high number of organizations correlates with a high level of differentiation and integration of the overall organizational pattern. In this section we deal with the structural differentiation in particular, whereas the functional differentiation is dealt with in section 4.

Structural differentiation expresses the structure of the organizational pattern in terms of the variety of *different types of organizations*. In this case we have distinguished four categories, based on (a) the *problem orientation*, (b) the *sectoral basis*, (c) the *group orientation*, and (d) the *geographical scope* of organizations.

3.2.1   Problem Orientation

Two different types of HIV/AIDS organizations can be distinguished: those organizations exclusively oriented towards the problem of HIV/AIDS – the exclusives – and those organizations for which the HIV/AIDS epidemic is just one of a string of problems. These organizations have been labelled as *inclusives*.[33]

In empirical real terms, inclusive organizations are in general organizations which existed at the start of the epidemic. Many of them do not consider themselves as HIV/AIDS organizations. Their orientation towards the HIV/AIDS problem could be described as *task-enlargement*. Only a few cases were found to be "older" organizations that had changed their problem orientation from inclusive to exclusive.[34]

Table 3.7:   **Interorganizational Differentiation by Problem Orientation – The Netherlands Compared with Six Other Countries in the European Region (1993)**

Country	Inclusive		Exclusive		Total	
	N	%	N	%	N	%
Netherlands	623	88	88	12	711	100
Switzerland	239	78	67	22	306	100
Belgium*	35	70	15	30	50	100
Austria	83	80	21	20	104	100
Sweden	45	71	18	29	63	100
Portugal	15	94	1	6	16	100
Hungary	2	29	5	71	7	100
Total	1,042	83	215	17	1,257	100

* Only *Flanders*.

Of the 711 organizations in 1993, 623 organizations (88%) were inclusive organizations and 88 organizations (12%) belonged to the category of exclusives. In other words, and only quantitatively speaking, the organizational response to the HIV/AIDS epidemic is dominated by the already existing organizational configuration. However, from an international comparative point of view, the absolute number of exclusive organizations in the Netherlands indicates a relatively high response coming from newly founded and HIV/AIDS-specific organizations. Almost 41% of all exclusive organizations in the seven countries of the European region (Table 3.7) are to be found in the Netherlands, followed by Switzerland with 31%.

3.2.2   Differentiation by Sector

In terms of the classic distinction between *state, private non-profit* and *market* (private for-profit), it would be interesting to ask oneself which sector in particular responds to the HIV/AIDS epidemic in the Netherlands. The role of market organizations in the HIV/AIDS policy domain is (still) very marginal (see Table 3.8). We have found only three market organizations so far. One of these organizations is a commercial firm (the Best Publishing Group) which runs a database (Gaytel) and an information magazine (AIDS info). This organization was founded by the homosexual movement, but has more developed into a commercial firm which sells information. The other organization is *Adviesburo Drugs August de Loor,* which is an example of the classic entrepreneur: an individual selling his knowledge and information from the complicated world of drug users to local and central governments.

The category of state organizations is also relatively minimally represented: only 3% of all organizations are central state organizations. If we include the peripheral state organizations, the total sum is still only 23%. The organizational pattern is clearly dominated by the private non-profit sector: almost 74% of all organizations involved in the HIV/AIDS policy domain belong to this sector. The private non-profit sector is, however, a very heterogeneous one. It is in particular in the context of managing the HIV/AIDS epidemic where it might be relevant to identify the different types of private non-profits. In this case we have made a distinction between *professional health and welfare organizations* (which have become the core institutions of the developed, institutionalized welfare state), *organized communities* and *organized groups at risk*. In the final section the different organizational types in the private non-profit sector as well as the state and market organizational types will be related to particular types of *governance*. This will reflect different views on the way the epidemic should in fact be managed.

**Table 3.8:   The Sectoral and Social Basis of Organizations in the HIV/
AIDS Policy Domain – The Netherlands (1993)**

	N	%
Sectoral basis		
State total	168	24
Private non-profit	526	74
Market	3	1
Other/unknown	14	2
Total	711	100
Social basis of private non-profits		
Professional health & welfare	310	59
Organized community	181	34
Organized group at risk	18	3
Other (mixed organizations)	17	3
Total	526	100

If, from this perspective, we look more closely at the composition of the non-profit sector, we can see that the private non-profit sector is dominated by the professionalized health and welfare institutions (59% of the sector and almost 44% of all organizations). Organized communities and organized groups at risk represent 34% and 3% respectively – of this particular sector however (Table 3.8). From an international comparative point of view, and compared to the other countries in the European Region (Table 3.7), the total number of community-based organizations and organized groups at risk is highest in the Netherlands.

3.2.3   Differentiation by Target Group Orientation

Apart from the social basis of organizations, the organizational pattern can be differentiated by the organizations' HIV/AIDS activities' target groups. We have made a distinction between three different categories of target groups: the *general public*, *groups at risk* and *professionals or workers in health care institutions*.[35] Table 3.9 gives an overview of services offered to the general public and to specific target groups. Five per cent of the organizations focus on the general public whereas the others mainly focus their activities on a particular target group. Most of these organizations (68%) are oriented towards particular groups at risk.

Table 3.9:   Organizational Differentiation by Target Group Orientation for HIV/AIDS-related Services – The Netherlands (1993)

Target Group	Number of Organizations	%
Public in general		
Everybody	32	5
Youth	6	1
Women	1	-
Subtotal	39	5
Groups at risk		
Persons with HIV/AIDS	189	27
People with or involved in HIV/AIDS	170	24
(IV)-drug users	72	10
Men with homosexual contacts	42	6
Haemophiliacs	3	-
Prostitutes	2	-
Parents of children at risk	2	-
Subtotal	480	68
Professionals		
Health care professionals	59	8
General practitioner/dentist	30	4
Everybody at work	17	2
Scientific community (researchers)	14	2
Subtotal	120	17
Other	66	9
Unknown	6	1
Total	711	100

3.2.4   Differentiation by Geographical Scope

The geographical scope of organizations shows a high regional response. Eighty-eight per cent of the organizations have a regional and/or local scope and only 12% of the organizations have a national one.

Table 3.10: Geographical Distribution (Provinces and Some Large Cities) and Organizational Density – The Netherlands (1993)

Region	Inclusives		Exclusives		Total		Organizational Density (a)	
	N	%	N	%	N	%	I	III
Province								
Southern-Holland	158	89	20	11	178	100	36.7	54.0
Northern-Holland	102	82	23	18	125	100	8.9	51.2
Gelderland	85	89	10	11	95	100	79.2	51.6
Northern-Brabant	63	86	10	14	73	100	69.5	32.5
Limburg	44	86	7	14	51	100	68.0	45.5
Overijssel	44	80	6	20	50	100	62.5	48.1
Utrecht	35	88	5	12	40	100	33.6	38.2
Groningen	16	89	2	11	18	100	54.5	32.4
Flevoland	9	82	2	18	11	100	50.0	45.2
Sealand	9	82	2	18	11	100	78.6	30.5
Friesland	9	100			9	100	33.3	14.9
Drenthe	9	100			9	100	128.6	20.1
unknown	41	100			41	100		
Total	624	88	87	12	711	100	27.6	46.7
large cities								
Amsterdam	39	74	14		53	100	4.2	73.6
The Hague	28	82	6		34	100	11.3	76.5
Utrecht	24	83	5		29	100	53.7	123,8
Rotterdam	15	75	5		20	100	15.2	33.6

a I = organizational density per 100 AIDS cases.
   III = organizational density per million inhabitants.

**Table 3.11: Interorganizational Differentiation by Type of Organization
and Geographical Orientation – The Netherlands (1993)**

Type of Organization	Geographical Orientation				Total	
	National		Regional/Local			
	N	%	N	%	N	%
Problem orientation						
Exclusive	16	18	72	82	88	100
Inclusive	47	8	576	92	623	100
Sectoral basis						
State total	19	11	149	89	168	100
Private non-profit	44	8	482	92	526	100
Market	2	67	1	33	3	100
Social basis of private non-profits						
Professionalized						
health & welfare	16	5	294	95	310	100
Organized community	20	11	161	89	181	100
Interorganizational						
organizations			17	100	17	100
Organized group at risk	8	44	10	56	18	100
Other			8	100	8	100
Unknown	6		6	100	6	100

The differentiation by type of organizations is summarized in Table 3.11. As one can see, the dominant level of organizational activity is on the regional/local level for almost all types of organizations. There are two exceptions: market-organizations and organized groups at risk, respectively 67% and 44% at the national level.

3.3 The Organizational Response over Time: 1980-1993

In the following tables and figures we shortly summarize the organizational response over time. The number of organizations performing HIV/AIDS activities gradually increased during the 1980s. This is illustrated in Figure 3.2.[36]

Figure 3.2 clearly illustrates that it was already in the years 1985-1987 that the majority of organizations started to offer HIV/AIDS services. This relatively early start can be largely explained by the initiatives of the informal predecessor (a mix of community-based organizations and representatives of health and welfare state professionals) of the National Committee on AIDS Control (NCAB), established by the government in 1987. AIDS activities on the regional level were strongly

**Figure 3.2:   Year HIV/AIDS Activities Began, by Number of
Organizations – The Netherlands (1994)**

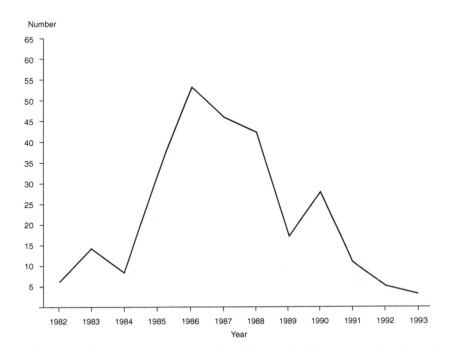

stimulated by this predecessor, as also illustrated in Figure 3.4. A large number of
regional organizations were established in the period of 1985-1987. One important stimulus has been the foundation of the so-called *"AIDS platforms"* in which
different types of organizations and professionals exchange and coordinate knowledge, experiences, policies and practices. These platforms have, in turn, stimulated
the entrance of many organizations in the HIV/AIDS policy domain at a regional
level.

By the time the NCAB was established, and subsidies became available, 45%
of the organizations had already started their AIDS activities. Six organizations
mentioned 1982 as the year in which they started their HIV/AIDS activities (of
which three organizations are in Amsterdam).

In Figure 3.3 the start of HIV/AIDS activities is divided by exclusive and inclusive organizations. The development of the organizational response differs between inclusive and exclusive organizations. The inclusive profile corresponds with
the general profile, which is not surprising given the high proportion of this type
of organization. Between 1986-1991 the number of newly founded exclusive organizations was approximately 15. From 1991 onwards there is a clear decline in
new exclusive organizations.

Figure 3.3: Year HIV/AIDS Activities Began, by Exclusive/Inclusive Organization – The Netherlands (1994)

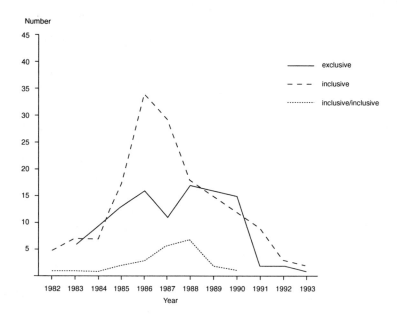

Figure 3.4: Year AIDS Activities Began, by Organizational Territorial Domain – The Netherlands (1994)

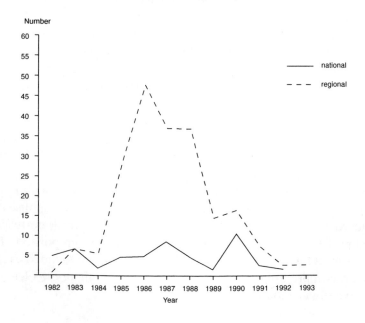

From Figure 3.4 we learn that national organizations started somewhat earlier with HIV/AIDS activities than regional organizations. 1990 is a year in which some national organizations started with AIDS activities. For regional organizations the majority started their HIV/AIDS activities in the mid-1980s.

Given the various regions in the Netherlands, Table 3.12 and Figure 3.5 demonstrate that although the epidemic predominates in Amsterdam, organizations are distributed all over the country. There is a variation in the number of organizations across regions, with a concentration of organizations in Amsterdam.

Table 3.12: Year HIV/AIDS Activities Began, by Region

	'82	'83	'84	'85	'86	'87	'88	'89	'90	'91	'92	'93	Total
Groningen				4	1		1	1	1				8
Friesland			1			2			1	1			4
Drenthe					1	1			1	1			4
Overijssel		1	1		5	2	5	1	2				17
Flevoland				2	2		1				1		6
Gelderland		2	1	4	3	7	4	4	5				30
Utrecht	1	2		2	2	5	3	1	2	1			19
Northern Holland	3	6	2	5	10	9	9	5	12	1	2		64
Southern Holland	1	1	1	7	10	14	7	2	3	4	3	2	55
Sealand						2	2						4
Northern Brabant	1		1	4	12	4	6	1		1		1	31
Limburg		1	1	5	8	1	4	2	1	1			24
Total	6	14	8	33	53	46	42	17	28	11	5	3	266

**Figure 3.5: Year HIV/AIDS Activities Began, by Large Cities –
The Netherlands (1994)**

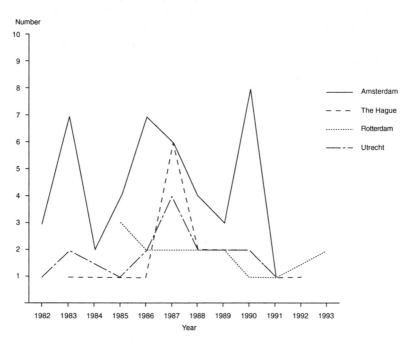

3.3 Summary and Conclusion

The general pattern and structure of the organizational response can be characterized by the organizational density, the structural differentiation and the development of the number of organizations. In 1993 the total number of HIV/AIDS
organizations was (estimated at being) 711. The number of organizations per 100
AIDS cases is 28. Compared to other European countries, the organizational density
is high both concerning the number of organizations per 100 AIDS cases and the
number of organizations per million inhabitants.

The structural differentiation is characterized by the different types of organizations, the high participation of one or the other subsector, differentiation in target
groups and the geographical scope of organizations. However, 12% of the organizations are exclusively involved with HIV/AIDS, which is a relatively high number
compared to other countries. The organizational response is largely dominated by
the already existing organizational structures. The organizational pattern is dominated by the private non-profit sector; however, this sector is a heterogeneous one.
A distinction can be made between professional health and welfare organizations
and organized communities and organized groups at risk, and most organizations
concentrate on a particular group at risk, and most have a regional or local scope
which indicates a more or less even distribution across the country.

The development of organizations shows an interesting and clear pattern over time. Most organizations began with AIDS activities between 1984 and 1990. It is interesting that a large part of inclusive organizations started earlier with HIV/AIDS activities than the exclusive ones.

4 Organizational Response: Functional Differentiation by Task and Goal

4.1 A Global Picture

The functional differentiation refers to the division of labour within the organizational pattern of HIV/AIDS activities. From this perspective, HIV/AIDS activities have therefore been put into distinctive subsectors which will be described in the following sections: Prevention (4.3.1), Care (4.3.2), Research (4.3.3), Control and Monitoring (4.3.4), Interest Representation (4.3.5), and Fund-raising (4.3.6).

In Table 3.13, all 711 organizations are classified by their most important HIV/AIDS activities. The number of organizations which provide HIV/AIDS activities differs profusely from subsector to subsector. Most of the organizations in the sample provide activities in the Care subsector, followed by Prevention. The subsectors Control and Monitoring, and Interest Representation take on a middle position. Only a small number of organizations perform mainly Research or Fund-raising activities.

Activities and Organization Resources

In this section, however, we will focus more specifically on the organizational response in terms of HIV/AIDS activities within the subsectors. For this purpose 288 organizations of the 711 organizations were approached to fill in a question-

Table 3.13: Organizations Providing HIV/AIDS Activities by Subsector (N=711)

Subsector	Number of Organizations[a]
Prevention	486
Care	590
Research	59
Control and Monitoring	210
Interest Representation	142
Fund-raising	16

a = organizations were allowed to provide more than one category of activities.

Source: *Managing AIDS in the Netherlands*: Dataset 3 (n=74).

Table 3.14: Managing AIDS in the Netherlands: Datasets

	Dataset 1	Dataset 2	Dataset 3	Dataset 4
Source	Questionnaire sent to all exclusive, all national, and to a sample of inclusive regional organizations	Remaining inclusive regional organizations: information filled in by ourselves, based on general, available information and/or from the extrapolation of the sample (Dataset 1)	Combination of Dataset 1 + Dataset 2 for a number of general variables	Selection of organizations from Dataset 1 for in-depth study
Total number of organizations (1993)	288	423	711	48

naire. This information is contained in Dataset 1 (Table 3.14). For the remaining 423 regional inclusive organizations, we have deduced some basic information from general sources and/or have extrapolated some other variables based on the filled-in questionnaires. This has resulted in Dataset 2. Datasets 1 and 2 have been combined for a number of general variables, resulting in Dataset 3. From the organizations in Dataset 1, 48 organizations were selected for in-depth study, based on interviews and the analysis of organizational documents (Dataset 4). The results in this chapter will mainly be based on Dataset 1, complemented occasionally with information from Dataset 4.

4.2 *HIV/AIDS Activities in General*

A first significant element of the AIDS sector is the number of activities organizations provide. The question is whether organizations perform just one HIV/AIDS activity or whether they provide a whole range of activities. It can be concluded that whenever organizations perform HIV/AIDS activities in the Netherlands, they usually perform more than one activity. Forty per cent of the organizations perform four or more activities. Five per cent of the organizations even perform ten or more. It must, however, be noted that a considerable number, i.e. more than a quarter of the organizations (28.6%), only offer one HIV/AIDS activity.

Table 3.15: Organizations Providing HIV/AIDS Activities by Subsector (N=288)

Subsector	Number of Organizations[a]	
Prevention	151	(52.4%)
Care	203	(70.5%)
Research	43	(14.9%)
Control and Monitoring	118	(40.9%)
Interest Representation	3	(12.2%)
Fund-raising	15	(5.2%)

a = organizations were able to provide more than one category of activities.

This illustrates that a large portion of the organizations is more or less specialized in and geared towards HIV/AIDS activities. Only a small number of organizations is multifunctional, with HIV/AIDS activities as one of a number of services. Eight organizations are active in at least five subsectors, i.e. five municipal health services, the Dutch gay interest organization: NVIH COC, an AIDS platform and a drug support organization.

Before studying the volume, structure and development of certain subsectors, look at a table of the number of organizations which perform activities in different subsectors; this is based on the sample of 288 organizations (Table 3.15).

4.3 Activities and Their Subsectors

4.3.1 Prevention

The first subsector, Prevention, consists of activities to inform the general public or specific groups at risk to educate these groups in preventive activities, and to train people to take preventive action either if directly exposed to risk of HIV infection or when training workers in how to cope with people who are HIV-infected.

More than half of a total of 151 organizations provide prevention activities. Two thirds of the organizations offering preventive activities perform just one or two activities and one third of the organizations have three or more. The mean number of activities is 2.3 per organization. Organizations which perform at least four prevention activities are mainly municipal health services. Ten per cent of the drug support organizations perform four or more activities. The other organizations all perform three or less prevention activities. The following table shows scores of organizations with different prevention activities.

Table 3.16 illustrates that all types of prevention activities – information, education and training – are being carried out, despite the variation between activities being minimal. Educational and Information Work scores highest, and the activity Hotline, the lowest.

A closer view on the different categories of organizations reveals some relevant differences between organizations. Municipal health services appear as the most specific prevention organization. They perform all types of prevention activities and they provide the largest number of prevention activities. They also carry out some drug-related prevention activities, which is not surprising as these organizations have a specific task delegated to them by the local/regional government.[37] Drug support organizations offer drug-related prevention. Health education organizations primarily produce information material, organize information campaigns and carry out educational and information work.[38] Organizations which represent groups at risk, whether an interest organization or a specific HIV/AIDS service organization, are also prominent. Their aim is to produce information material and provide education activities. Typical health care organizations like for mental health care, social work and home care, as well as hospitals and nursing homes are present in this subsector for their training of health care professionals.

Table 3.16: Organizations and Specialized Prevention Activities

(n=288)	Number of Organizations	Per cent
Hotline	34	11.8
Production of information material	53	18.8
AIDS information campaigns	61	21.2
Educational and information work	81	28.1
Drug-related prevention	60	20.8
Training of volunteers / health care professionals	53	18.4
Total activities	342	

Source: *Managing AIDS in the Netherlands*: dataset 1 (n=288).

4.3.2 Care

The Care subsector comprises medical (ambulatory) care (AIDS-specialized medical care, home care, hospices[39], voluntary HIV-testing and counselling), psychosocial care (psychological help for PWAs/HIV+s and face-to-face counselling), social services (buddy systems, referral services and food banks). In this subsector, there is a considerable difference between the activity and its weight of importance.

203 organizations offer one or more health care and/or social service activities. 90% of these organizations perform one to three activities and 10% of these organizations carry out four to six activities in this subsector. There is an average of 1.5 activities per organization. These are again mainly municipal health services (40%). Table 3.17 shows the number of organizations per activity.

The variation in number of organizations per activity is larger than for the Prevention subsector. It is striking that 30% of the organizations provide psychological help for seropositives and face-to-face counselling, while other services like food banks and home care services score very low.

Governmental organizations like municipal health services as well as most types of non-profit organizations are strongly represented in this subsector, whereas interest organizations/service-providing organizations of groups at risk/social groups are less so.

Looking at the activities individually, one can observe a differentiation in activities for the different types of organizations.

Municipal health services perform a variety of activities, mainly individual consulting activities and voluntary HIV-testing and counselling. They also seem to have a large hand in buddy projects. Ambulatory mental health care mainly concerns providing psychological help to seropositives and persons with AIDS. Social work and home care services, like mental health care, also give psychological help to seropositives (72%), and like municipal health services they also largely provide face-to-face counselling activities (64%) and cooperate in buddy projects (52%). Surprisingly enough, they are not involved in home care facilities.[40] Drug support organizations and consultation bureaus for alcohol and drugs are mainly engaged in psychological help and face-to-face counselling, one third in (AIDS-specialized) medical care. Hospitals and nursing homes are generally provided for by AIDS-specialized medical care centres and hospices/shelters. Interest/patient organizations and groups at risk/community organizations are mainly involved in providing psychological help, face-to-face counselling and cooperation/buddy projects.

A few additional remarks should be made to this subsector. Firstly, the subsector's pronounced involvement in psychological help can be explained by the large participation of ambulatory mental health care and social work agencies. For these organizations, this activity belongs to their original organizational task. The ques-

Table 3.17: Organizations and Care Activities

Activities	Number of Organizations	%
AIDS-specialized medical care	55	19.1
Psychological help for seropositives	86	29.9
Face-to-face counselling	86	29.9
Home care services	7	2.4
Hospices, shelters	31	10.8
Voluntary HIV-testing and counselling	49	17.0
Buddy system	46	16.0
Referral services	44	15.3
Food bank	2	0.7
Total	406	100

Source: *Managing AIDS in the Netherlands*: Dataset 1 (n=288).

tion remains, however, as to whether they consider this type of activity as HIV/ AIDS-specific and different from their other organizational activities. Second, the high number scored on face-to-face counselling can be explained by the vague description of this type of activity. This activity not only involves case management, but also information and counselling on different subjects which could concern the HIV-infected person. This means that persons take time to inform and consult clients in different types of organizations. This is true for municipal health organizations, social work agencies, drug support organizations, hospitals and service-providing organizations of groups at risk. Third, the large number of organizations which report having buddy systems does not mean there are many different buddy systems in the Netherlands, i.e. several organizations can be involved with the same buddy system within a certain region. Fourth, food banks are hardly relevant according to AIDS patients and seropositives in the Netherlands.

4.3.3   Research

Three general categories of research have been distinguished, namely epidemiological research, social research and (bio/basic) medical research. Table 3.18 illustrates the number of organizations per type of research activity.

Table 3.18: Organizations and Their Research Activities

Activities	Number of Organizations	% of (n=288)
Epidemiological research	23	8.0
Social research	8	2.7
(Bio)medical research	12	4.2
Total	43	

Source: *Managing AIDS in the Netherlands*: Dataset 1 (n=288).

Twenty-three organizations (8%) reported epidemiological research as an activity, twelve organizations reported (bio)medical research (4%), and eight organizations (3%), social research.

Of the above activities, 50% of the epidemiological research is done by municipal health services. This can be explained by the fact that this activity is largely linked to the HIV test and to the responsibility these institutes have to monitor public health. Hospitals and local councils also report it as one of their organizational activities. (Bio)Medical research is mainly reported by hospitals (one might ask, however, how far [scientific] research is a core organizational activity or not). Social research is mainly done by research organizations.

4.3.4   Control and Monitoring

This subsector includes three different HIV/AIDS activities. The first activity, AIDS Policy Coordination and Implementation, is a broad category for it consists of both policy coordination and implementation.[41] The second and third categories, being the control of blood plasma, and HIV-screening, etc., are monitoring activities which concern blood supplies.

Thirty-seven per cent of the organizations surveyed are active in AIDS policy coordination and implementation. Only 3% of the organizations are active in the control of blood/plasma product safety and 8% in HIV-screening, testing and identification.

Organizations which are most active in this subsector are AIDS platforms and municipal health services, respectively 36 and 29%. Table 3.21 illustrates the number of different categories of organizations per activity.

From the perspective of separate activities, all AIDS platforms and municipal health services are involved with the activity: AIDS policy coordination and implementation. AIDS policy coordination of organizations on the regional/local level was formulated as one of the main AIDS platform goals on their foundation. Municipal health services were subsidized by the health department to create AIDS policy coordination institutes and they are as such responsible for the AIDS platforms. Some interest or patient organizations and groups at risk or community organizations also reported performing AIDS policy coordinating activities. Even a small number of health and welfare organizations, ambulatory mental health care, social work and home care, and drug support organizations, hospitals/nursing homes consider themselves to perform AIDS policy coordination activities. The control of blood plasma is carried out by blood banks/laboratories and hospitals. HIV-screening, testing and identification is done by half of the municipal health services, a few drug support organizations, and some hospitals/nursing homes.

A large part of the organizations in this sector, i.e. 39%, are exclusively committed to AIDS. This is due to the large number of AIDS platforms which perform AIDS policy coordination activities and were founded as exclusive HIV/AIDS organizations.

Regarding the geographical scope, 86% of the organizations are regional and 14% of them, national.

4.3.5   Interest Representation

Two different sub-categories were distinguished in this category. One being for activities organized for or oriented towards target-groups, like self-help activities, legal advice and counselling for insurance/welfare entitlements. And the other being

Table 3.19: Organizations and Their Control and Monitoring Activities

Activity	Number of Organizations	% of N=288
AIDS policy coordination and implementation	107	37.3
Control of blood/plasma and product safety	9	3.1
HIV-screening, testing, identification	22	7.6
Total	138	

Source: *Managing AIDS in the Netherlands*: Dataset 1 (n=288).

the pure form of interest representation like political lobbying and civil and human rights protection against discrimination (Table 3.22).

There is some variation in the number of activities. Self-help and counselling for insurance/welfare entitlements score highest. One organization – the gay in-

Table 3.20: Subsector Activities by Type of Organization

Societal sectors	Category of organization/ functional type	Number of organizations in Dataset 1	Number of organizations in Subsector	%
Governmental	Municipal health service	40	34	85
	aids platform	44	43	98
	Local/regional council/ governmental organization	10	6	60
Non-profit organizations	Ambulatory mental health care	24	1	4
	Social work & home care	26	3	12
	Drug support	33	10	30
	Hospital & nursing home	50	9	18
	Laboratories/ bloodbanks	4	4	100
Groups at risk/ community organizations	Gay/HIV/buddy service	17	3	17
	Interest/patient representation	11	3	27
	Other	29	2	20
	Total	288	118	41

Source: *Managing AIDS in the Netherlands*: Dataset 1 (n=288).

terest association: NVIH COC – reports offering legal advice. The largest part of the organizations in this subsector (89%) perform just one or two activities; 11% of the organizations perform three or more. The mean number of activities is 2.1 per organization.

As was to be expected, most interest/patient organizations are involved in this subsector. Remarkably, however, a relatively large number of non-profit organi-

Table 3.21: AIDS Policy Coordination and Implementation Activities by Types of Organizations

Type of organization	AIDS policy coordination and implementation	Control of blood/plasma and product safety	HIV-screening, testing and identification
Municipal health service	32	1	14
AIDS platform	43		1
Local councils/ governmental organization	6		1
Ambulatory mental health care	1		
Social work & home care	3		
Drug support	9		2
Hospital & nursing home	5	4	3
Laboratories/ blood banks		4	1
Gay/HIV/buddy service	3		
Interest/patient representation	3		
Other	2		
Total	107	9	22

Source: *Managing AIDS in the Netherlands*: Dataset 1 (n=288)

zations – health care and welfare organizations – provide these types of activities. Governmental organizations – municipal health services – and AIDS platforms are less involved here than in other subsectors.

The most represented type of organization is the interest organization of the risk-group and patient. They appear in all categories and perform the largest total number of activities. Viewed per activity, civil/human rights protection and political lobbying score highest. Drug support organizations and social work agencies score relatively high in self-help, which would be rather remarkable as they cannot perform self-help in a strict sense. This can be explained by the fact that they supervise or support self-help groups. One should perhaps question the self-help activity quoted and its relevance in these cases. Counselling for insurance/welfare entitlements can be seen as a classic task for the social work agency. This is also true for drug support organizations which can be seen as providing social work for a specific target group. Not surprisingly, municipal health services score low in this subsector. However, some institutes consider self-help an activity, e.g. social work agencies. It seems that municipal health services and social work agencies are the most fit organizations to pick up the threads, i.e. some extra tasks in cases or calamities like a new disease such as AIDS with nothing to aid the problem.

4.3.6   Fund-raising

This subsector consists of fund-raising activities and general support activities for other organizations/persons (Table 3.23).

Table 3.22: Interest Representation and Self-help Activities

Activities	Number of organizations	% of N=288
Self-help groups	22	7.6
Counselling for insurance/ welfare entitlements	25	8.7
Civil/human rights/ protection against discrimination	14	4.9
Political lobbying	16	5.6
Legal advice	1	0.3
Total	78	

Source: *Managing AIDS in the Netherlands*: Dataset 1 (n=288)

Table 3.23: Organizations and Support Activities

	Number of organizations	% of N=288
Fund-raising	8	2.8
Support activities	7	2.4

Source: *Managing AIDS in the Netherlands*: Dataset 1 (n=288)

This is the smallest of all subsectors in terms of numbers of organizations. Seven organizations record giving support activities to other organizations and eight record escalating fund-raising activities for HIV/AIDS.

4.4   Resources

4.4.1   Resources of Organizations in General

The resources an organization has, can give one an indication of the number of HIV/AIDS activities an organization can perform. These resources mean the number of employees – this includes both paid personnel and volunteers – and financial resources. These three types of resources can only partly be described by the

Table 3.24: Organizations and the Number of Paid Personnel for HIV/ AIDS Activities (n=115)

Number of HIV/AIDS paid personnel	Frequency	(Total number)	Valid %
1	41		34.8
2	22	(44)	19.1
3	8	(24)	7.0
4	9	(36)	7.8
5	7	(35)	6.1
6-10	8	(60)	1.1
11-20	3	(31)	0.3
21-30	2	(48)	0.2
94	1	(94)	0.1
Total	101 organizations	(423) persons	
0	14		12.2
-9	175		24.5

organizations which provide HIV/AIDS activities.[42] The next table shows the number of paid personnel according to HIV/AIDS activities for a limited number of organizations.

The number of paid personnel on HIV/AIDS is low compared to the high number of organizations which provide HIV/AIDS activities. The average number of paid personnel is 3.7 per organization. The number of paid persons working on HIV/AIDS ranges from 0 to 25. A remarkable fact is that 36% of these organizations only have one person who works on AIDS. There is one organization which is an exception to the rule. This organization has indicated its paid HIV/AIDS personnel as being at 94 persons. However, one should point out the fact that it is not calculated in full-time equivalents but in the number of persons.

Forty-six organizations reported having a number of volunteers. The average number of volunteers according to these organizations is 12. The number of volunteers ranges from one to 55. There is also one big exception here: one organization has 126 volunteers. In contrast to paid personnel for AIDS, it is remarkable

Table 3.25: Organizations and the Number of Volunteers for HIV/AIDS Activities

Number of volunteers	Frequency	Total number	Valid %
1	2	2	3.1
2	10	20	15.4
3	3	9	4.6
4	1	4	1.5
5	3	15	4.6
6-10	9	76	13.9
11-20	6	93	9.1
21-30	4	99	6.1
31-40	2	70	3.1
41-50	3	145	4.5
51-60	2	107	3
126	1	126	1.5
Total	46 organizations	766 volunteers	
0	19		29.2
-9	223		

Source: *Managing AIDS in the Netherlands*: Dataset 1 (N=288)

Table 3.26   Organizations and the Annual Budget for HIV/AIDS Activities

Annual budget	Frequency	Valid %
500-10.000	12	18
10.000-20.000	5	8.5
20.000-30.000	5	7.5
30.000-40.000	6	9
40.000-50.000	4	6
50.000-60.000	3	4.5
-		
100.000-500.000	23	34.6
500.000-1.000.000	2	3
1.000.000-2.000.000	4	6
2.000.000-3.000.000	2	3

Source: *Managing AIDS in the Netherlands*: Dataset 1 (N=288)

that most of the organizations have two or more volunteers. One should point out here, however, that the total number of volunteers for HIV/AIDS far exceeds the total number of paid personnel.

Only 66 organizations were able to specify their annual budget on AIDS. This annual budget ranges from Hfl 500 ($290) to 3,000,000 ($1,740,000). More than 50% of the organizations have a relatively small annual budget on AIDS, namely between Hfl 500 ($290) and 60,000 ($34,800). Of these organizations, 35% receive between Hfl 100,000 and 500,000 and 12% of the organizations have an annual budget for AIDS of between Hfl 1,000,000 ($580,000) and 3,000,000 ($1,740,000).

4.5   Summary and Conclusions

The organizational response demonstrates strong functional differentiations. Organizations usually provide more than one activity. Multifunctional organizations are: municipal health organizations, AIDS platforms, NVIH COC, and drug support organizations.

The majority of organizations are active in the field of health care and social services (Care) and/or prevention, information and education (Prevention).

Given the differentiation in exclusive and inclusive organizations, the largest numbers of exclusive organizations are to be found in the subsectors of Fund-raising and Control and Monitoring.

Given the differentiation in governmental, private non-profit organizations, and groups at risk/community organizations, a slight difference becomes apparent.

Governmental organizations are most strongly represented in the subsector of Control and Monitoring and lowest in the Care subsector. Non-profit organizations are most strongly represented in the subsector of Care. Groups at risk/community organizations come most to the fore in the subsectors of Interest Representation and Prevention.

Given the geographical differentiation, the subsectors of Control and Monitoring, and Care have the largest percentage of organizations on a regional level.

With respect to resources, the pattern is varied. The number of paid personnel for HIV/AIDS activities is low compared to the total number of paid personnel, as well as related to the total budget. At the same time, a relatively large number of volunteers are involved in this sector. The annual budget for HIV/AIDS activities varies between a relatively large budget of more than one million Dutch guilders for only a few organizations and a relatively small budget of less than half a million for the majority of organizations.

5   Organizational Responses: A New Division of Labour

In this section we will describe the organizational response from a different angle. The central question here is:

> Does the organizational response to the HIV/AIDS epidemic follow the existing organizational structure and dominant type of governance, or are new types of organizations and types of governance evolving?

To answer this question, we must reformat the described organizational data.

Firstly, we must define the distinction between the inclusive and exclusive organizations, and, secondly, a distinction must be made between two types of organizational response which have been labelled top-down and bottom-up. The top-down organizational response is located in the existing institutionalized welfare state structure. It includes all those organizations which have a recognized and formalized task within the welfare state: both public organizations and professional welfare organizations. The bottom-up organizational response has its roots outside the formalized welfare state structure and includes organized risk-groups, organized communities and market organizations.

If the organizational response to the AIDS epidemic only followed the existing organizational density and regulative response, one might expect the "traditional" welfare state response based on inclusive and top-down organizational structures. On the other hand, the AIDS epidemic has a number of particular characteristics which need a different approach, i.e. needing to deal with the specificity of the disease and groups at risk. Instead of inclusive and top-down, in our opinion, the AIDS epidemic stimulates the opposite response seen in exclusive and bottom-up organizations.

5.1 Inclusive and Exclusive Organizational Responses

As has already been described, the HIV/AIDS problem in the Netherlands has not only been integrated in activities of the existing organizational structure but has at the same time resulted in problem-oriented organizations, in so-called "exclusives". Organizations are divided between 623 and 88 respectively. The inclusive organizations dominate the organizational response in almost every country (in our research project). However, the number of exclusive organizations is – at least in some countries – remarkable. So far, there seems to be a correlation between the number of inclusives and the establishment of the new exclusives: High numbers of inclusives correspond with relatively high numbers of exclusives. In this sense, this seems to be an indication – at least in the Netherlands – for the correlation between organizational density and new organizational initiatives (as has been discussed in organization sociological literature). The number of 88 exclusive organizations is at least an indication that the then existing organizational configuration at the beginning of the epidemic was unable to cope with the problem.

5.2 Top-down and Bottom-up Responses

So far we have used the traditional organizational differentiation between state, private non-profit and private for-profit (market). We will now use the more differentiated model of top-down and bottom-up organizations.

With respect to the question "How does one manage the HIV/AIDS epidemic?", the different organizational types can be related to particular commonly discussed types of governance. These reflect different views about the way the epidemic should be managed. The choice for the bureaucratic state organization expresses the belief in a hierarchical solution; in the end, the use of mandatory measures is legitimated. On the other end of the organizational scale in this context, we find the market organization, which symbolizes the belief in individual, free and rational choice. The other three organizational types – the organized community, the organized risk group and the professionalized welfare organization – waver between these two types. The organized community and the organized group at risk reflect altruism and solidarity as motives for intervention. The professional organization is the dominant type of the modern, complex society. It reflects the belief in organized expertise, i.e. in the expert system. Problem solutions are in this case in the hands of specialized professionals.

Notwithstanding the fact that the private non-profit sector is dominated by the professional health and welfare institutions, we can at the same time notice a relatively high involvement of organized communities and organized groups at risk in the organizational response to HIV/AIDS.

Compared to the other countries, the Netherlands combines a high score of organized communities with a relatively low proportion of organized groups at risk.

This can be explained by the fact that the main groups at risk – such as homosexuals and drug users – were already organized before the epidemic broke out. These organized communities expanded and added HIV/AIDS programmes to their activities. In other countries we see the opposite development: the epidemic has stimulated the collective action and formal organization of these groups (such as homosexuals in Austria).

The relatively strong position of organizations from the homosexual community – homosexual organizations as well as a number of organizations of people with HIV/AIDS, which are often closely related to the homosexual communities – has clearly something to do with the particularities of the epidemic. However, the relatively high risk for this community cannot sufficiently explain the relatively strong organizational response. In this case, some of the particular organizational preconditions outlined above can explain this particular organizational response: Firstly, the size of the group at risk, and, secondly, the level of social cohesion.

5.3 *Conclusion*

So far, the AIDS epidemic has not only mobilized the existing organizational and/ or regulative capacities of the different societies, but it has also stimulated new organizational initiatives: group and/or problem-oriented organizations, this development has been labelled as the bottom-up response. The persistency of the problem, the need to change behaviour, the embeddedness of risk behaviour within the private spheres and particular cultures, modern states being unable to intervene, the limits of professional expertise, are all factors which have stimulated new concepts and approaches. This explains the relatively important increase in organized communities, organized groups at risk and exclusive HIV/AIDS organizations in the last decade in most countries. The rise in community organizations seems to support the opinion that it is too easy to define these community values and structures as pre-modern and pre-industrial. With respect to the AIDS epidemic, our findings show that not only the traditional community organizations (e.g. Red Cross, churches, etc.), but also a number of modern community organizations and communities at risk have entered the AIDS policy domain: homosexual, haemophiliac, IV-drug user organizations, etc. The rise in these organizations not only reflects the still existing organizational capacity of this so-called "traditional" sphere in modern welfare states, but also shows a new functional institutional choice for a modern health problem. In the case of HIV/AIDS, organized risk groups seem to be important intermediaries for a prevention policy in utilizing the experience of risk. These organizations can develop a culture of solidarity which could help to create a culture of responsibility between infected and non-infected members of the group. Such solidarity can then strengthen the development of group activities in addition to regulating effects regarding behaviour. In general, the AIDS epidemic has stimulated an alternative approach to health and welfare problems.

Instead of the task-differentiated approach, the epidemic has stimulated an integral approach, which also seems important for other welfare areas.

The intriguing question is whether these new organizational responses will result in a "new division of labour" and in its counterpart "a new organic solidarity", to quote Durkheim. Will these different organizational responses lead to new interorganizational and so-called horizontal and cooperative relations between public and private, or to competing, conflicting or parallel "sectors"? So far, there are in fact indications of new organizational public/private structures. The various regional and local AIDS platforms are a good example. In these "horizontal cooperative policy structures" different types of organizational approaches (experts, state organizations, organized communities and organized risk groups) work together by exchanging information, experience, knowledge, resources and programmes to cope with this modern problem. These modern horizontal policy structures might be a fruitful and new approach which goes beyond the classic either/ or choice of hierarchy or market, public or private, rational choice or altruism.

What we can learn from the analysis of the organizational response to the HIV/ AIDS epidemic done so far is that modern societies not only need but are also able to produce various types of complementary organizational structures with different modes of governance to deal with modern social problems effectively and adequately. The central question is whether these new "joint-ventures" of different intervention strategies and institutions will survive and grow in the near future. From a recent study by McKinney among HIV/AIDS joint-ventures in the UK and the Netherlands we may learn that it is still unclear as to which direction the old and new organizational answers might take (McKinney, 1995).

Notes

1   Stuurgroep Toekomstscenario's Gezondheidszorg (STG) (Steering Committee for Future Scenarios regarding Health Care), 1992: 59.
2   *Nota inzake het Aidsbeleid* (TK, 1986-1987, 19218, nr. 2:3). In other sources, early 1982 is mentioned as the year of the first registered AIDS case (WHO, *AIDS Surveillance in Europe*).
3   Houweling et al., 1987.
4   Jager/Poos/Houweling et al., NTG, nr. 51, 1990.
5   Stichting AIDS Fonds, *AIDS-bestrijding*, March 1996, nr. 27: 10.
6   As defined in the public discourse and official policy documents.
7   For the time being, and for the sake of argument, we assumed the dialectical relation between the social definition of subgroups and subepidemics on the one hand, and the policy and organizational response on the other.
8   R. Coutinho, 'Een terugblik vanuit het beleid', p. 14 in: Herman Vuijsje/Roel Coutinho (ed.) (1989) *Dilemma's rondom AIDS*. Amsterdam/Lisse.
9   B. de Vroom (1991) *AIDS en gedragsregulering. Dilemma's en mogelijkheden van overheidsingrijpen en categorale zelfregulering.* Leiden, pp. 3-4.

10 STG, 1992: 64.
11 STG, 1992: 71. It has also been reported that a number of the foreign prostitutes are from the Dominican Republic and Cape Verdian Islands, i.e. countries with a high incedence rate among the heterosexual population.
12 STG, 1992: 57.
13 Olson, 1965; Dunleavy, 1988.
14 STG, 1992: 57.
15 Anneke van den Hoek (1990) *Epidemiology of HIV infection among drug users in Amsterdam.* Amsterdam.
16 STG, 1992: 76, 77.
17 Hans Warmerdam/Pieter Koenders (1987) *Cultuur en Ontspanning. Het COC 1946-1966.* Utrecht.
18 NCAB, *AIDS-Bestrijding*, October 1990.
19 Stichting AIDS Fonds, *AIDS-Bestrijding*, March 1996, nr. 27: 10
20 STG, 1992: 67.
21 STG, 1992: 67. This is not seen as representative of the whole population however.
22 STG, 1992: 77.
23 STG, 1992: 59.
24 GG&GD Amsterdam, *Factsheet AIDS and Drugs Amsterdam*, July 1992.
25 GG&GD Amsterdam, 1992; Buning, 1990; Toet/Van der Ven, 1989: 26 (STG, 1992: 58).
26 STG, 1992: 63.
27 GG&GD Amsterdam, 1992.
28 STG, 1992: 63.
29 STG, 1992: 74; Smit/Rosendaal, 'Hemofilie en AIDS', pp. 47-67 in Vuijsje/Coutinho (ed.), 1989, op.cit.
30 The year 1993 has been chosen for statistical and comparative reasons (with respect to the organizational response).
31 The public response was in other words primarily related to reproachable behaviour of individuals and groups as was the case for leprosy in the Middle Ages: "The evil of leprosy was regarded as a punishment sent by God, against which human resistance was of no avail. Whoever was struck by this punishment was considered impure and sinful, and was treated as such – with stigmatization and ostracism (...). The treatment of lepers was not based upon any precise knowledge of the nature of transmission of the disease but rather on disgust and fear" (Goudsblom, 1986 32: 165-166).
32 Both in written douments and interviews.
33 The category also includes the inclusive-inclusives: organizations not performing particular AIDS activities, but mentioned as part of the HIV/AIDS policy network.
34 For instance, the Schorerstichting is an example of this type of goal displacement.
35 In certain circumstances these workers are also defined as groups at risk.
36 The year when HIV/AIDS activity started in organizations was filled out by 44% (243) of all surveyed organizations. It nevertheless gives a figure of the growth of the number of organizations.
37 And drug support organizations started relatively late with the coordination of their HIV/AIDS activities; there was therefore a difference in opinion about the treatment of drug users. Organizations which originally focused on the therapeutic treatment of

drug users were found to be up against low threshold help. Needle-exchange and the free distribution of condoms did not match this vision. For this reason some municipal health authorities responded by claiming that these activities were also on offer.

38 Some large national health education organizations have the specific task to produce information material for specific target groups.

39 Nursing homes filled in "hospice" as their specific activity.

40 Here, it can be concluded that home care is underrepresented in the questionnaire for it is a core activity for some of their organizations.

41 Advice counselling, and monitoring are usually included in this category as no separate categories for these types of activities exist.

42 It must be stressed that only a part (n=115) of the organizations was able to quote its resources on AIDS. Other organizations were facing problems by doing this mainly because their HIV/AIDS activities are integrated in other organizational activities. However, the answers of those who did respond to this question can give one an indication as to the resources available to organizations involved with HIV/AIDS activities.

References

Bayer, Ronald (1989) 'AIDS, Privacy, and Responsibility', *Daedalus, Journal of the American Academy of Arts and Sciences* 118-3.

Brinkman, L.C. (1988) 'De rol van de overheid bij de bestrijding van AIDS', p. 91 in Nederlands Gespreks Centrum, *AIDS, moraal en maatschappij*. Utrecht/Antwerpen.

Bunning, E. (1990) *De GG&GD en het drugprobleem in cijfers deel IV*. Amsterdam: GG&GD.

CBS (1994) *Statistisch Jaarboek*.

Coutinho, R. (1989) 'Een terugblik vanuit het beleid', in Herman Vuijsje/Roel Coutinho (ed.), *Dilemma's rondom AIDS*. Amsterdam/Lisse.

Dunleavy, P.D. (1988) 'Group Identities and Individual Influence: Reconstructing the Theory of Interest Groups', *British Journal of Political Science* 18 (January): 21-49.

European Centre for the Epidemiological Monitoring of AIDS (1992) *AIDS Surveillance in Europe*, Quarterly Report No. 33.

Friedman, Lawrence M. (1985) *Total Justice*. New York: Russell Sage Foundation.

GG&GD Amsterdam (1992) *Factsheet AIDS and Drugs Amsterdam*. July.

Goudsblom, Johan (1986) 'Public Health and the Civilizing Process', *The Millbank Quarterly* 64 (2): 161-188.

't Hart, Piet (1990) 'Bestrijding van cholera in de negentiende eeuw. Een ziekte van de armen?', *Intermediair* 49: 59-63.

Hendriks, A. (1991) *AIDS, HIV Prevalence and AIDS/HIV Policies in Europe; A Survey*.

Hoek, Anneke van den (1990) *Epidemiology of HIV Infection Among Drug Users in Amsterdam*. Amsterdam.

Houweling, H. et al. (1987) 'Epidemiologie van AIDS en HIV infecties in Nederland; huidige situatie en prognose voor de periode 1987-1990', *Nederlands Tijdschrift voor Geneeskunde* 131 (19): 818-824.

Jager, J.C. c.s. (1990) *Nederlands Tijdschrift voor Geneeskunde* 51, December.

Kattouw, M./Nijboer, J.F. (1990) 'AIDS in het strafrecht. Hoe crimineel is AIDS?', pp. 5-23 in J.K.M. Gevers/S.M.S.M. van de Goor/J.F.L. Roording/H.D.C. Roscam Abbing, *AIDS in het recht*. Nijmegen.

Kamerstukken 19218, *Nota inzake het AIDSbeleid* (TK, 1986-1987).

Marin, Bernd/Kenis, Patrick (1989) *Managing AIDS. The Role of Private Nonprofit Institutions in Public Health and Welfare Policy, Research Design*. Vienna: European Centre for Social Welfare Policy and Research.

McKinney, Martha M. (1995) *A Time to Gain, A Time to Lose: New Directions for Western European HIV/AIDS Alliances*. Research Monograph. Department of Health and Human Services, May.

NCAB, *AIDS bestrijding* (different years).

NVHP (1992) *Hemofilie en AIDS*. September.

Olson, Mancur (1965) *The Logic of Collective Action. Public Goods and the Theory of Groups*. Cambridge/London: Harvard University Press.

Smit/Rosendaal (1989) 'Hemofilie en AIDS', pp. 47-67 in Vuijsje/Coutinho (eds.), op.cit.

STG / Stuurgroep Toekomstscenario's Gezondheidszorg (1992) *AIDS in Nederland tot 2000*. Houten/Zaventem: Bohn/Stafleu/Van Loghum.

Swaan, Abraham de (1989) *Zorg en de Staat*. Amsterdam.

Toet/Van der Ven (1992), p. 58 in STG / Stuurgroep Toekomstscenario's Gezondheidszorg, *AIDS in Nederland tot 2000*. Houten/Zaventem: Bohn/Stafleu/Van Loghum.

Vroom, B. de (1991) *AIDS en gedragsregulering. Dilemma's en mogelijkheden van overheidsingrijpen en categorale zelfregulering*. Leiden.

Vroom, B. de (1993) 'AIDS: nationale patronen van organisationele respons', pp. 183-214 in Jacques van Doorn/Pauline Meurs/Ton Mijs (eds.), *Het organisatorisch labyrint*. Utrecht: AULA.

Vroom, B. de/Kester, C.C.M. (1992) 'AIDS en beheersing van risicogedrag', pp. 163-186 in N.J.H.Huls (ed.), *Sturing in de risicomaatschappij*. Zwolle: Tjeenk Willink.

Vroom, Bert de/Kenis, Patrick (1994) Managing HIV/AIDS Through Organizational Responses. Findings from a Cross-national Study. Revised version of paper prepared for the 1994 Annual Meeting of the American Sociological Association, *The Challenge of Democratic Participation*, 5-9 August, 1994, Los Angeles, California. A German translation has been published in Adalbert Evers/Thomas Olk (eds.), *Wohlfahrtspluralismus*. Opladen: Westdeutscher Verlag (1996).

Warmerdam, Hans/Koenders, Pieter (1987) *Cultuur en Ontspanning. Het COC 1946-1966*. Utrecht.

WHO (1988) *Health Legislation and Ethics in the Field of AIDS and HIV Infection*.

WHO (1990) *Current Status of HIV/AIDS Prevention and Control Policies in the European Region*.

CHAPTER 4

The Role of Non-Profit Organizations in Managing HIV/AIDS in Sweden[1]

Dagmar von Walden Laing
Victor A. Pestoff

1 Institutional, Policy and Epidemiological Context

In 1982 the disease, that was later to be labelled AIDS, was diagnosed for the first time in a Swedish hospital. Although the number of patients was rather low in the first years, the reports from the USA were carefully monitored by the health authorities, by specialist groups within the medical profession and by the voluntary organization whose members were most closely affected to begin with – the Swedish Federation for Gay and Lesbian Rights, RFSL. All three groups were involved from early on in what we in this study will call HIV/AIDS-related activities.

In May 1985, the government decided to form the National Commission on AIDS within the Ministry of Health and Social Affairs as a "consensus platform", where representatives from the two major political parties (later from all political parties), relevant ministries and government agencies, regional and municipal governments and legal and medical experts could meet. Special "reference groups" were attached to the commission, one of them consisting of representatives from relevant private non-profit organizations (PNPOs).[2]

The responsibilities of the commission were to:
* coordinate the work in all spheres of society in order to limit the spread of AIDS;
* monitor and initiate research and other relevant measures;
* assess the need for information and initiate this to groups at risk, health care personnel, the public at large, etc.;
* assess and call attention to the need of immediate action, e.g. initiate legal changes;
* assess the urgent need of resources.[3]

The establishment of such a commission within a government department was a unique move since the responsibility for all these activities would normally have rested with the National Board of Health and Welfare, where a group of medical experts had been meeting regularly since December 1982, and where a "reference group" of representatives for the concerned private non-profit groups was consulted from 1984 onwards (Lewin, 1987). The feeling of urgency and the public concern forced the government to act, after a proposal made by the National Board of Health and Welfare and one of its major scientific experts, H. Wigzell. The main advantage of the new organization was that decisions could be made quickly, without the delay caused in a regular bureaucracy, according to Gertrud Sigurdsen, then Minister of Health and Social Affairs and the chair person of the commission from its start until 1991. From the time when all political parties were represented in the commission, debates could take place there and consensus be reached before proposals were introduced into the *Riksdag*, which also helped to pave the way for speedy results.[4]

The National Commission on AIDS was dissolved on 1 July 1992, when its main functions were taken over by the new National Institute of Public Health. After 10 years, AIDS had lost its unique label and become one of the many public health concerns.

1.1   The National AIDS Programme

In April 1986, the government presented the first complete action plan for the fight against AIDS for consideration in the Riksdag.[5] The main points were:
- information and psychosocial support to risk groups;
- action in order to limit the spread among homo- and bisexual men;
- increased support for and treatment of drug addicts;
- urgent investigations into how to intensify research on AIDS.

Additional funds were immediately set aside for implementation of the action plan, and in the years that followed, the plan continued to play the role of a specific programme with separate financing from the annual government budget. When the National Commission on AIDS was dissolved in 1992, the new coordinating body, the National Institute of Public Health, continued to receive funding specified for the HIV/AIDS programme. As part of the 1986 plan, extra financial support was also allocated to the three major urban areas – Stockholm, Gothenburg and Malmö – in order to support the increased demands for preventive measures and medical care where the largest number of HIV-positive persons were to be found. Later the recipients of this extra funding were only specified to be "certain counties and municipalities". For the amounts specifically budgeted for the fight against AIDS, see Table 4.1.

Table 4.1:   Government Allocation for the Fight Against AIDS, Fiscal Years 1986/87-1993/94 (in 1,000 SKr)

| | | | Special AIDS Programme | |
Year	Total	Total*	For PNPOs*	Urban Areas
1986/87	125,000	75,000	n/a	50,000
1987/88	80,000	80,000	n/a	0
1988/89	230,000	145,000	10,787	85,000
1989/90	226,000	106,000	11,825**	120,000
1990/91	193,500	73,500	11,980	120,000
1991/92	193,500	73,500	16,019	120,000
1992/93	192,720	72,720	18,205	120,000
1993/94	185,220	65,220	n/a	120,000
Total	1,425,940	690,940	68,816	735,000

*   Incl. drug treatment; see also Table 4.10.
**   Excl. immigrant organizations.
Source: *Regeringens propositioner* (Government Bills) 1985/86:171, 1986/87:100 app. 7, 1987/88:79, 1988/89:100 app. 7, 1989/90:100 app. 7, 1990/91:100 app. 7, 1991/92:100 app. 6, 1992/93:100 app. 6. Eva Ekdahl, The National Institute of Public Health, *Personal Communication.*

The first national information campaign was organized in 1987 by the National Commission on AIDS. Three main objectives were spelled out:
• decrease the spread of infection;
• counteract prejudice and misunderstanding about the disease;
• counteract unjustified fear and anxiety.
Over the period March 1987 to November 1988, SKr 49.3 million ($ 6,162,500) were spent on campaigns targeting 11 specified groups, including printed material, films, etc. This two-year campaign was thoroughly evaluated by the National Audit Bureau in 1989.[6] Further major campaigns, focusing on different groups and built on varying themes, have been launched virtually every year since then.

The structure of the national health care and social welfare systems is an important factor for understanding the development of HIV/AIDS activities in any country. However, the efforts of the state in developing preventive measures and in financing and organizing care for the HIV-infected is not sufficient. In Sweden, as in most countries, a large number of voluntary organizations have become involved in activities aiming at preventing the spread of the HIV infection and in making life easier for those already infected.

In a separate section of the 1986 action plan, the government emphasized that the need for psychosocial support to groups at risk could best be met by voluntary organizations, among persons with common backgrounds and situations. The relevant organizations engaged in the reference group of the National Commission on AIDS were described as partners in the prevention work. Specific tribute was paid to the early initiatives with contact groups for support and counselling, arranged by the Federation for Gay and Lesbian Rights. The purpose of our research has been to study the role of PNPOs in managing HIV/AIDS in Sweden.

From an organizational-structural perspective, Swedish, private non-profit organizations are often built up in the traditions of democratic, popular movements. Traditions from the temperance movements originating in the early 1800s as well as from non-conformist churches and the labour movements of the mid-1800s, are noticeable in the way new groups have developed in later years, including the ease with which they have been accepted as valuable partners to the state. Some associations for the handicapped are old, but as a political force they became more noticeable in the 1970s. Sweden became a country of immigration after the Second World War. Organizations where immigrants met and worked in order to safeguard their interests also functioned as a means of keeping in touch with the language and culture of their country of origin.[7]

Private non-profit organizations, PNPOs, are to a varying degree financed by government grants, on the national as well as the regional and local levels. Certain types of organizations, e.g. for the handicapped, can apply for an annual grant covering the costs of administration and general activities if they meet certain standards and have a democratic membership structure. Other grants can be awarded for specified projects, e.g. information campaigns or support to specific target groups. From 1966/67, project grants were awarded to non-profit organizations for defined activities aimed at groups of immigrants. After proposals from the Royal Commission on Immigration, grants were allocated "in support of the activities of immigrant and minority associations", beginning in 1975/76.[8] The context in which the need for HIV/AIDS-related activities affected the private non-profit organizations in the early 1980s included the availability of government grants for drug prevention and drug treatment programmes, for the general activities of a few established patient organizations and specific project grants given to various charities.

The rules and regulations attached to AIDS financial support have been changing over the years. The allocation of grants to non-profit organizations was originally organized by the Ministry of Health but later, during the years 1988-1991, a separate unit within the National Board of Health and Welfare took this over from the National Commission, as well as some other administrative tasks. Earmarked money for setting up therapeutic communities for HIV-infected drug addicts was recorded in the specific AIDS grant one year, but moved to another part of the budget the next. From 1990, SKr 14 million ($ 1,750,000) was granted – outside the special

AIDS budget – to the Prison and Probation Authorities for the development of HIV/AIDS programmes among drug-using offenders.

HIV/AIDS was considered an infectious disease from the outset. One important part of the Swedish HIV/AIDS strategy which came into effect in September 1985, was the government's decision to apply the Control of Infectious Diseases Act of 1968 to HIV/AIDS, thus making HIV infection a notifiable disease. This made it possible to follow the epidemiological development in a unique way and was later codified in the 1989 Prevention of Infectious Diseases Act. Unlike most countries, not only cases of full-blown AIDS, but also diagnosed HIV infection, now have to be reported. Every physician who undertakes an HIV test, has to report sero-positive cases to the National Bacteriological Laboratory/the Swedish Institute for Infectious Disease Control, which coordinates the epidemiological work. The reporting is done in such a way that the individual cannot be traced, but enough information is given to allow for statistical follow-ups (sex, year of birth and when possible, route of transmission) – see section 1.4 below for the details of the development of AIDS and HIV in Sweden from 1983 to 1992.

1.2 Major Issues of Conflict in Public Debate

Swedish political life is often characterized by its tendency to seek consent rather than conflict. The general development of a Swedish AIDS policy is a good example of how the consensus can be managed. From 1985 to 1992 it was coordinated by the National Commission on AIDS, working within the Ministry of Health and Social Affairs and chaired for most of the time by the responsible minister herself. The commission, with the status of an advisory body, included representatives from all political parties. They prepared matters to be presented to the Riksdag and consensus was reached beforehand, in all cases but one – namely, the question of whether clean syringes and needles should be supplied to intravenous drug users in order to prevent HIV/AIDS being transmitted via shared, infected tools. This matter brought about one of the most heated debates related to the disease in Sweden.

Two additional questions have been subject to much debate; in the mass media, within the groups concerned, and also within the National Commission on AIDS, where the reference group representatives of the gay community in particular have been active. One is the consequence of making HIV/AIDS a notifiable disease which results in the option to isolate a virus carrier without symptoms in hospital if he/she does not follow the given directives to prevent transmission. The other, the closure of "sauna clubs" or the Swedish equivalent of gay bathhouses, is of minor interest as a matter of principle, but still mirrors difference in attitudes.

1.2.1 Syringe Exchange Schemes

The first time the syringe exchange issue was discussed by the Riksdag was in early 1987 when the government proposal on AIDS appropriations was presented. Two

MPs, one from the Swedish Liberal Party and one from the Centre Party, proposed different ways of making needles and syringes available to drug addicts in order to stop the spread of HIV through the communal use of infected tools. The liberal proposal, where the government should allow doctors to prescribe and supply needles and syringes, caused an extensive discussion in the Standing Committee on Social Affairs, including a statement that no law forbids doctors to prescribe the equipment. The committee decided that there was no reason for the Riksdag to evaluate the matter, since the National Board of Health and Welfare as the proper authority in this case, had already accepted that the Lund Project for clean syringes and needles was being carried out by doctors, acting in accordance with the "science and experience" requirement. It was stressed, however, that the programme in Lund should remain the only programme of this kind, lest the restrictive drug politics be jeopardized.

In February 1989, the government reported to the Riksdag on the Lund Test Project. The National Board of Health and Welfare had evaluated the project which had been going on since the end of 1986. In 1988, about 150 clients were involved in Lund, and another programme which started in Malmö in August 1987, involved some 500 addicts. A survey on 29 hospital departments treating patients with infectious diseases all over the country, revealed that at least eight other hospitals were running programmes where needles and syringes were supplied to drug addicts. In most places, the programmes were run in cooperation with psychiatric departments, social welfare authorities and drug prevention teams.

In the report from the National Board, brief information was also given on what was going on in other countries in Europe. Experiences from programmes in Britain (England and Scotland) together with the Lund-Malmö findings, constituted the base for the proposal that a three-year trial period with controlled syringe exchange programmes should begin.

Intravenous heroin use is primarily apparent in the Stockholm area and in the southern province of Skåne. It was therefore proposed that these regions should be included in the three-year programme and that two more regions, with a low HIV-incidence, should take part. The National Board would issue detailed guidelines and set up a special steering committee including expertise in medical and social sciences.

From the time the Evaluation Report was made public in November 1988, until the Riksdag decision was made in April 1989, there was a lively public debate on the matter. Those opposing the project claimed that allowing needles and syringes to be supplied in the proposed way would counteract the strict Swedish drug policy, and imply that IV-drug use was acceptable. According to one source, the social services section within the National Board of Health and Welfare was strongly opposed to the proposed project, it even encouraged the opposition and played a part in the creation of a national association called Social Workers Against AIDS

(Gould, 1994). This association, or rather action group, was dissolved after about a year of activity. However, the divided views within the National Board mirrored the division between the medical and the social work professions, also noticeable in the general debate.

The social-democratic government proposed a trial period, limited in scope: including only enough places and participants that were necessary as a base for the evaluation, and under no circumstances carried out in more than four places. Furthermore, supplying free needles and syringes would not be allowed outside the organized trial programme. Within the programme, only those who were prepared to get in touch with social authorities in order to undergo treatment for their addiction should be admitted to the syringe exchange projects.

When the Riksdag Standing Committee met in April 1989, they had a number of proposals from the opposition parties and individual members of the Riksdag to consider. The Committee recommended that the Riksdag should accept a limited test programme in three places, excluding the Greater Stockholm area. The need for careful control and scientific design was stressed. After a vivid debate in the Riksdag, the recommendation of the Standing Committee was accepted.

1.2.2   HIV-testing, Anonymity and the Issue of "Forced Care"

Making HIV/AIDS a notifiable disease by making the Infectious Diseases Act applicable, meant that the mandatory reporting of positive cases, contact-tracing and other measures intended to safeguard public health, had to be carried out in the cases where HIV-testing led to a seropositive answer. The physician in charge of the testing is responsible for counselling the patient and for the contact-tracing in order to test persons with whom the patient has been in contact and who might have acquired the disease. Part of the counselling is aimed at preventing the patient from spreading the infection further. This includes advice on the responsible practice of "safe sex" and the duty to inform present and future partners about the infection.

Informed consent before testing is required since all testing is voluntary, except for persons approached because somebody carrying the virus has revealed that he/she might have transmitted the infection to, or acquired it from them.[9] The law on medical records did not originally allow for a patient to stay anonymous in relation to his/her doctor however, which caused an outcry from the gay community especially. This was partly changed when a new law regarding HIV-testing came into force on 1 July 1987. Now samples may be coded if the patient wants to be anonymous, but complete anonymity lasts only as long as the result is seronegative. If positive, the Infectious Diseases Act takes over and the medical record, which stays with the investigating doctor, has to be completed.

One much debated ingredient of the Infectious Diseases Act is the option to isolate a virus carrier without symptoms in a hospital if he/she does not follow the directives given by the physician in order to prevent transmission. The decision is taken by an administrative court after a proposal made by the county medical officer, to whom the treating physician is obliged to report. Every county medical officer (25 in all) has this regulative function, but so far it has been a major subject of controversy only in the Stockholm area – where 18 persons were isolated by July 1993, most of them drug addicts and/or prostitutes, but also some African refugees who have not "adjusted" to the Swedish rules.

The procedure, that a patient can be isolated in a hospital against his/her will as "a last resort", if he/she continues a behaviour that may result in a further spread of the infection, has been accepted for a long time for other communicable diseases, including venereal; but the fact that there is no adequate treatment available for HIV carriers made the question of forced isolation highly controversial. The gay community and spokesmen for human and civil rights have opposed the fact that detention could be enforced without regular court proceedings. However, equally strong is the opposition from within the medical profession, where some doctors working with AIDS patients refer to the Council of Europe's recommendation R89 on ethical issues, which has not been ratified by Sweden, according to which forced isolation in this form is not acceptable. They claim that HIV-positive persons with a lifestyle that involves exposing others to the disease could be tried according to the penal code. A strong argument for substituting partner notification for contact-tracing and abolishing the administratively enforced isolation, is that these coercive measures destroy the trust which is a necessary component in the relationship between the patient and his/her doctor (Berglund, 1993).

1.2.3   Closure of the "Sauna Clubs"

The closure of the so-called "sauna clubs" in June 1987, was motivated by the risks connected with the sexual practices among their homosexual customers. The clubs, the Swedish equivalent of the "gay bathhouses", as described by other countries, were meeting places for homosexual men, and arranged in such a way that temporary, sexual contacts between anonymous customers were facilitated. The National Board of Health and Welfare, supported by the National Commission on AIDS, had initiated the new legal measures in an attempt to decrease the spread of HIV among gay men.[10]

Due to the urgency, a hearing on the matter had been substituted for the normal procedures of a "remiss" of the proposed act to concerned authorities and organizations. Among those invited to take part in the hearing were experts from government agencies, legal experts and representatives of private non-profit organizations, specifically the Swedish Federation for Gay and Lesbian Rights (RFSL), the Swedish Association for Sex Education (RFSU) and Swedish Physicians Against AIDS.[11] Before the legal steps were initiated by the National Commission on AIDS, RFSL had offered to take steps in order to influence the way the clubs were being run and also got economic support for this activity. The idea was that information to the customers and to the proprietors should encourage safer sex practices and that way, have a preventive effect. No results were obvious, however, and in the debate during the hearing, the majority of those present agreed that the clubs should be closed.

Those representing RFSL, Swedish Physicians Against AIDS and the Gay Men's Health Clinic at the hearing, argued that if the clubs were closed, new, hidden meeting places which were not available for scrutiny would be set up and the dangerous practices would continue. The clubs could be a valuable place for dissemination of information on safer sex, and the effective measure should be to enforce change in the way the clubs were arranged and run, by penalizing unacceptable practices. The majority, however, saw this as impossible to control and the government proposal was accepted in the Riksdag. The law took effect on 1 July 1987.

1.3 HIV/AIDS and the General Health and Welfare System

In Sweden, everybody who is resident in the country has access to social services and to the public health care system, which includes all kinds of health care provisions. Government administration and services are separated into three geographical planes: national, regional, and local/municipal – all three allowed to levy taxes in order to provide their services. The division of responsibilities between the three levels is laid down by the law. Almost all hospitals and a widespread network of health care centres are organized by the regional governments and mainly financed by the national and regional budgets. Private practitioners also supply both general and specialized medical care, with the patient's costs subsidized to a large extent by the social security system. Social security provisions include subsidizing medical care and pharmaceuticals, as well as payments of pensions and benefits during sick leave or unemployment. Social services aimed at all groups in society who need support, financially or similarly, are the responsibility of the local/municipal government.

All welfare provisions are, of course, available to HIV/AIDS sufferers as well as to anybody else. Certain services are, however, of specific importance. At the national level, the responsibility for the prevention of communicable diseases rests on the National Board of Health and Welfare and the National Bacteriological Laboratory – the latter was replaced by the Swedish Institute for Infectious Disease Control in July 1993.

At the regional level, the 23 county councils and three of the municipalities supply health care for all inhabitants within their areas. This includes preventive measures and medical care, with hospital departments for infectious diseases as well as for genito-urinary medicine located in every county. Units for prevention of infectious diseases, directed by the county medical officer, are mandatory in each county, according to the Prevention of Infectious Diseases Act. For a graphical representation of counties, see Appendix 2. The 295 municipilaties are in charge of the local social services, including prevention and non-medical services related to drug abuse.

1.4 Epidemiological Development

In Sweden, like most countries in Northern Europe, the earliest and still to date, the largest number of AIDS cases were identified among homosexual and bisexual men. Infection via blood products and blood transfusion appeared after a couple of years, but although the spread via intravenous drug-taking was reported already in 1985 soon after HIV-testing had started, no AIDS patient with such a background was reported until 1988. Table 4.2 provides the statistics of AIDS cases by route of transmission, reported between 1983 and 1993.

**Table 4.2:   Number of AIDS Cases Reported 1983-1993,
            by Route of Transmission**

Year	Homo-/ Bisexuals	IVDU*	Blood products	Hetero- sexuals	Mother to child	Other	Total	Cumu- lative
1983	6						6	6
1984	10						10	16
1985	21		3	2			26	42
1986	41		6	1			48	90
1987	51		10	7	1		69	159
1988	61	5	16	13	2		97	256
1989	89	5	14	12		1	121	377
1990	89	7	9	23	1	2	131	508
1991	86	20	6	23	1	1	137	645
1992	77	19	5	24		2	127	772
1993	90	33	3	49		1	176	948
Total	621	89	72	154	5	7	948	
%	65.5	9.4	7.6	16.2	0.5	0.7	99.9	

*   Intravenous drug users.

Source: The National Bacteriological Laboratory, *Personal Communication.*

Figure 4.1: Number of New AIDS Cases Reported per Year, 1983-1993

New AIDS Cases per Year

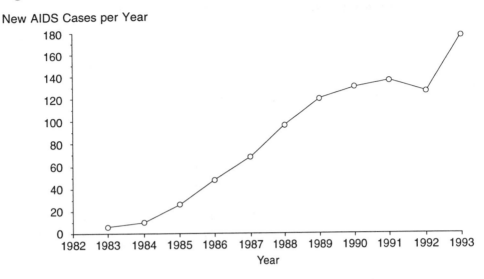

The number of new AIDS cases reported annually, increased at an even pace between 1984 and 1989. From 1990 the curve levelled off, and in 1992 there was even a temporary decrease in number compared to the previous and following years as seen in Figure 4.1.

The cumulative figures represented in Figure 4.2 illustrate the rather stable increase from 1988 and onwards.

**Figure 4.2: Number of AIDS Cases Reported 1983-1993
(Cumulative Figures)**

AIDS Cases, Cumulative

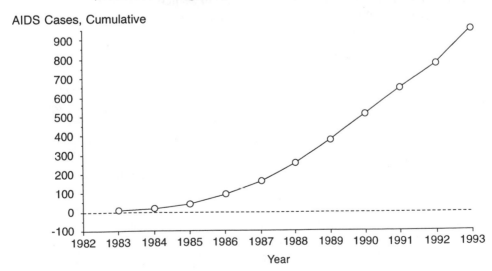

Table 4.3:   Number of HIV-positive Cases Reported 1983-1993 by Route of Transmission

Year	Homo-/ Bisexuals	IVDU*	Blood products	Hetero- sexuals	Mother to Child	Other	Total
1983	6						6
1984	10						10
1985	133	142	19	21			315
1986	559	204	149	53	1	1	967
1987	184	98	10	101	4		397
1988	159	45	8	92	2	2	308
1989	139	44	5	109		6	303
1990	111	43	1	169	4	6	334
1991	107	31	3	179	8	1	329
1992	98	26	2	210	6	7	349
1993	115	25	3	229	3	8	383
Total	1,621	658	200	1,163	28	31	3,701
%	*43.8*	*17.8*	*5.4*	*31.4*	*0.8*	*0.8*	*100*

*   Intravenous drug users.
Source: The National Bacteriological Laboratory, *Personal Communication.*

The statistics of recorded HIV-positive cases by route of transmission and year when the report reached The National Bacteriological Laboratory, are found in Table 4.3.

Notice that before 1985, when testing methods came into use, only AIDS cases were reported. The high number reported in 1986 depicts the effects of encouraging persons with risky behaviour to be voluntarily tested, once the methods became generally available in 1985. Since then, testing has been carried out free of charge on a large scale. Added to the voluntary testing done on the individual's initiative, is a large number of tests which are carried out in different screening programmes. Local health care centres, clinics for venereal diseases and drug treatment centres offer testing. Testing is offered routinely to pregnant women at maternity health clinics, and accepted by almost 100,000 women every year. At STD clinics,[12] 25,000 patients are tested annually. Refugees seeking asylum are offered HIV-testing as part of their general health tests, and although they represent a considerable proportion of the heterosexually transmitted HIV-positive cases in Sweden, the result of it is not permitted to affect the outcome of their asylum applications. People detained within the prison and probation system are also given the option of being tested, and among the drug users who were detained in Stockholm awaiting trial 1987-1991, approximately 68% accepted the offer of an HIV test. Blood donors are routinely tested at every donation, adding up to approxi-

Figure 4.3: Number of New HIV-seropositive Cases Reported 1983-1993

New HIV Cases per Year

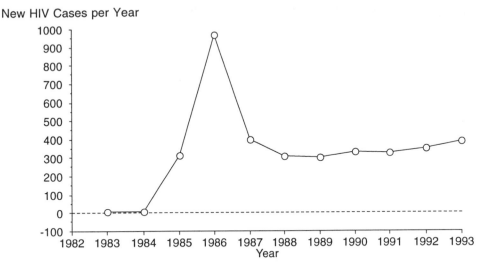

mately 590,000 tests annually, and non-identifiable blood samples collected at hospital laboratories, received for routine analysis, have been tested in order to get information on the HIV status in hospital populations. The rather stable number of HIV cases reported annually from 1988 is illustrated in Figure 4.3.

Trends and predictions regarding the development of the HIV epidemic are built on information from the compulsory reporting of HIV-positive cases. The general opinion among Swedish specialists is that the epidemiological situation with regard to the spread of HIV is stable. The number of unknown HIV-positive cases does not exceed 10% of the number identified, i.e. approximately 300. Since immigrants from high endemic risk areas constitute more than half the total number of infected heterosexuals, and more than half the total number of Swedish heterosexual carriers were infected outside the country, these two groups are the ones "most likely to disrupt the equilibrium", according to experts from the National Board of Health and Welfare (Malmquist/Ramgren, 1992).[13] After the peak year, 1986, the number of new HIV-positive cases reported per year has declined in all categories except the heterosexually infected and transmission from mother to child. From 1990, the number of annually reported, heterosexually infected, HIV cases is considerably higher than those among homo- and bisexual men. In 1990-1993, heterosexual transmission was reported in 787 cases, compared to 431 cases in homo- and bisexual men, a ratio of almost 2 to 1. The corresponding comparison with HIV-infected drug users shows a ratio of 6.3 to 1.

Women with HIV infection and AIDS constitute an increasing part of the total, along with the growing number of heterosexually transmitted cases. From the early part of the epidemic and up to 1993, approximately 30% of those infected via IV-drug use were women. Blood transfusion led to HIV infection among women in

Table 4.4:   Gender and Number of Heterosexually Transmitted AIDS and HIV-infected Cases Reported 1985-1993

Year	AIDS cases			HIV-positive cases		
	Women	Men	Total	Women	Men	Total
1985	0	2	2	9	12	21
1986	1	0	1	21	32	53
1987	1	6	7	43	58	101
1988	5	8	13	45	47	92
1989	6	6	12	56	53	109
1990	10	13	23	69	100	169
1991	9	14	23	101	78	179
1992	5	19	24	97	113	210
1993	18	31	49	114	115	229
Total	55	99	154	555	608	1,163
%	*36*	*64*	*100*	*48*	*52*	*100*

Source: The National Bacteriological Laboratory, *Personal Communication.*

45 cases, while transfusion and other blood products infected as many as 155 men, since haemophilia is a "male condition". With the spread through heterosexual transmission, the proportions changed, as seen in Table 4.4.

2   Mapping the Services and Development of Organizational Responses to HIV/AIDS

The Swedish part of the Managing AIDS Study covers 18 public bodies representing the three governmental levels, and 45 private non-profit organizations. In this report, the activities carried out by these 63 units are often described in relation to their legal status – public or private non-profit – and also divided according to their basic purpose or orientation. Organizations or units specifically set up to work with HIV/AIDS-related activities are called exclusives, i.e. they were started exclusively for combating HIV/AIDS, whereas those with a wider purpose, carrying out HIV/AIDS activities as part of a larger programme, are called inclusives, i.e. they include combating HIV/AIDS among their other activities. We refer to this as their organizational orientation.

2.1   Number of Organizations

The organizational orientation of the 18 selected public bodies and all 45 Swedish voluntary organizations providing one or more HIV/AIDS-related activities at the time of the study, are presented in Table 4.5.

Table 4.5:   Number of Organizations by Legal Status and Orientation

	Exclusives	Inclusives	Total
Public (Sample)*	3	15	18
Private Non-Profit (Total)	15	30	45
Total	18	45	63

*   See section 2.1.1 for the sample of public bodies.

New organizations specializing in HIV/AIDS work, exclusives, have been formed on the regional government level as well as within the private non-profit sector from 1982 onwards.[14] For Swedish circumstances, an extraordinary large number of new voluntary organizations working exclusively with HIV/AIDS, have been formed. Already existing organizations with other activities on their agenda, inclusives, have started dealing with HIV/AIDS activities at different points in time. Out of the 63 organizations in this study, 18 are exclusives and 45, inclusives. Only one sixth of the public bodies included in our sample are exclusives, but as much as one-third of the PNPOs.

2.1.1   Public Bodies

It was clear from the outset that not every public body engaged in HIV/AIDS activities would be included in the Swedish study. All county councils have the same responsibilities for health care, although the HIV/AIDS work varies according to the prevalence of the disease in the particular region. The social welfare work in the municipalities has the same make-up everywhere, but the mix differs depending on demographic structure and social circumstances. We decided to select 18 public bodies as a sample, to represent the different levels of government activities in the HIV/AIDS field to compare them with the activities undertaken by the private non-profit sector (Appendix 3). They were selected either because they were considered important and significant, or because they helped to illustrate the wide scope of existing activities. It was not our intention to give a complete picture of public efforts.

Of the 18 public bodies selected, 5 are found at the central government level, 11 are county councils, and 2 are municipalities, although one of the municipalities (Gothenburg) has the additional responsibilities of a county council. Some of these public entities have been formed specifically for HIV/AIDS work, although most of them are units within larger agencies, hospitals or other health care organizations performing a wider range of activities.

The three main coordinating bodies – the National Board of Health and Welfare, the National Bacteriological Laboratory and the National Commission on AIDS/ the National Institute of Public Health – evidently had to be included in the study. The National Board of Occupational Safety and Health was chosen as an example of an authority where the HIV/AIDS question could be integrated into their general programmes. This way, information could be disseminated to a large population. Finally, the Drug Treatment Group within the National Prison and Probation Administration is of special interest as the Swedish authorities were aware of HIV/AIDS as a specific problem in prisons at an early stage.

The county councils dominate, with 11 out of the 18 public bodies that have been selected for the study. Their responsibility for public health, including the prevention of infectious diseases, and to supply health and medical care, including hospitals, makes them especially important. The units for the prevention of infectious diseases in the three main city regions, Stockholm, Gothenburg and Malmö, were included because of the relatively high number of HIV/AIDS cases there. Two other counties, Uppsala and Norrbotten, with different demographic structures, were selected for comparison. Since the responsibilities and tasks of these units are clearly expressed in the Prevention of Infectious Diseases Act, the recorded activities are likely to be valid for most other counties. Other county council units, representing different types of activities, have been selected to illustrate the wide range of responses on the county level. Hospitals and other health care facilities are included only if they run outreach activities, with HIV/ AIDS-relevant functions outside the institution. Medical research is included only if it has a social and/or epidemiological profile. Two units from the municipal level have been chosen, one for its county-like responsibilities (Gothenburg) and the other as an example of the municipality's responsibility in coordinating preventive work. Among the selected bodies, are two units within hospital departments for infectious diseases in the Greater Stockholm area. They have been working with AIDS patients from the outset, serving the region with the highest number of HIV-infected persons, and both having extensive contacts with the HIV-infected population. Three other specialized units were included in the study. One is the Gay Men's Health Clinic in Stockholm, a unit contained in the major STD clinic in Stockholm, which played an important role in the early identification of AIDS cases and in the safe-sex education efforts directed towards men who have sex with other men. Other units are the Psychosocial Centre for Gay and Bisexual Men with HIV-related Problems and the Drug Treatment Centre in Lund, which runs Sweden's only major needle and syringe exchange programme for IV-drug users.

At the local level, cities/municipalities are in charge of the prevention and treatment of drug abuse through their local social welfare boards. A more or less close cooperation exists between the local social welfare fieldworkers and the medical drug treatment centres, normally located at a general or psychiatric hospital. Only one local social welfare authority has been included in the study.

2.1.2 Private Non-Profit Organizations

In this study, 30 inclusive non-profit organizations were identified, which undertake HIV/AIDS-related activities as part of a more differentiated programme. Only 20 of those have been in existence prior to 1982. Of the remaining 10, three immigrant organizations were founded in 1982, when HIV/AIDS is unlikely to have influenced their decisions. Seven organizations founded in 1988-1990, representing high-risk groups (gays, drug prevention or treatment initiatives, and immigrants from high endemic risk areas), might have been initiated at least partly as a result of the HIV/AIDS situation.

In response to the special needs of different groups affected by the HIV infection, 15 voluntary organizations included in the study have been formed specifically in order to work with HIV/AIDS. A few such organizations that were formed early on in the period, later dissolved. The 45 PNPOs included in the study are listed in Appendix 4.

Structurally, organizations engaged in HIV/AIDS-related activities can be divided into four groups.

A. Unitary associations working independently, some of them at the national level, but often as local organizations which might cooperate with peer associations in other places. Some of these associations have individual members, others are organized in other forms; examples are Noah's Ark and Positiva Gruppen.

B. Foundations (*Stiftelser*), which can be distinguished from associations, in that they have no members. They are often formed by organizations rather than by individuals. In contrast to the three other types, a foundation does not claim to have a democratic structure. Board members are often appointed by the founding individuals or organizations according to rules in written statutes. The aims and functions of the foundations differ from organizing therapeutic communities for drug addicts, like Vallmotorp, or providing educational activities, like Kontrapunkt, to fund-raising for research, as the Foundation of Sighsten's Friends Against AIDS.

C. National associations are organized as popular movements with local societies, sometimes working together on a regional level, and with a national central board elected by an assembly of delegates from the local associations, meeting at regular intervals. Typical examples are the Swedish Federation for Gay and Lesbian Rights (RFSL), and the Swedish Association for Help and Assistance to Drug-Abusers (RFHL).

D. Federations are often peak organizations for independent organizations with certain common interests. Their member organizations are often national in scope, sometimes themselves structured as national associations with local societies. The national board of a federation is also elected by delegates in an assembly, but the

Table 4.6:   Number of Private Non-profit Organizations by Organizational Structure and Orientation

	Exclusives	Inclusives	Total	%
A. Unitary associations	10	7	17	37.8
B. Foundations	4	7	11	24.4
C. National associations	0	10	10	22.2
D. Federations	1	6	7	15.6
Total	15	30	45	100

national board does not have the same strong coordinating and directing function as in a national association. Examples are the Federation of Kurdish Associations in Sweden, the Federation of African Associations in Sweden.

For the distribution of the 45 private non-profit organizations included in the study according to organizational structure and orientation, see Table 4.6.

The structural profile of exclusive organizations is dominated by the 10 unitary associations; five of them work only on the regional or local level, three are only nationally active, and two work mainly locally. However, these two are also involved with national activities. The single federation, and three out of the four foundations are national in scope, while one foundation, the most influential of them all, is active on all geographical levels.

All four organizational structures are represented among the inclusives. National associations, the most common structure, are by definition active on both the national and local levels. The federations report in some cases only national activity, but some of them also register regional and/or local activities, although these are probably carried out by their member organizations. Four unitary associations are active only nationally, one only regionally, whereas two report activities on more than one level. Three foundations work only nationally, two regionally and two on several geographical levels.

On the whole, organizations working exclusively with HIV/AIDS, i.e. exclusive organizations, tend to cover a more narrowly defined geographical area, whereas almost two-thirds of those with broader aims, the inclusives, are represented on more than one geographical level. Table 4.7 summarizes the geographical scope of the activities undertaken by exclusive and inclusive organizations respectively.

The internal structure of the private non-profit organizations can of course be described in various ways. One significant feature is whether it is based on individual membership or not. Out of the 45 Swedish non-profit organizations, 29 have individual members. Less than half of the exclusives are individual member-based organizations, while more than two-thirds of the inclusives are based on individual

Table 4.7: Number of Private Non-profit Organizations by Geographical Scope and Orientation

	Exclusives	Inclusives	Total
Single level	11	11	22
Multiple levels	4	19	23
Total	15	30	45

membership. For the distribution of non-member and membership organizations between exclusives and inclusives, see Table 4.8.

One significant feature of the organizations built on individual membership, related to their being national associations, although not totally explained by it, is that they are active on more than one geographical level, to a larger extent than those without members. Nearly two-thirds of those with individual members are active on more than one level, while only one-third of organizations lacking individual members are active on multiple levels. This difference is shown in Table 4.9.

Table 4.8: Number of Private Non-profit Organizations by Membership and Orientation

	Exclusives	Inclusives	Total
Individual Members	7	22	29
No Individual Members	8	8	16
Total	15	30	45

Table 4.9: Number of Private Non-profit Organizations by Geographical Scope and Membership

	Individual Members	No Individual Members	Total
Single Level	11	11	22
Multiple Levels	18	5	23
Total	29	16	45

2.1.3   Public Support to the Private Non-Profit Sector

The private non-profit organizations were – and still are – seen as important partners in the effort to inform and educate both the general public and specific target
groups about HIV/AIDS. Special grants for this purpose, as well as for the psychosocial activities pointed out early on in the government programme, are still
allocated every year. These grants have increased considerably in the last three years.
The sums granted to non-profit organizations from the specific AIDS programme
appropriation for the fiscal years 1988/89-1992/93 can be seen in Table 4.10.

Some organizations, which received government grants for their general activities before the AIDS alert, were seen as particularly valuable in their role as AIDS
prevention bodies, and were granted larger sums than before from the old sources.
For this reason, funding to voluntary organizations working with IV-drug addicts
increased in 1990. The annual organizational grant to the Federation for Gay and
Lesbian Rights was at the same time doubled from SKr 500,000 ($ 62,500) to 1
million ($ 125,000).[15] Furthermore, organizations engaged in psychosocial HIV/
AIDS activities are also partly funded by the regional and/or local governments.

Three organizations – Noah's Ark/Red Cross Foundation, The Swedish Federation for Gay and Lesbian Rights (RFSL) and the Swedish Association for Sex Education (RFSU) – are the major recipients, answering for more than two-thirds of the
total sum of nearly SKr 70 m. ($ 8,750,000) allocated to private non-profit organiza-
tions from the specific AIDS appropriation. They are presented briefly below.

**Table 4.10: Government Grants to Private Non-profit Organizations for
HIV/AIDS Information and Psychosocial Work, 1988/89-1992/
93 (in 1,000 SKr)**

Year	Noah's Ark/ Red Cross	RFSL	RFSU	HIV/AIDS organizations	Immi- grants	Others	Total
1988/89	4,600	1,850	1,430	500	35	2,372	10,787
1989/90	4,900	3,588	1,039	750	n/a	1,548	11,825*
1990/91	4,160	2,552	2,500	765	481	1,522	11,980
1991/92	5,385	2,610	2,694	1,650	2,431	1,249	16,019
1992/93	6,220	3,330	2,990	3,030	2,294	341	18,205
Total	25,265	13,930	10,653	6,695	5,241	7,032	68,816
Percentage 1988-92	*36.7*	*20.2*	*15.5*	*9.7*	*7.6*	*10.2*	*100*

*   Excluding immigrant organizations.
Source: Eva Ekdahl, The National Institute of Public Health, *Personal
Communication*, August 1993.

Noah's Ark/Red Cross Foundation is the major exclusive organization in Sweden, managing a broad spectrum of HIV/AIDS activities. The organization was initiated in the mid-1980s by gay physicians in Stockholm. In 1987, Noah's Ark was established as the headquarters of the Swedish Red Cross's HIV engagement. Although the HIV-positive homo- and bisexual men were the first to benefit, Noah's Ark now acts as an educational and care centre involving different groups of HIV-positive persons, e.g. haemophiliacs infected by blood products and immigrants from high endemic risk areas. Noah's Ark also targets partners and family members as well as the general public. Its special education is aimed at health care personnel. In 1990, the total budget of Noah's Ark was SKr 18 million ($ 2,250,000), of which approximately 22% came from the national government, 28% from the regional, and 17% from local governments. The rest (33%) came from voluntary sector contributions and service fees.

RFSL was founded in 1950 and started its HIV/AIDS activities as early as 1980, being aware of the development of the mysterious "gay disease" in the United States. Information was transferred to the regional gay support groups, and in November 1982 the Gay Men's Health Clinic started, initiated by physicians within the organization in cooperation with the Stockholm County Council and the National Bacteriological Laboratory. This clinic was later integrated into a genito-urinary department of a county council hospital. In January 1983, when the American Gay community was still fiercely divided on the issue as to whether blood donors should be asked about their sexual affinity (Bayer, 1989), RFSL issued an appeal to homo- and bisexual men in Sweden not to give blood (RFSL, 1988). In 1990, RFSL's budget totalled SKr 13.5 million ($ 1,687,500), almost all of it (99%) came from public sources. The national government contributed 40% or SKr 5.4 million ($ 675,000), of which SKr 3.6 million ($ 450,000) from the special AIDS appropriation and the rest from other parts of the national budget. Regional governments contributed 40% and local authorities 20%. Most of these contributions can be viewed as linked to the role RFSL plays in the HIV/AIDS area – the organization's total budget did non exceed SKr 1 million ($ 125,000) before 1985.

RFSU started in 1933 as a family planning organization. Over the years, RFSU has had a great impact on the development of openness in Swedish sex education, availability of contraceptives and generally in sex policy matters. With 14 local branches and 4 clinics open to the public, RFSU is available for counselling all over Sweden. Two local branches have organized specific HIV/AIDS projects. In a special project called "the tramp bag",[16] RFSU supplies young persons travelling abroad for summer holidays with information on HIV/AIDS and condoms free of charge. In 1990 approximately 25% of the total budget of SKr 10 million ($ 1,250,000) was devoted to HIV/AIDS work.

2.2 Number of Activities

For this study, 26 different HIV/AIDS-related activities were identified and included in the survey. Two additional types of activities, not initially included, were reported by the Swedish organizations themselves.

The number of HIV/AIDS-related activities carried out by a single organization varied between 1 and 17, with higher mean and median figures for exclusive organizations than inclusives, as seen in Table 4.11. Public organizations also have somewhat higher median and mean scores than PNPOs.

Table 4.11: HIV/AIDS-related Activities per Organization: Range, Median and Mean by Legal Status and Organizational Orientation

	Number of organizations	Number of activities per organization		
		Range	Median	Mean
Public*				
Exclusives	3	3-10	9	7.5
Inclusives	15	2-12	4	4.8
Private Non-Profit				
Exclusives	15	2-16	5	6.5
Inclusives	30	1-17	3	4.3

*   See section 2.1.1 for the sample of public bodies.

Table 4.12: Number of Activities and Expected Frequency by Legal Status and Organizational Orientation

	Number of Activities (Expected frequency)		
	Exclusives	Inclusives	Total
Public*	22	72	94
	(15)	(77)	(92)
Private Non-Profit	98	130	228
	(77)	(153)	(230)
Total	120	202	322
	(92)	(230)	(322)

*   See section 2.1.1 for the sample of public bodies.

In Table 4.12, the total number of reported activities is presented by legal status and organizational orientation. The observed frequencies are compared to the expected frequencies, calculated as the number of activities one could expect to find in each group, if the activities were statistically independent of the legal status and orientation.

The total number of activities is distributed between public and private non-profit organizations in proportion to the number of organizations studied. Therefore, the figures for the observed and the expected frequencies are close to each other. The comparison by organizational orientation, on the other hand, shows that the organizations working exclusively with HIV/AIDS perform a greater number of activities than expected, whereas the number of activities carried out by the inclusives is lower than the expected frequency. This observation is valid for both the public and the private non-profit organizations. The difference between exclusives and inclusives may be explained by the fact that inclusives, with a lot of other activities than the HIV/AIDS-related ones in their programmes, get into the HIV/AIDS sphere in order to perform specific activities related to their own overall aim rather than to the overall national HIV/AIDS management objective. In this context, it must be stressed that all figures relating to private non-profit organizations show the total number of activities that are carried out by these kinds of organizations in the country, whereas the activities reported for public bodies represent only a small number, related to the selected number of units. All public/private comparisons, therefore, have to be related to the number of organizations studied.

2.3 Development

The development of organizations working in the HIV/AIDS field can be divided into three time periods, 1980-84, 1985-89 and 1990-92. We refer to organizations started in these three periods as "early movers", "meeting the challenge", and "latecomers" respectively. The number of organizations having started HIV/AIDS-related activities is shown for different years in Figure 4.4.

"Early movers" were in the main, already existing organizations; either public health care organizations, as hospital departments and the National Bacteriological Laboratory, or the homosexuals' voluntary organizations. The development of HIV/AIDS programmes followed the same pattern in both public and private non-profit organizations until 1989, but after that, no new and significant public organizations were formed. The number of organizations starting their HIV/AIDS programmes during each of the three periods, divided according to legal status, is shown in Table 4.13.

Figure 4.4: Year HIV/AIDS Programmes Started

Number of Organizations
Starting HIV/AIDS Activities

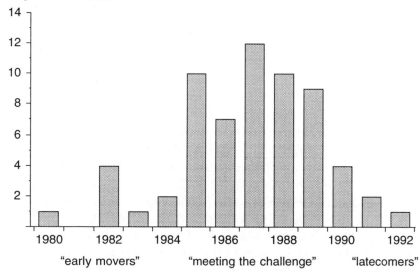

"early movers"   "meeting the challenge"   "latecomers"

Table 4.13: Number of Organizations Starting HIV/AIDS-related Activities by Period of HIV/AIDS Involvement and Legal Status

	1980-84	1985-89	1990-92	Total
Public*	5	13	0	18
Private Non-Profit	3	35	7	45
Total	8	48	7	63

*   See section 2.1.1 for the sample of public bodies.

Before 1985, three existing private non-profit organizations became involved in information activities, mainly aimed at their own members. During the years 1985-1989 the interest of the general public grew, and the question of how to prevent the further spread of the infection became acute, as did the need for psychological and social support for those identified as HIV-positive. During this period, about 40 inclusive and exclusive private non-profit organizations started HIV/AIDS-related activities. A few of these new, exclusive organizations later ceased to exist, but 12 of the HIV/AIDS-specific organizations from this period are still active and included in the study.

During the last three years, only seven additional organizations have become involved in HIV/AIDS activities, three of them working exclusively in this field. The number of new HIV/AIDS-related initiatives has been diminishing since 1990. The explanation for this might be that the need for specific measures has been made oblivious now; but it could also be related to changes in the public funding policy. Another interpretation is that we have reached a stage of "normalizing", when the specific problems and needs generated by the disease have been properly identified and activities have been established in organizations that can deal with them on a permanent basis.

The number of organizations becoming involved in HIV/AIDS activities during each of the three periods, divided according to organizational orientation, is shown in Table 4.14. The two exclusives that started during the first period were both initiated by professionals. One started as a coordinated private/public effort and was later integrated as a specific HIV unit in a public STD clinic. The other is a private non-profit organization initiated by physicians. Neither of the organizational orientations show divergent patterns of involvement.

The development of HIV/AIDS-related activities by private non-profit organizations shows no clear relation to the annual number of new AIDS cases reported, nor with the annual number of new HIV cases reported as seen in Figure 4.5. However, we see a dramatic peak in the number of new HIV cases reported in 1986 when HIV-testing became generally available, which at the time could have been interpreted as a shocking trend. The number of PNPOs, regardless of their organizational orientation, shows a relatively early development of HIV/AIDS-related activities. Most of them initiated their HIV/AIDS activities in the period 1985-89. They were clearly meeting the challenge in a way which probably contributed directly to staving off the spread of the virus.

Table 4.14: Number of Organizations Starting HIV/AIDS-related Activities by Period of HIV/AIDS Involvement and Organizational Orientation

	1980-84	1985-89	1990-92	Total
Exclusives	2	13	3	18
Inclusives	6	35	4	45
Total	8	48	7	63

Figure 4.5: Number of HIV/AIDS Cases and Organizational Development, Private Non-profit Organizations 1980-1992

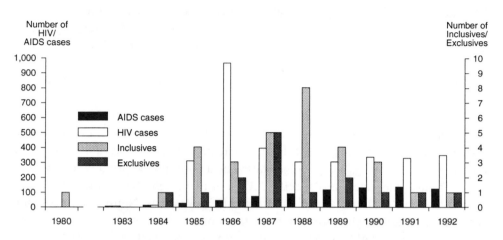

2.4 *Organizational Responsiveness, by Those Groups Most Affected*

The way in which the HIV infection has been transmitted has, to a large extent, determined which existing voluntary organizations have become involved in HIV/AIDS work, and which target groups the new organizations focus on. The existing organizations for homosexuals started early to disseminate information to homo- and bisexual men in order to teach them how to avoid risk behaviour. Fairly soon, existing organizations active in drug politics and drug treatment also became involved. All in all, 11 of the 30 organizations involved in multiple areas of operation, belong to one of these two groups.

Newly initiated organizations, undertaking support activities, have also to a certain extent been formed by, or are aiming at, groups defined by the routes of transmission. This applies to groups exhibiting risky behaviour such as men having sex with men, or persons injecting drugs intravenously. Other organizations focus on those infected via blood transfusions, or other blood products. Among the 15 organizations working exclusively with HIV/AIDS, five are in fact targeting such groups, and at least three others have been initiated by circles close to such groups.

Immigrant organizations form another large group which are active in the dissemination of information. Government grants have been given for HIV/AIDS information projects and in 1992, 11 immigrant organizations were engaged in such work directed at their own ethnic or language groups. The general characteristics of the 45 private non-profit organizations are summarized in Table 4.15.

Table 4.15: Number of Private Non-profit Organizations Involved in HIV/ AIDS Activities by Organizational Feature and Orientation

	Exclusives	Inclusives	Total	%
Immigrants	0	11	11	24.4
Support PWA* in general	10	0	10	22.2
Drug abuse	1	7**	8	17.8
Homosexuality	2	4	6	13.3
Charity organization, church-affiliated or secular	0	5	5	11.1
Blood/blood products	2	1	3	6.7
Other	0	2	2	4.4
Total	15	30	45	99.9

* PWA = Persons with AIDS. Two of these organizations were initiated by gay interest groups, but support PWAs in general.
** One of these targets immigrants in particular.

Outreach is the unique feature of PNPOs in managing AIDS. Three groups of organizations serving the homosexual community, the drug addicts and those who acquired the virus via blood products, will be used to illustrate this function. They all contribute to the implementation of government policy, to a large extent financed by government grants.

2.4.1   Homosexuality and Managing AIDS

The appearance of a fatal disease, initially striking primarily homo- and bisexual men, has highlighted the different ways in which homosexuality is viewed in different countries. In the Swedish context, the organizational response to the disease from the gay community, as well as from the state, is best viewed in relation to the development of public policy and societal attitudes from the late 1970s onwards.

Sexual relations between persons of the same sex were illegal in Sweden until 1944. From that year, homosexual relationships were allowed between consenting adults, but with a higher minimum age stated than for heterosexual couples. In 1978, the same minimum age (15 years) was set for voluntary homo- and heterosexual relationships. In the WHO "International Classification of Diseases" from 1966, homosexuality was considered a "sexual anomaly" under the heading "Mental Disorders". In 1979, this diagnosis was deleted from the Swedish classification by the National Board of Health and Welfare as being an irrelevant clinical concept.[17] In 1978, a government commission was set up to investigate the situation for homosexuals in Swedish society. Two surveys were carried out, aimed at both the general public and homosexuals themselves. The conclusions from the surveys were that two factors were decisive in the social situation of homosexuals. One was that "the silence surrounding homosexuals and homosexuality is virtually total. Homosexuality is not a natural part of society; it is not present as a social and cultural institution". The other was that "there exists a social prohibition or taboo on homosexuality, which is reinforced by the fact that it is viewed as pure sexuality".[18]

In the report, a number of anti-discriminatory measures were proposed, and the importance of equal treatment for homo- and heterosexual persons was stated. This included a wide range of situations such as employment, housing, military service, education,[19] culture and health care. Amendments to the Instrument of Government and the Penal Code were proposed, asserting that discrimination based on sexual proclivity would be illegal in the same way as discrimination is when based on race, colour, creed or ethnic origin. The importance of the homosexuals' own organization, for the individuals, as well as for their situation in society, was acknowledged, and motivated the proposal for economic support to gay organizations working on a nationwide basis.

The most widely debated item in the proposed package of changes presented by the commission was whether two persons of the same sex should be allowed to marry. The conclusion was that this would require a different way of defining marriage. On the other hand, the legal status that already existed for persons of the opposite sex, cohabiting under forms resembling those of marriage, ought to be also accepted for homosexual couples, wanting to make a home and live together. A new law to that effect, came into force in January 1988 – no changes were made in anti-discrimination laws.[20]

There was still an open question as to whether Sweden would follow Denmark's example and introduce a law of "registered partnership", giving the homosexual relationship the same status as that of a married heterosexual couple. The National Board of Health and Welfare, which was given the coordinating responsibility in matters concerning homosexuality through a government decision in December 1987, opened the matter officially in a letter to the government in June 1990. A new committee was set up and in June 1994, the Riksdag accepted the new law, by which the same rules that apply to marriage will also be valid for homosexual couples, with a few exceptions, e.g. adoption.[21]

How does this fit into the question of how to manage AIDS? First of all, the Swedish public policy on homosexuality grew, to a large extent, out of the proposals by the government commission set up in 1978, before the HIV/AIDS crisis was on the agenda. Some of the activities proposed by the commission, particularly education and information on homosexuality to children, professional groups and the general public, have probably been reinforced by the HIV/AIDS information, though not always in a positive way for the gay community. However, one important aspect has been crucial for the role of PNPOs in managing AIDS; the recognition of the gays' own organizations as important vehicles for change towards improved social conditions for themselves. Thanks to this, and to the concomitant economic support, RFSL established itself more vigorously, and was able to act on the information from peer groups in other countries at a very early stage. This major gay organization contributes to the implementation of public polices, with both information and psychosocial support, and at the same time has gained more strength to promote its own political objectives.

Several other PNPOs with more specialized gay membership work more or less unnoticed by the general public and the political establishment. The support organization for HIV-positive gay men, Positiva Gruppen, fits into the psychosocial objective however, and receives an annual government grant.

2.4.2　Intravenous Drug Abuse, Prevention and Treatment

The Swedish drug policy has been a concern of public debate for the last 25 years, but no major changes were implemented until 1981, when the rule of "Compulsory Care of Adult Misusers" in special therapeutic communities (LVM homes) was accepted under certain conditions. As part of the national HIV/AIDS prevention programme, major sums have been spent on the expansion of compulsory care programmes for drug abusers. From 1 July 1988, a new law states that the consumption of illegal drugs is a criminal offence. The maximum penalty was tightened up in 1993, from a fine to a maximum of six months imprisonment. One major argument for this was that the harsher penalty also allows for imposing treatment in LVM homes.[22]

The number of active intravenous drug users (IVDUs) in Sweden is estimated at 7,000-10,000, approximately 1,500 use heroin and the rest of them take amphetamines (Tunving, 1991). Amphetamine abuse was recognized early on in Sweden, and became the subject of much debate in the 1960s, when related drugs such as Ritalina and Preludine were still considered as being effective and acceptable in the treatment of depression and obesity (Bejerot, 1968).

The conflicting views on how to balance HIV/AIDS prevention against restrictive drug policies have been described in section 1.2.1. Another issue, which never grew to the same proportions, was whether the so-called methadone programme should be extended and made available on a larger scale. In this programme, heroin addicts are given methadone, a synthetic narcotic drug, as a substitute for heroin. The programme is intended to help heroin addicts to quit heroin and become more readily socially rehabilitated. After 20 years of a restricted programme in one place in the country, covering a maximum of 150-200 clients, an extension of the programme was accepted in 1988. For the moment, the National Board of Health and Welfare has set the limit to 450 clients, but in fact, only about 300 are in actual treatment in three different places. Stockholm has approximately 75% of the methadone clientele of which more than 50% are HIV-positive.

The gay community is in most countries well organized, with active members able to take part in policy advocacy and debates. They can speak for themselves and function as a more or less strategic opinion-forming pressure group. The drug users on the other hand, as long as they are drug-dependent, are rarely in such a physical and psychological state that they can work with endurance in projects aiming at bettering their social situation. They have to rely on family and friends, social workers and health professionals, to speak for their cause. However, former drug dependants who have managed to return to a drug-free or methadone-stabilized life, are excellent advocates for improved drug treatment and changed drug policies and so are the parents, sisters and brothers of those who have demonstrated the evils of drugs.

Three PNPOs were formed in the 1960s with varying degrees of social support to drug dependants, opinion formation and political lobbying in drug issues on their programmes. Two of these, the Swedish Association for Help and Assistance to Drug Abusers (RFHL) and the Swedish National Parent Organization Against Drugs (FMN), are also involved in HIV/AIDS prevention and/or services. The third one, the National Federation for a Drugfree Society (RNS), exclusively advocates political means to keep drugs away, without including HIV concerns on its agenda. All three organizations are to a large extent financed by government grants.

RFHL characterizes itself as primarily an organization for drug treatment, offering help to drug abusers. With 4,000 members and functioning as an umbrella for foundations administering 15 therapeutic communities, RFHL has an important role as a complement to the public health and social welfare system. The organization's function as policy advocate is also very important. It has taken an active part in the drug policy debate, in favour of making needles and syringes available, hesitant to the methadone programmes, critical to the present form of compulsory isolation of HIV-positive IVDUs.[23]

FMN, with approximately 10,000 members started as, and still to a certain extent is, an organization for parents and others concerned with the drug abuse of family members. Counselling and self-help groups for parents and others involved, advocating early intervention when youngsters start trying drugs, providing information in schools, for health care professionals, etc., are all important. FMN together with RNS advocate a restrictive drug policy, taking a strong stand against making needles and syringes easily available, accepting coercive measures as necessary in drug treatment, and they do not object to the rules of the Prevention of Infectious Diseases Act.

RFHL and FMN lobby extensively, have formal as well as informal connections in the government and the Riksdag and influence the restrictive views which are obvious within the political parties.[24] Although they both see HIV/AIDS, to some extent, as their concern in dealing with their prime clientele, their involvement is by no means as strong as that of RFSL. The drug prevention programmes of RFHL and FMN, as well as parts of their therapeutic communities, have been strengthened through increased government funding, thus functioning in a two-step HIV/AIDS prevention capacity. The specific psychosocial goal in the public HIV/AIDS policy is probably better met, however, through initiatives aimed at the specific target group, HIV-positive drug users or ex-users.

CONVICTUS started in Stockholm in 1986 as a buddy system and self-help group, a reaction to lacking psychosocial support for former addicts who were diagnosed with HIV and had nowhere to go with their concerns. In 1992, the organization had 200 members, 50% of them were HIV-positive. Leisure time activities are arranged for members and other visitors to their centre. Ex-addicts and persons on methadone programmes are welcome to take part, active drug abusers as well, as long as they are not under the current influence of drugs. The organization works in close contact with the hospital-based drug treatment centres in order to offer their services to new groups. One particular problem has been how to reach female drug users. The organization was started and originally run by men, and women apparently did not feel welcome. In 1991 a separate programme started, with a project designed as a "programme for girls". This is now established as a permanent part of the organization's activities.

Those working with HIV-positive drug addicts and ex-addicts are convinced that they need to work separately from the rest of the HIV-positive community. Their multi-problem status aggravates their situation and other criteria have to be met when it comes to dealing with their problems. Clearly both the older, established inclusive organizations, and the younger, exclusive ones, play important parts in implementing the public HIV/AIDS policy regarding prevention/information and psychosocial support.

2.4.3 Blood Products and "the Innocent Victims"

HIV transmission through blood and blood products has hit two distinctly different groups, however, both with one thing in common besides the disease: the fight for economic compensation.

The approximately 600 *haemophiliacs* and about 800 persons with another co-agulation factor disorder are registered in three treatment centres, located in the major cities: Stockholm, Gothenburg and Malmö. Some of those with major disorders are dependent on regular treatment with blood products containing the coagulation factor component that is missing in their own blood. Others with a milder form of the disorder need treatment in connection with accidents or for surgery. Amongst the *c.* 400 in these groups, who were registered at the treatment centres, and known to have received blood products before the testing of donors and heat-treatment of the blood components started in 1985, 88 HIV-positive cases were identified before December 1989. In all, 103 HIV-positive cases infected by blood products were registered by December 1991 (Malmquist/Ramgren,1992: 36-38).

Although blood donors were notified and recommended already in 1983 not to give blood if they belonged to certain, stated risk groups, *blood transfusions* with HIV-infected blood could not be effectively prevented until the testing of all donated blood started in 1985. Identifying those who had received contaminated blood was, however, dependent on the follow-up of persons found to be HIV-positive and blood donors, in which cases recipients could be traced via the blood banks. The total number of registered persons who had become HIV-infected via blood transfusions was 94 as of December 1992, 6 of them reported in 1990-92 (Malmquist/ Ramgren,1992).[25]

The Swedish Haemophilia Society is an interest organization for haemophiliacs, founded in 1964. In the early stages of HIV awareness, the society was engaged in information activities addressing their own members. Later, when the Noah's Ark/ Red Cross Foundation was established, a subgroup within the foundation took over the task of supplying psychosocial support for HIV-positive haemophiliacs. The two organizations cooperate, both of them receive government financial support for projects aimed at this particular group, and besides the activities of a psychosocial nature, lobbying for financial compensation has been a major task. A separate foundation for blood product infected persons, the PSB Foundation, was founded in 1991 with information and buddy support on its programme.

The Friendship Association NU was initiated in 1987 by hospital staff working with the blood transfusion transmitted patients at one of the hospitals in the Greater Stockholm region. Involving both patients and their families, and open for participants from the whole country, the number of people involved is still rather limited. The main activity has been to lobby for financial compensation and other forms of support.

The common goal for the organizations for blood product HIV-transmitted persons, has been to get recognition for the view that the health care system is responsible for their disease. Since blood products for treatment of the coagulation disorder are monitored by the Medical Products Agency and administered by the public health care institutions, and blood transfusions are given within the national health care system, the state – so was the argument – should take the responsibility for any harm caused by the treatment. The public opinion has accepted these groups as being "innocent victims" of a fatal disease, whereas other victims, homosexuals and drug users, seem to some extent to be thought of as being partly responsible for the effects due to their respective lifestyles.

The county councils, responsible for health care, and the pharmaceutical companies, producing the coagulation factor products, accepted the responsibility and paid, through their insurance arrangements, compensation to all blood product infected patients, in two stages during the period 1986-1990. The amounts were calculated according to indemnity principles, and varied according to age and family situation. For example, a 30-year-old person was paid around SKr 250,000 ($ 31,250). A further SKr 200,000 ($ 25,000) was paid in 1991 to each affected person, half the sum from the government, half from the same sources as the previous payments.[26] In 1993 the Riksdag decided that health care, dental care and pharmaceuticals should be supplied free of charge to those who had acquired HIV within the Swedish health care system through blood products.[27]

The situation for the blood product infected HIV-positive person is in many ways different from that of the homosexual or the IV-drug user, as the number of infected is limited and will not continue to grow. There is no need for group involvement in preventive measures or information activities, since the prevention has been organized within the health care system. Psychosocial support is strongly needed, and has to a certain extent been arranged by the organizations, with government financial support. But the main concern (lobbying for economic compensation) is unique for this group, and has – after a long period of struggle – been met with what seems to be a reasonable amount of understanding from the authorities.

2.4.4   Heterosexual Transmission – A New Threat

The question whether HIV can be transmitted via heterosexual contact was the subject of much debate during the first years of HIV/AIDS research. Even though AIDS patients claimed that they were neither homo- nor bisexual, nor IV-drug users, nor had received blood products, there was some doubt about their truthfulness. Gradually, however, the warning had to be accepted; heterosexual sex could prove fatal as HIV could be transferred in either direction during vaginal sex. In Sweden, the first heterosexually infected AIDS cases were reported in 1985, and by the end of 1992, 932 persons had been identified as HIV-positive.

Three organizations included in our study work exclusively with women or have special programmes for women, i.e. the International Organization for Immigrant Women, the Women's Forum and Convictus, which has a special programme for women drug abusers. Two or three organizations work with persons of both sexes, and sometimes have programmes specifically directed towards women, e.g. PLUSS and Noah's Ark. All the rest of the PNPOs, except those for gay men, deal with men and women on equal terms, but provide no special programmes for women.

The need for those infected via heterosexual transmission to meet other people in the same situation was recognized by Noah's Ark – the major exclusive HIV/AIDS organization – where they could meet and find support. However, unlike the gay community, or those with a common economic cause like haemophiliacs, the heterosexually infected persons lacked an organizational base of their own. Furthermore, the fact that a substantial proportion was made up of refugees or immigrants from various countries with different cultural backgrounds, also meant that there was no solid base for any formal organization. In 1991, however, the PLUSS Association was formed. It is open to everybody, irrespective of how he/she acquired the virus and has become a natural forum for heterosexually infected persons, but only had 50 members in 1992.

It was mentioned in section 1.4 that immigrants from high endemic risk areas constitute more than half of the heterosexually infected group in Sweden. A growing number of immigrant organizations introduce HIV/AIDS information in their programmes. Eleven are included in this study, and others have become involved after 1992. The government response to this development has been rapidly increasing financial support to immigrant organizations, the total rising from SKr 35,000 ($ 4,375) in 1988/89 to almost SKr 2.3 million ($ 287,000) in 1992/93 (see Table 4.10 for details).

3 Subsectoral Response

The activities carried out by the organizations involved were divided into the following six subsectors:
• Prevention, Education and Information;
• Care;
• Interest Representation;
• Policy Coordination and Monitoring;
• Research;
• Support activities.

3.1 Responsiveness, by Legal Status and Organizational Orientation

The extent to which organizations are involved in activities from the different subsectors is clearly related to their legal status and organizational orientation, as can be seen from Table 4.16.

Table 4.16: Number of Organizations Active in Different Subsectors by Legal Status and Organizational Orientation

	Public*		Private Non-Profit		Total	%
	Exclusives	Inclusives	Exclusives	Inclusives		
Prevention, Education and Information	3	14	12	28	57	90.5
Care	3	5	8	14	30	47.6
Interest representation	1	0	12	13	26	41.3
Policy coordination & monitoring	1	12	0	4	17	27.0
Research	2	6	0	2	10	15.9
Support activities	0	0	7	2	9	14.3
n	3	15	15	30	63	

* See section 2.1.1 for the sample of public bodies.

A division of labour is particularly obvious, in that the subsectors *policy coordination & monitoring* and *research* are mainly public concerns, whereas *interest representation* and *support activities* (mainly fund-raising activities) are almost entirely provided by the private non-profit organizations.

Prevention, Education and Information is clearly a shared interest where all but six organizations take part in some such activities. Not surprisingly, given the fact that the government grants are specifically aimed at private non-profit organizations involved in these activities, information and education engages the highest number of voluntary organizations: 40 out of the 45. About half of the 45 participate in some form of care, and the same is true for interest representation. Nine organizations are active fund-raisers for their own activities, or in order to support activities run by others.

"Care" as subsector in a Swedish context, conventionally implies public services within the health or social service sectors. Why then, do so many private

Table 4.17: Number of Activities in Different Subsectors by Legal Status and Organizational Orientation

| | Number of Activities (Expected frequency) | | | | | |
| | Public* | | Private Non-Profit | | | |
	Exclusives	Inclusives	Exclusives	Inclusives	Total	%
Prevention, Education and Information	8	36	36	69	149	46.3
	(7)	(35)	(35)	(71)		
Care	7	14	26	29	76	23.6
	(4)	(18)	(18)	(36)		
Interest representation	3	0	29	24	56	17.4
	(3)	(13)	(13)	(27)		
Policy coordination	1	15	0	4	20	6.2
& monitoring	(1)	(5)	(5)	(9)		
Research	3	7	0	2	12	3.7
	(0)	(3)	(3)	(6)		
Support activities	0	0	7	2	9	2.8
	(0)	(2)	(2)	(4)		
Total	22	72	98	130	322	100
	(15)	(77)	(77)	(153)	(322)	
n	3	15	15	30	63	

* See section 2.1.1 for the sample of public bodies.

organizations perform caring activities in a country with regional governments responsible for all kinds of health care, and local governments responsible for social services? The fact that the private non-profit organizations in this study are so engaged in "care" activities will be discussed further in section 3.3.2.

The distribution of the total number of registered activities in subsectors also shows the high priority given to information (see Table 4.17). Almost half of the activities (46%) belong to this subsector. This is obviously a result of two parts of the AIDS strategy. One is that public education and information to specific groups – professionals as well as persons at risk – will have an effect on behaviour, and so prevent the spread of the virus. The other is that information activities will help to counteract the fear and prejudice, and so minimize the stigma attached to the infection.

In comparing the actual figures with the expected frequency, it becomes obvious that activities within the subsector *Prevention, Education and Information* is distributed evenly in relation to legal status and organizational orientation. *Care* on the other hand is more common than expected among exclusives, in both the public and private non-profit sectors. The activities in the subsectors *policy coordination & monitoring* and *research*, as mentioned earlier, are primarily undertaken by public bodies. Both subsectors will be presented in greater detail in Table 4.22. It is obvious that the coordinating role is carried out mainly by inclusives, implying that it has been taken up by units already in force when the HIV/AIDS problem arose. *Interest representation* and *support activities* are almost entirely private non-profit undertakings and are more often initiated by exclusives than by inclusives. These latter two subsectors are jointly presented in Table 4.23 below.

3.2 "Early Movers" and "Latecomers"

Initiatives within the HIV/AIDS field, taken on early by voluntary organizations, mainly included information activities within a peer group and interest representation. Public bodies were involved in the care of the first patients diagnosed with AIDS, quality control of blood and epidemiological research. However, the "early movers" have gradually also taken on other activities.

Organizations starting their HIV/AIDS-related activities during the first period, 1980-84, registered a high number of activities in 1992. One intriguing observation is that early movers are of a higher frequency than expected for all subsectors of activities. The explanation is that five out of eight organizations of the first generation working with HIV/AIDS were public institutions that came into early contact with patients affected by the virus, and which still carry a large part of the HIV/AIDS work load. The National Bacteriological Laboratory and four hospital departments demonstrate how the Swedish HIV/AIDS work was integrated from the very start into the existing institutions, a fact that has obviously also influenced the shape of the policies concerning care and epidemiological control that has developed over the years.

Table 4.18: Number of Activities in Different Subsectors Reported in 1992, by Organizational Development

| | Number of Activities (Expected frequency) | | | | |
	"Early Movers"	"Meeting the Challenge"	"Latecomers"	Total	%
Prevention, Education and Information	28	110	11	149	46.3
	(19)	(113)	(17)		
Care	18	46	12	76	23.6
	(10)	(58)	(8)		
Interest	10	40	6	56	17.4
representation	(7)	(43)	(6)		
Policy co-ordination	7	13	0	20	6.2
& monitoring	(3)	(15)	(2)		
Research	6	6	0	12	3.7
	(2)	(9)	(1)		
Support activities	2	7	0	9	2.8
	(1)	(7)	(1)		
Total	71	222	29	322	100
	(41)	(245)	(36)	(322)	
n	8	48	7	63	

The other three "early movers" are private non-profit organizations; two interest organizations for gay and lesbians, and one opinion-forming group of physicians. These organizations are obviously involved in two of the subsectors reporting higher than expected numbers of activities, information and interest representation. In Table 4.18 we can see the overall activity pattern as it was in 1992. Organizations founded in 1990 or later, are not engaged in research, policy coordinating functions or fund-raising activities, which implies that there might have been a balance between demand and supply in these subsectors by then.

3.3 Single HIV/AIDS-related Activities

The existing programmes and activities related to HIV/AIDS, carried out by public and private non-profit organizations in Sweden, cover the whole spectrum as identified at the outset of the study. In this section, the reported frequency of separate activities is presented by legal status and organizational orientation. Expected frequencies have been computed in order to highlight which activities are specifically related to different organizational characteristics.

Table 4.19: Number of Separate Information Activities by Legal Status and Organizational Orientation

	Public*		Private Non-Profit			
	Exclusives	Inclusives	Exclusives	Inclusives	Total	%
Educational and information work	2	9	11	22	44	29.5
Production of information material	1	6	7	14	28	18.8
Training of volunteers & health care professionals	3	7	5	9	24	16.1
Hotline	2	4	7	7	20	13.4
AIDS information campaigns	0	4	4	11	19	12.8
Drug prevention	0	6	2	6	14	9.4
Total	8	36	36	69	149	100
Expected frequency	*(7)*	*(35)*	*(35)*	*(71)*	*(149)*	
n	3	15	15	30	63	

*   See section 2.1.1 for the sample of public bodies.

3.3.1   Prevention, Education and Information

Prevention and information activities of all kinds are shared between public and private non-profit organizations, both exclusive and inclusive ones, to a degree close to the expected frequencies, as seen in Table 4.19. It is often said that private non-profit organizations have a tendency to initiate activities of sorts than can attract financial support. No doubt, the government plan of action at an early stage set the pattern for what kind of HIV/AIDS-related activities would be funded when carried out by the third-sector organizations. However, information is seen as an important preventive measure in the public sphere too.

3.3.2   Care

Private non-profit organizations report a surprisingly high number of caring activities, as has been previously mentioned. The figures for single activities show a distinctive pattern, however (Table 4.20). Medical care and home care are almost exclusively public concerns. Shelter/housing facilities, food banks and buddy systems are exclusively private. Other activities, which could be grouped under the label "psychosocial services" are shared between public and private organizations.

Four organizations reported activities not originally included in the study. Three of them engage in recreational activities for HIV-positive persons. One church-

Table 4.20: Number of Separate Caring Activities by Legal Status and Organizational Orientation

	Public*		Private Non-Profit			
	Exclusives	Inclusives	Exclusives	Inclusives	Total	%
Care/psychological support to persons with AIDS	2	3	4	8	17	22.4
Face-to-face counselling	0	3	4	9	16	21.1
Buddy system	0	0	8	6	14	18.4
Referral services	2	2	5	2	11	14.5
AIDS-specialized medical care	1	3	0	0	4	5.3
Other	0	0	2	2	4	5.3
Voluntary HIV-testing and counselling	1	2	0	1	4	5.3
Home care services	1	1	1	0	3	3.9
Shelter, housing facilities	0	0	1	1	2	2.6
Food banks	0	0	1	0	1	1.3
Hospices	0	0	0	0	0	0.0
Total	7	14	26	29	76	100.1
Expected frequency	*(4)*	*(18)*	*(18)*	*(36)*	*(76)*	
n	3	15	15	30	63	

*   See section 2.1.1 for the sample of public bodies.

affiliated charity organization has taken the lead in providing day care and family support to families with HIV-infected children. One particular note has to be made of the absence of hospices for AIDS sufferers. This particular form of institution originally aimed at the care of terminally ill cancer patients, but did not exist in Sweden until recently. Instead, the terminal (or with the latest terminology, the continuing) care has been carried out in general hospitals or long-term hospitals, in cooperation with home care teams. No specific hospices for AIDS patients have been opened so far.

The exclusives report a higher than expected number of separate caring activities. This is apparently an area where the need for specialized organizations has been strongly felt. The involvement of new organizations in HIV/AIDS-related activities has not meant that totally new kinds of services have been offered, however, but rather an increase in the output of already existing kinds of caring activities (Table 4.21).

Table 4.21: Number of Separate Caring Activities Reported in 1992, by Organizational Development

	Number of Activities		
	"Early Movers"	"Meeting the Challenge"	"Latecomers"
Care/psychological support to PWAs	4	10	3
Face-to-face counselling	3	10	3
Buddy system	1	10	3
Referral services	2	8	1
AIDS-specialized medical care	4	0	0
Other	0	3	1
Voluntary HIV-testing and counselling	3	1	0
Home care services	1	2	0
Shelter, housing facilities	0	1	1
Food banks	0	1	0
Hospices	0	0	0
Total	18	46	12
Expected frequency	*(10)*	*(58)*	*(8)*

All four organizations that provide AIDS-specialized medical care started their activities in the early period, 1980-84. So did three of four organizations active in HIV-testing. This is, of course, mainly explained by the fact that the public response to HIV/AIDS has been, to a large extent, organized within existing frameworks. Medical care was automatically integrated into hospitals and clinics run by the county councils; making HIV/AIDS a notifiable disease meant that it could be handled according to the Infectious Diseases Act necessitating only a few legal changes, such as the one related to the keeping of medical records. This means that the administrative apparatus was already in shape. The profile of organizations starting HIV/AIDS work in 1990-92 is very different. With the exception of one organization providing housing, all other reported activities could be labelled as "psychosocial services". Again, this is one of the areas where the government grants were made available to voluntary organizations from the very start of the national AIDS programme.

3.3.3 Policy Coordination & Monitoring and Research

Policy coordination and monitoring as well as research are subsectors dominated by the public authorities (Table 4.22). The private non-profit organizations contribute to some degree with social research and coordination/implementation of policies within their own peer groups.

Table 4.22: Number of Separate Activities in Policy Coordination & Monitoring and Research by Legal Status and Organizational Orientation

	Public*		Private Non-Profit			
	Exclusives	Inclusives	Exclusives	Inclusives	Total	%
Policy coordination & monitoring						
AIDS policy coordination and implementation	0	9	0	4	13	43.3
HIV-screening, testing, identification (contact-tracing)	1	5	0	0	6	20.0
Control of blood/plasma product safety	0	1	0	0	1	3.3
Research						
Epidemiological/ social research	2	6	0	2	10	33.3
Total	3	21	0	6	30	99.9
Expected frequency	*(1)*	*(7)*	*(7)*	*(15)*	*(30)*	
n	3	15	15	30	63	

*   See section 2.1.1 for the sample of public bodies.

Blood banks are organized by the county councils, mainly located in larger hospitals. The National Bacteriology Laboratory, now replaced by the Swedish Institute for Infectious Disease Control, had an advisory function and in that capacity it issued early warnings about the risks of an infected blood transmission with the then unknown pathogen causing AIDS. All blood donors were informed in 1993 via their blood centres and warned not to give blood if they belonged to any of the known high-risk groups. Commercial blood products such as Factor VIII, which is a necessity for haemophiliacs, have to be approved by the Medical Products Agency, a government body which was not included in the study.

Out of the six public units reporting that they are active in HIV-screening, testing and identification (contact-tracing), only four perform all these functions. Three of these are specialized HIV units in hospitals and one is a unit working exclusively with psychosocial support for gay and bisexual men with HIV-related problems. Of the other two, one is a county medical officer, whose responsibility starts if the testing physician does not manage to fulfil all the steps in contact-tracing and testing of the contacts, the other is the National Bacteriological Laboratory, responsible for certifying positive test results.

3.3.4 Interest Representation and Support Activities

The separate activities listed under this heading are all very clearly the responsibility of private non-profit organizations rather than the public institutions included in the study (Table 4.23).

One public unit, the psychosocial centre, reports activities within this subsector. As part of their psychosocial approach, they support the clients in organizing self-help groups and offer various types of counselling. Otherwise, counselling for insurance or welfare entitlements and legal advice are available in public institutions in Sweden, but in the terminology of this study these would be called "inclusive

Table 4.23: Number of Separate Interest Representation and Support Activities by Legal Status and Organizational Orientation

	Public*		Private Non-Profit			
	Exclusives	Inclusives	Exclusives	Inclusives	Total	%
Interest representation						
Civil and human rights/ protection against discrimination	0	0	11	10	21	32.3
Self-help groups of people with HIV/AIDS	1	0	7	5	13	20.0
Political lobbying	0	0	4	5	9	13.8
Legal advice	1	0	4	2	7	10.8
Counselling for insurance/ welfare entitlements	1	0	3	2	6	9.2
Support activities						
Fund-raising for HIV/AIDS programmes	0	0	7	2	9	13.8
Total	3	0	36	26	65	99.9
Expected frequency	*(3)*	*(15)*	*(15)*	*(31)*	*(65)*	
n	3	15	15	30	63	

*   See section 2.1.1 for the sample of public bodies.

inclusives", meaning that they are available to HIV/AIDS sufferers on the same terms as to anybody else and, therefore, not included in the study.

The high proportion of interest representation and fund-raising activities among exclusive organizations compared to the inclusives, implies that new organizations have started in order to meet these particular needs of HIV-seropositive and AIDS-affected persons. Since fund-raising is normally done to support activities that fall short of government funding, it is obviously an activity for private non-profit organizations. Among the nine organizations active in fund-raising, three exclusives classify this as their main activity in order to support other organizations. The other six, both exclusives and inclusives, raise funds in order to finance their own activities.

4   Policy Implications

4.1   The National Style of Organizational Response

The first 10 years of HIV/AIDS management in Sweden are characterized by a strongly centralized coordination of planning and financing. The formation of a National Commission on AIDS within the Ministry of Health and Social Affairs gave prominence to the problem, as well as easy access to the political agenda. The Swedish tendency to seek consent rather than conflict was obvious in that different kinds of expertise and all political parties were represented on the commission. The debates could take place within this limited group before proposals were formalized and presented by the government.

The basic principles of the Swedish AIDS policy came from the public health sector and the pattern was set by including HIV/AIDS among the notifiable diseases regulated by the Infectious Diseases Act. Voluntary HIV-testing made easily available – anonymously only as long as the test proves negative – together with mandatory reporting of positive cases and contact-tracing, are the main public health measures used. Since the Swedish health care system is supposed to provide the whole population with all kinds of care – including preventive medicine, health education and public health services – public bodies are automatically expected to take on such activities as: research, monitoring, HIV-testing and care. Most of the organizations active in these sectors of activity were there already, able to include their concern about a new disease in their regular organizational pattern. A few new bodies were initiated to meet specific needs, such as support to home care staff or psychosocial support to HIV-positive gay men.

One of the reference groups attached to the National Commission on AIDS from the start, included representatives for private non-profit organizations whose members have a special interest in the HIV/AIDS problem, such as the homosexual community, organizations dealing with drug misuse and the haemophiliac society. This kind of formalized representation by voluntary organizations, allowed to have a say at an early stage but not necessarily being part of the decision-making public body, is common in Sweden.

Information to the public and to the different groups at risk is the second leg in the Swedish HIV/AIDS policy. Financial support to voluntary organizations active in information or psychosocial support to specific target groups, have developed as an important complement and supplement to the information campaigns organized by public bodies, and to the public health care system. The variety of PNPOs taking on such activities reflects the Swedish pattern with a large proportion of the population being involved in formal organizations. Not only groups at risk of becoming personally affected with the disease – as the bi- and homosexual men, the drug users or the recipients of blood products – got involved at an early stage. Also charity organizations such as the Swedish Red Cross, the City Mission of Stockholm and Caritas Sweden take part in information and caring. One very significant part of the Swedish organizational response is the fact that immigrant organizations are so active in HIV/AIDS information. One quarter of all PNPOs identified in our study belong to this group.

4.2 The Organizational Response and the Health and Welfare System

Examining the frequency of various types of activities from a developmental perspective, we find that all types of activities have been developed by organizations that started their HIV/AIDS work in the early 1980s. Both public and private non-profit "early movers" are engaged in more activities than expected across the board. Most of them are inclusives, which explains the early start, and their early involvement gave them an opportunity to influence the further development of the Swedish AIDS policy, which in many ways is based on existing organizational structures, such as the health care system, the public health principles for the prevention of infectious diseases and the public financial support of voluntary organizations.

The inclusive, private non-profit organizations, which started HIV/AIDS activities early, were already active in areas where persons with high-risk behaviour were to be found. During the last 10 years, they have established themselves as major actors in the field. New PNPOs have been formed at a unique pace, in many cases working with a specific target group defined by the route of virus transmission. Inclusive public bodies that started their HIV/AIDS activities early, are part of the general health care system, and they integrated their HIV/AIDS activities as a natural part of their existing programmes. Some units, like the Gay Men's Health Clinic, were formed as outreach units linked to existing agencies.

Prevention, Education and Information, Care, Interest Representation, Policy Coordination & Monitoring, Research and Support Activities, all quickly became the focus of Swedish organizations. Many of these activities were later extended and further developed, but at a somewhat slower pace in the late 1980s, while the pace of development slowed down even more in the 1990s.

4.3 Division of Labour between Different Types of Organizations

At a general level of analysis of HIV/AIDS activities and organizations in Sweden, and borrowing from the distinction of organizational orientation employed by this project, we found that exclusive organizations are more engaged in HIV/AIDS-related activities than inclusive organizations. Regardless of whether they were public or private organizations, exclusives had both higher median and mean scores in terms of activities than inclusives. In addition, both types of exclusives had much higher activity scores than the "expected frequencies". This appears logical, since exclusives were created explicitly for the sole purpose of working with HIV/AIDS. By contrast, inclusives were neither created solely for, nor do they devote themselves entirely to, working with HIV/AIDS. Thus, we can conclude that our distinction between these two types of orientations is meaningful and important in the Swedish context. Moreover, we can note that exclusives bear a much greater relative burden of HIV/AIDS activities. This seems to be related to the singularity and intensity of their purpose, which results in a much greater fervour of engagement in providing HIV/AIDS activities.

Turning to the more specific types of HIV/AIDS activities undertaken by Swedish organizations, we note a lot of variation between organizations, both with respect to their legal status and organizational orientations. The largest category seen from the number of HIV/AIDS activities, Prevention, Education and Information, demonstrates a relatively even distribution among all organizations, i.e. all types and orientations of organizations are equally engaged in such activities. This is not so surprising, given the Swedish policy emphasis on prevention and information. Private non-profit organizations are readily given grants for information projects. The approach differs, however, between the public and the private non-profit involvement. Major information campaigns, targeting the population at large and subgroups like young people, health care personnel, etc., have been organized by government agencies, whereas PNPOs have concentrated on information to specific groups at risk, like homo- and bisexual men, IV-drug addicts and travellers. Thus, in this area private non-profit organizations are both a supplement to and a complement to public bodies in their efforts. Private non-profit organizations reach out to groups not always reached by public campaigns, bringing information to new groups.

This balanced engagement does not hold true for any other type of activity. Private non-profit exclusives are clearly overrepresented in the provision of care and social services, while both types of inclusives are less engaged in such activities. Again this might be explained by the singularity of purpose and closeness between organizations and their clients/members that is unique to exclusive private non-profit organizations. Noticeable is the difference in separate caring activities reported by private non-profit organizations compared to the public units. The private initiatives can to a large extent, be referred to as "psychosocial services", a field stressed in the national policy papers as an area where the private non-profit contributions can be of specific value. Here too, these organizations both complement and supplement the activities of public bodies, reaching groups and persons not accessible through public efforts of providing care and social services. This, however, means that private non-profit organizations also provide an alternative channel of delivering such services which is preferable in the eyes of many HIV/AIDS-infected persons.

Private non-profit exclusives are clearly more engaged in interest representation than other categories of organizations. It seems reasonable that public bodies do not become equally engaged in such activities. Similarly, private inclusives have several sets of clients to which they must cater, and cannot demonstrate the same singularity in lobbying for any single subgroup. Moreover, when it comes to support activities such as fund-raising, exclusive non-profit organizations are more engaged in providing such services than all other categories of organizations in Sweden, while public bodies are completely absent. Thus, we find that private non-profit organizations are clearly an alternative to public bodies, rather than a complement to them in terms of lobbying and support activities.

When it comes to policy coordination, public bodies clearly dominate and private non-profits contribute little. It is mainly the inclusive public bodies that are engaged in such activities, perhaps because of their broader range of responsibilities than public exclusives. Similarly, when it comes to research activities, which require extensive funds and an appropriate organizational structure, we note that public bodies of both orientations clearly dominate this type of activity in Sweden, and private non-profit organizations only make a marginal contribution. Therefore, public financial support goes to public bodies when it concerns research on HIV/AIDS. Both research and policy coordination & monitoring activities, are completely absent from the programmes of private non-profit exclusives. Thus, we find that private non-profit organizations can neither be a supplement to public bodies nor provide an alternative to them in terms of research, policy coordination and monitoring.

In terms of differences in the activities of the Swedish organizations in relation to legal status and organizational orientation, we can note the following profiles:

a) Public exclusives are more involved in care and research than other types of activities.

b) Public inclusives are more engaged in research and policy coordination than other types of activities, less engaged in care, but not at all in interest representation and support activities.

c) Private non-profit exclusives are more engaged in care and social services, interest representation and support activities than other activities, and completely absent from research and policy coordination.

d) Private non-profit inclusives are less engaged in care and social services, research and policy coordination than in other activities.

Turning to developmental aspects of HIV/AIDS activities in Sweden, we can note that relatively more public bodies became engaged in the early 1980s than private non-profit organizations, while several of the latter became engaged first in the 1990s. This lends support to the idea that private non-profit organizations mobilize resources to meet shortcomings in the activities of the public sector, particularly in terms of lobbying for improvements in, or for more HIV/AIDS care and service activities for specific groups. No similar differentiation is found in terms of the development of activities by exclusive or inclusive organizations.

The value of private non-profit organizations in giving information and psychosocial support to groups at risk of acquiring HIV, was stressed when the first national HIV/AIDS programme was accepted by the Riksdag in 1986. This interest in cooperation between the state and the voluntary organizations has been repeated constantly over the years, and the effect is obvious. Out of the 45 PNPOs included in the study, 40 are active in prevention. The 24 PNPOs active in care and/or social services share between them 55 separate activities, of which all but 12 can be characterized as psychosocial. The general tendency among PNPOs to select activities which can attract outside financing is clearly present in managing HIV/AIDS.

4.4 Private Non-Profit Organizations in Public Health and Social Welfare

In some countries, private non-profit organizations have for a long time been seen as a means for providing more efficient welfare services than either public or private for-profit channels. This opinion has gained ground in Sweden, during recent years.[28] The volunteer aspect of PNPOs gives rise to expectations of less costly services compared with public or private for-profit provisions, which in turn, can relieve heavily burdened public budgets (Kramer, 1981). When a representative for the Swedish government described the plans for a more active role for the voluntary sector in the Swedish welfare mix, however, he stressed that the reason for this is ideological – increasing the spirit of community – rather than economic (Hedman, 1993).

Looking at the case of HIV/AIDS, the issue has not so much been whether PNPOs could help to increase efficiency and cut costs, but rather whether they could contribute to greater effectiveness in achieving the goals of public health and welfare by mobilizing their outreach function. The way PNPOs manage to facilitate the outreach functions is particularly crucial when public health and social welfare services are faced with crisis situations. In the case of HIV/AIDS, high risk groups might be reluctant to work directly as "individuals" or in groups with the public authorities because of the stigma attached to their group.

The increasing number of heterosexually infected HIV-positive persons of both sexes during later years has so far been met with a rather low profile response. In a situation where the number of infected cases discovered each year in the heterosexual population is twice as high as among homosexual/bisexual men, one would expect a more diversified organizational response and more financial support to different types of voluntary organizations, i.e. those catering specifically for the heterosexual population. Immigrant organizations have in fact received increased priority since 1991/92. Furthermore, RFSU provides information to young persons travelling abroad, in an attempt to prevent Swedish young people from catching the infection. However, we lack evidence of other PNPO activity directed towards heterosexual persons at risk, e.g. tourists and business travellers. The growing instance and awareness of "female HIV/AIDS" justifies the question about an appropriate organizational response to meet the growing number of affected women. The PLUSS Association may have an important role to play in the future, but so, too, do women's organizations in general, although the latter seem relatively passive when compared to other groups studied here. Immigrant organizations in particular, need to be encouraged to look at the needs of their countrywomen in this respect.

Private non-profit organizations can sometimes either function as a complement or a supplement to public bodies in terms of undertaking HIV/AIDS activities. However, they clearly serve as an alternative to public bodies in terms of providing other activities. Nevertheless, no matter which role they play, they play it in their unique capacity of reaching out to HIV/AIDS-infected persons, something which is completely beyond the nature and means of public bodies. Thus, from an overall perspective, private non-profit organizations are at once complements, supplements and alternatives to the public sector, but in no way do they compete with them.

Notes

1   The study "Managing AIDS" has been supported financially by the National Board of Health and Welfare (1990-91) and the Swedish Council for Social Research (1992-93).
2   See Appendix 1 for details.
3   Minutes from meeting with the Swedish Government, 5 September 1985.
4   Gertrud Sigurdsen, Minister of Health and Social Affairs 1982-1991, Interview 6 November 1992.
5   *Regeringens proposition 1985/86:171 om särskilda medel för bekämpningen av AIDS.*
6   *Informationskampanjen om HIV/AIDS – samhällsinformation som styrmedel.* Riksrevisionsverket, Stockholm, 1989.
7   *Folkrörelse & Föreningsguiden.* Civildepartementet, Stockholm, 1986.
8   *Invandrarutredningen 3. Invandrarna och minoriteterna.* SOU 1974: 69, Stockholm, 1974. *Invandrar- och minoritetspolitiken.* SOU 1984: 58, Stockholm, 1984.
9   Another deviation exists in that a victim of rape can demand an HIV test to be carried out on the rapist, if he does not accept to have it done voluntarily.
10 *Regeringens proposition 1986/87:149. Socialutskottets betänkande SoU 1986/87: 38. Riksdagens protokoll 1986/87: 135.*

11 RFSL = Riksförbundet för sexuellt likaberättigande, The Swedish Federation for Gay and Lesbian Rights.
    RFSU = Riksförbundet för Sexuell Upplysning, Swedish Association for Sex Education.
12 STD = Sexually Transmitted Diseases.
13 Håkan Wrede, Secretary, The National Commission on AIDS, Interview, 11 September 1992.
14 The three public "exclusive" bodies in the study are: Huddinge hospital support unit for home care; Stockholm's county council psychosocial centre for gay and bisexual men with HIV-related problems; Gay men's health clinic.
15 *Regeringens proposition* 1988/89: 100, *Bilaga* 7, pp. 157-161.
16 *Luffarpåsen.*
17 *Förslag till lagstiftning om registrerat partnerskap.* Letter to the Government from the National Board of Health and Welfare, 14 June 1990.
18 *Homosexuella och Samhället.* SOU 1984: 63, Stockholm, 1984.
19 The Commission was of the opinion that the way the subject "love and marriage" is taught in the middle school, could counterbalance discrimination and contribute towards a more open and socially acceptable way of treating homosexuals. Its opinion was that "the National Swedish Board of Education must evolve suitable forms of more actively stimulating individual schools and teachers to improve the way in which they teach their pupils about homosexuality".
20 *Regeringens proposition* 1986/87: 124. *Socialutskottets betänkande* SoU 1986/87: 31. *Riksdagens protokoll* 1986/87: 136.
21 *Äktenskaps- och sambofrågor.* Lagutskottets betänkande 1992/93: LU36. 'Partnerskapslag delade partier', *Dagens Nyheter*, 8 June 1994.
22 *Åtgärder mot bruk av narkotika samt ringa narkotikabrott.* Justitieutskottets betänkande 1992/93: JuU 17.
23 Arne Bogren, interview as part of the "Managing AIDS" project.
24 Gould, Arthur, ibid.
25 Also information from the National Bacteriological Laboratory.
26 *Pressmeddelande*, Socialdepartementet, Stockholm, 21 February 1991.
27 *Proposition* 1992/93: 178, Stockholm, 18 February 1993.
28 *Folkrörelseutredningen.* Kommittédirektiv, Civildepartementet, dir. 1986: 17, Stockholm, 1986. *Ju mer vi är tillsammans.* Folkrörelseutredningen, SOU 1987: 33-35, Stockholm, 1987. *Mål och resultat.* Folkrörelseutredningen, SOU 1989:39, Stockholm 1989.

References

Bayer, Ronald (1989) *Private Acts, Social Consequences. AIDS and the Politics of Public Health.* New York: The Free Press, pp. 72-85.
Bejerot, Nils (1968) *Narkotiafrågan och samhället.* Stockholm.
Berglund, Ove (1993) 'Byt ut smittskyddsläkaren!', *Dagens Nyheter*, 6 July.
Gould, Arthur (1994) 'Sweden's Syringe Exchange Debate: Moral Panic in a Rational Society', *The Journal of Social Policy,* Loughborough University.
Hedman, Kurt (1993) *The Third Sector – A Developing Force in the Swedish Society.* Paper given at the conference on "Well-being in Europe by Strengthening the Third Sector", Barcelona, May.

Kramer, R. (1981) *Voluntary Agencies in the Welfare State*. Berkeley: University of California Press.
Lewin, Barbro (1987) *AIDS-delegationen. En studie i den svenska förvaltningspolitikens omvandling*. Term Paper, Uppsala University.
Malmquist, H./Ramgren, O. (eds.) (1992) *HIV/AIDS in Sweden*. Stockholm: The National Board of Health and Welfare.
RFSL (1988) *Säkrare sex. En sammanställning av teorier och studier av sexuella beteenden bland män som har sex med andra män*. Stockholm, p. 69.
Tunving, Kerstin (1991) 'Finland och Island skonade – men narkotikamissbruket utbrett i övriga Norden', *Läkartidningen* 88 (15): 1413.

Appendix 1:   The National Commission on AIDS; Reference Group of PNPOs

In April 1989, the following organizations and authorities were represented or invited to participate in the reference group dealing with matters concerning private non-profit organizations.

PNPOs engaged in HIV/AIDS Activities

Convictus
The Friendship Association NU
National Federation for a Drugfree Society, RNS
Noah's Ark – Red Cross Foundation
NORNA Foundation
Positiva Gruppen – The Swedish Organization for HIV-positive Gay Men
The Swedish Association for Help and Assistance to Drug-Abusers, RFHL
Swedish Association for Sex Education, RFSU
The Swedish Federation for Gay and Lesbian Rights, RFSL
The Swedish Haemophilia Society, FBIS
Swedish National Parent Organization Against Drugs, FMN

Labour Market Organizations

Confederation of Professional Employees, TCO
Swedish Confederation of Professional Associations, SACO
Swedish Trade Union Confederation, LO

Public Organizations

Gay Men's Health Clinic, Stockholm
Ministry of Health and Social Affairs
National Board of Health and Welfare

Appendix 2:   Sweden and its Counties

AB = Stockholm
BD = Norrbotten
C   = Uppsala
OG = Gothenburg
MM = Malmö

Appendix 3:   Public Bodies Selected for the Study

National Government

National Bacteriological Laboratory
National Board of Health and Welfare
National Board of Occupational Safety and Health
National Institute of Public Health, HIV/AIDS Programme
National Prison and Probation Administration, Drug Treatment Group

Local and Regional Government

Danderyd Hospital, Dept. of Infectious Diseases, HIV-unit
Gothenburg Environmental and Health Protection Agency, HIV-unit
Huddinge Hospital, HIV-unit
Huddinge Hospital, Support Unit for Home Care
Malmö Regional Centre for Infectious Disease Control
Norrbotten County, Dept. of Epidemiology and Control of Infectious Diseases
St Lars Hospital Drug Treatment Centre, Lund
Stockholm City Social Welfare Authority, Aids-unit
Stockholm County Aids Prevention Programme
Stockholm County, Gay Men's Health Clinic
Stockholm County, Psychosocial Centre for Gay and Bisexual Men
    with HIV-related Problems
Uppsala County Medical Officer
Uppsala University Hospital, Dept. of Infectious Diseases

Appendix 4:   Private Non-profit Organizations

Exclusives

Art Against Aids
Body Positive South
Convictus
Foundation Sighstens Friends Against AIDS
The Friendship Association NU
National Coalition for HIV-positives in Sweden
Noah's Ark Malmöhus
Noah's Ark North-west Skåne
Noah's Ark Visby
Noah's Ark Östergötland
Noah's Ark – Red Cross Foundation
The PLUSS Association

The PSB Foundation
Positiva Gruppen, The Swedish Organization for HIV-positive Gay Men
Swedish Physicians Against AIDS

Inclusives

Africans Against AIDS
Arab Information and Cultural Centre
The Association of Kontrapunkt
Caritas Sweden
City Mission of Stockholm, Day Care Centre and Family Support
    for HIV-positive Children
City Mission of Stockholm, ESSEM-Centre
Ecumenical Christian Homosexuals (EKHO)
Eritrean Community in Sweden
Federation of African Associations in Sweden
Federation of Chilean Associations in Sweden
Federation of Kurdish Associations in Sweden
Federation of Yugoslav Associations in Sweden
Gay Conservatives
Gay Physicians
The International Organization for Immigrant Women
Kongo-Zaire Committee
The National Federation of Immigrants in Sweden
National Society of Finns in Sweden
SIMON, Immigrants in Sweden against Drugs
The Swedish Association for Help and Assistance to Drug Abusers (RFHL)
Swedish Association for Sex Education (RFSU)
The Swedish Federation for Gay and Lesbian Rights (RFSL)
The Swedish Haemophilia Society (FBIS)
Swedish National Parent Organization Against Drugs (FMN)
The Swedish National Union of Students (SFS)
The Swedish Red Cross
Swedish Save the Children
The Vallmotorp Foundation
The Vardi Foundation
The Women's Forum (Institute for Drug Abuse Issues)

CHAPTER 5

Managing AIDS in Flanders

Koen Matthijs
Hilde Degezelle

1   Institutional, Policy and Epidemiological Context

1.1   Public AIDS Policy in Flanders[1]

It is beneficial to have some knowledge of the Belgian political structure in order
to truly comprehend the first part of this study. The Belgian state was federalized
in the last decade and this reform had a significant effect on all the different existing
kinds of policies. The power which the national institutions originally had diminished whereas the importance of the Communities increased. This incurred several conflicts between competencies, which meant that it was difficult to build up
a coherent policy. These difficulties are clearly apparent when analysing the AIDS
policy.

The AIDS virus was discovered in 1981 in the USA and it was in 1983 when
Belgium introduced an AIDS policy; this functioned on different state levels. The
agreement was that personally-linked matters, e.g. prevention, health care, etc.,
had to be treated regionally[2] whereas matters like the regulation of blood banks,
screening and some kinds of research were federal (i.e. national) concerns.

In what is to follow, we look at the AIDS policy at each level. We firstly describe the responses given by the Belgian Federal Government. These are important because they are the same for all Belgian Communities and they give us a view
of how and when a country like Belgium reacted to the phenomenon of AIDS. We
then describe the Flemish situation in more detail – the federal, regional and local
dealings with HIV/AIDS.

1.1.1 Federal Government Response

Today, there are six ministers who have various competencies in different aspects of the AIDS policy on a federal level.[3] The most important ones are the Minister for Social Integration, Public Health and the Environment, who is responsible for the organization and monitoring of blood banks, screening, etc., and the Minister for Social Affairs, who is responsible for the AIDS reference centres (AIDS-Referentie Centra)[4] and for the reimbursement of funds for HIV-testing carried out by the National Sickness and Invalidity Insurance (RIZIV)[5,6]. Since the modification of the Constitution in 1988, there has been a definitive division of tasks between the Federal Government and the Communities. The competencies of the federal ministers are rather meagre when it comes to matters concerning prevention as they no longer have any say in it. Nevertheless, they still determine part of the Belgian AIDS policy and have an important responsibility concerning the monitoring of the blood banks, screening, etc.

In general, we can consider the original Belgian response to AIDS as being an institutional one. A whole set of institutions and committees were created during the 1980s. However, most of them have stopped being actively involved – although they were never abandoned – due to the governmental changes which took place (state reforms, elections, etc.). Only two of these institutions still operate today. A short description of the most important ones follows.

THE NATIONAL SCIENTIFIC AIDS COMMITTEE

In 1983 the National Scientific AIDS Committee (Nationale wetenschappelijke AIDS Commissie) was founded as part of the Supreme Health Council (Hoge Gezondheidsraad). The Supreme Health Council is composed of 40 professional academics, who are nominated by the Minister for Public Health. A few of them make up the AIDS Committee. The original task of the Committee was to give scientific and technical advice to the ministry and to control the effectiveness of the blood tests and the accuracy of HIV-positive tests. It also had to follow up the development and care given to those infected with the virus as well as to their relatives and personal contacts.

Nowadays, the AIDS Committee meets every three months to take note of and discuss all reported HIV/AIDS cases. It also monitors the AIDS reference centres, which are responsible for HIV-testing and screening.

THE COUNCIL FOR THE COORDINATION OF THE COMBAT AGAINST AIDS

Until 1988, the AIDS Committee only gave medical advice to the Ministry of Public Health; however, it was transformed into the High Council for the Coordination of the Combat against AIDS (De Hoge Raad voor de Coördinatie van de AIDS-bestrijding) by Royal Decree on 18 March 1988. This Council has functioned more or less independently and has had a more general approach to the problem of AIDS and its coordination.[7] It has also developed a more global view of the topic. Different working groups were set up which had to give information and advice concerning their fields of work. The Council has been an important instrument for the reference centres by defining the tasks of the Centres and by dividing up the budget, however, it has few further concrete directives.

This institute could not function as effectively as it had hoped because of the unclear task definition of the Council and the unclear statute with regard to the policy.[8] The Council was founded to bring more coordination into the Belgian AIDS policy. Seen constitutionally however, it is, in this case, not possible for a national institution to issue any binding measures with regard to community policy. So the Council for the Coordination of the Combat against AIDS can only give advice on federal matters, but cannot coordinate the whole policy. In 1989 the greatest part of the federal budget for AIDS policy was passed on to the communities responsible for prevention and health promotion. As the Council was a federal institute, it could not continue.

Today, the Council for the Coordination of the Combat against AIDS still officially exists, although the last time they met was in 1991.

THE INTERMINISTERIAL AIDS COMMITTEE

The Interministerial AIDS Committee (Interministeriële AIDS Commissie) was founded on the decision of the Council of Ministers in December 1986. Its main goal was to coordinate the combat against AIDS by delegating members of the different responsible ministries to stand on the Committee. This Committee was therefore a political one. Each minister could convene with the Committee when faced with a policy problem on AIDS in his/her department. At that time, the Committee met and discussed the problem on the basis of the expert advice of the Council for the Coordination of the Combat against AIDS.

Another task of the Interministerial AIDS Committee was to give some concrete proposals to the Council of Ministers regarding federal AIDS matters. Its most important accomplishment was the first national AIDS information campaign in 1987.

Since the modification of the Constitution in 1988, the competencies of the Federal Government have diminished, and as a result, the Interministerial AIDS Committee has stopped meeting since 1991.

THE AIDS REFERENCE CENTRES

At the moment, the AIDS reference centres are the most important bodies at the federal level. There are eight of them spread throughout the whole country.[9] Since 1985, different types of AIDS tests have been carried out in Belgium. All blood that has been collected in blood banks has to be monitored and screened for HIV.

To check and confirm these results, the original tests are rescreened by the AIDS reference centres. Fundamental scientific research as well as epidemiological studies are also carried out in the respective laboratories of the reference centres.

The AIDS reference centres were set up in 1986 as part of some existing clinics or laboratories and the Ministry for Public Health subsidized them. Due to the federalization, they became a matter for the communities which meant that The Council for the Coordination of the Combat against AIDS lost its right to decide on the subsidies to be allocated to the reference centres.

A year later, the government decided to make the reference centres part of a federal matter of concern again. Today, they are the responsibility of the Ministry for Social Affairs. At the moment, however, there are discussions concerning the present statute of the reference centres.

1.1.2 Responses of the Flemish Community

On the community level, it is the Minister for Employment and Social Affairs of the Government of Flanders who is accountable for the preventive health policy.[10] This minister takes all the decisions regarding AIDS, i.e. from topics regarding AIDS campaigns to the issuing of grants. He/she is assisted by an administration, a Scientific Steering Committee on AIDS, the IPAC and the VIG.[11] In the second part of this section we describe these different bodies and their respective orientations and in the final part we cast a glance at the financing of the AIDS policy. However, first of all, we try to outline some of the policy lines of the Minister of the Government of Flanders responsible for AIDS prevention.

POLICY LINES

At the beginning, there was no clear line in the Flemish AIDS policy. AIDS prevention was seen as a small part of the health policy and had no budget of its own. AIDS organizations were annually subsidized and grant allocation was, in fact, a very slow process with no clear principles. This made it very difficult to develop projects or to work out long-term initiatives. Various small initiatives were set up throughout the country, which worked side by side. However, they had no idea about what was happening in any other organization beside their own.

Through the foundation of the Scientific Steering Committee, and, later on, of the Provincial AIDS Coordination Committees and the IPAC, the Government has tried to establish some coordination between the multitude of AIDS organizations and numerous AIDS projects. However, because of the lack of financial resources and unclear task definitions, these organizations could not effectively function.

A real move in the right direction came about through the foundation of the VIG by the Government in 1991. The IPAC became a statute within the VIG and fell back (only receiving a basic subsidy) and was therefore not able to continue its work effectively.[12] In November of that same year, the Government fell, and the elections distorted the former political landscape. A new minister was put in charge of the matter of preventive health policy; she continued the policy initiated by her predecessor.

From that moment onwards (1992), the Flemish AIDS policy began to take shape. AIDS organizations became involved in the planning of the policy, and a new, extensive policy note[13] attested to an integrated approach on the subject of AIDS prevention. The different intiatives became integrated in the overall AIDS policy and it was no longer possible to start all kinds of activities without explanation. A thorough analysis of the existing projects, organizations and epidemiological figures was made in order to look for gaps in the offer of HIV/AIDS activities with a view to planning a more efficient AIDS policy.

One of the priorities of the new minister was to involve all different policy-makers by bringing them together in one consultative body. The AIDS Unit (AIDS-cel) was planned to be founded as a new coordinating body.[14] This unit has not yet been put into operation however.

A real improvement was that from 1993, AIDS prevention and care became a separate item on the budget of the Flemish Government. The new system orders the granting of subsidies on a three-year basis so that organizations have more guarantees for receiving their expected grant, which brings in some continuity in working and planning.

Of course not every idea which appears in the proposal has already been realized, but one may conclude that a big step has been taken in the direction of a co-ordinated AIDS policy in the Flemish Community.

THE INSTITUTIONS

The Scientific Steering Committee
As we have seen, the Scientific Steering Committee was one of the first organizations which had an advisory function with regard to AIDS prevention. This Committee was made up of experts from all scientific disciplines concerned (medical, juridical, ethical and psychosocial) as well as some representatives of the Flemish Community from the areas of administration and policy-making. It was housed in the Institute of Tropical Medicine, and its main task was to scientifically support all prevention and educational activities. The Committee was also responsible for building up a documentation centre and had an important advisory function regarding all aspects of the AIDS problem – serving the Ministry and its Public Health Sector. The Committee received little feedback and, until 1992, this organization mainly gave advice on formally presented projects for a period of one year. In addition to this, it also played a role in organizing some media campaigns.

After the foundation of the VIG, which meant an important reformation of the Flemish health care sector, the approval of projects occurred on the advice of the

Scientific Council of the VIG through the Scientific Council of AIDS. This is one of the reasons why, nowadays, the Scientific Steering Committee no longer assembles.

The IPAC

In November 1987, the IPAC was founded on the initiative of Peter Piot at the Department of Microbiology at the ITG.[15] It was set up as an executing organ by the Scientific Steering Committee to take over some of their tasks. From then on, the IPAC was responsible for the coordination of the AIDS policy in Flanders and for the documentation centre. The IPAC also housed the secretariat of the Scientific Steering Committee, and carried out its instructions.

In addition to the IPAC, the PACCs[16] (Provinciale AIDS Coördinatie Comités) were set up in each province of Flanders. These committees had to coordinate and support the local prevention activities concerning AIDS, and were headed by the local health inspectors. Unfortunately, most of these committees did not get off the ground.[17]

The first structured initiative on the level of consultation by the IPAC is to be found in the body of the AIDS Consultation (AIDS-overleg) which began in September 1988. Its members meet every two months as a forum for all exclusive and inclusive AIDS organizations and PACCs. Their meetings encourage mediation between the field organization, their coordinating bodies and the government. The AIDS Consultation can be seen as one of the most important realizations of the IPAC; it still stands today.

After the foundation of the VIG and the corresponding health sector reforms, the IPAC became an independent organization and fell back to receiving a basic subsidy like a statute. Consequently, problems arose and the IPAC criticized these reforms, because, firstly, they took place without consulting any organizations in the field and, secondly, no specific separate AIDS unit was foreseen, which will be explained more fully below. In 1991 the IPAC ran into trouble when it lost money and could therefore not continue its work.

In 1992, the objectives of the IPAC again became more clear. In cooperation with the VIG, the IPAC is now responsible for the coordination of all AIDS matters within the field of health. Its duties can be summarized using three keywords: advice, service and coordination. It has an advisory function to the responsible minister, offers service with its documentation centre and has a coordinative function with the AIDS Consultation by supporting and coordinating activities and projects. To realize these different functions, the IPAC works with a number of working groups.

The VIG

The VIG (Flemish Health Promotion Institute) is a cooperative body of 11 organizations which work in the field of health promotion in the Flemish Community.

It was set up in 1991 by order of the Flemish Executive, and was asked to assist the minister of the Government of Flanders responsible for health policy at that time in his tasks of coordination, organization and evaluation of the whole field of health promotion. The VIG also has a Council of Administration (Raad van Beheer) and a Scientific Council at its disposal so that it can reach its aims more effectively. The latter is composed of different functional working groups which are specialized in particular areas of interest, e.g. AIDS. These working groups evaluate presented projects and give advice to the Minister on the priority proposals.

The VIG was founded to solve some problems existing in the field of prevention and health. As previously mentioned, there was neither a clear subsidizing system for organizations which wanted to start up prevention activities in the field of AIDS, nor was there any guarantee that this agreement would continue for any length of time longer than one year. The lack of any coordination was another widespread problem. Consequently, the following changes were implemented to correct these problems.

Firstly, a difference was made between funds and projects. Organizations could be funded for a maximum of five years whereas projects could only be funded for a maximum period of three years.

Secondly, organizations wcre put into three different categories (A, B or C), each with its own separate subsidy. To be regarded as fitting into category A means that an organization stays relatively independent from the VIG, although it must continually cooperate with the VIG and other organizations. An organization of the B or C category is obliged to house its "social seat" and activity centre in the buildings of the VIG and to put 30% of its personnel at the disposal of the VIG.

By placing the different organizations within this structure, one can have an overview of the multitude of organizations recognized by the state.

Finally, the VIG has also written a "Strategical Plan for the Promotion of Health" in which it describes the priorities for the policy concerning health promotion in Flanders.

1.1.3 Financing

SCIENTIFIC RESEARCH

Until 1992, the annual budget for AIDS prevention in Belgium (Flanders) was no isolated item on the global budget for health promotion. An exception was made for scientific research as this was in connection with the "Research Programme: AIDS", which was approved by the National Council in December 1990. This programme was sanctioned by both the Flemish and the French-speaking Communities and spreads over a period of four years (1991-1994). The research programme on AIDS can be seen as an agreement to conduct the research programme in cooperation with the NFWO (Nationaal Fonds voor Wetenschappelijk Onderzoek)[18], the Belgian nation-state and the communities; it concentrates on scientific research of all kinds. The total budget foreseen for this programme in Flanders amounts to BFr 187,974,000 (US$ 5,342,114). From this total amount, the Flemish Government has to put up an annual BFr 25,000,000 (BFr 100,000,000 in total). Only 19% of this budget, however, is spent on evaluating or supporting current prevention projects. Another 31% is used for behavioural-scientific research.

PREVENTION PROJECTS

The following table gives us some figures on the financing of AIDS prevention activities in Flanders.

From 1991 onwards, the budget foreseen for AIDS prevention has significantly increased. These grants are divided between several target groups (not included in the table). We will not analyse this allocation in detail as there was no pattern in it until 1992.[19] It is the Flemish Government's intention to spend the sum of BFr 100 million ($ 2,860,000)[20] over a period of three years (by 1995).

Table 5.1:   Subsidies for AIDS Prevention Paid by the Flemish Community

Year	BFr (in thousands)	US $ (in thousands)
1987	500	15
1988	5,393	155
1989	14,634	418
1990	5,500	160
1991	15,783	450
1992	21,237	610
1993	47,000	1,340
1994	62,900	1,800

Source: *AIDS in Vlaanderen*, Beleidsnota (Policy Note), 1993, p. 17, 55.

1.2 Major Issues of Conflict in Public Debate

At the beginning, and during the political changes, there were a lot of discussions going on about the allocation of responsibilities. For example, the first AIDS campaign was organized by the national Government, although the Communities were generally seen as being responsible for matters of prevention. Even the AIDS Reference Centres – which were originally national concerns, then regional, and then national ones again – show us the typical Belgian conflicts in the division of labour.

A second problematic issue is caused by the difficulties between the field of HIV/AIDS and the IPAC on the one hand, and the IPAC and the minister on the other. The IPAC is sandwiched between these two demanding forces and does not have the financial power to answer to both of their needs. Its position, with respect to the VIG, is neither always very clear.

Sometimes there is not even a clear division of tasks between the different advisory bodies.

However, the IPAC does also cause a few bottlenecks of its own:[21]
- The disunity of the policy competencies on all different levels (local, provincial, community, national, European, international).
- The difficulties in talking about issues like sexuality, relationships, safe sex, etc.
- The invisibility of the AIDS problem (where the HIV-positive person is not visibly suffering).
- The very unclear structures and advisory organs.
- The fragmentary treatment of the AIDS problem.

1.3 Epidemiological Development

The epidemiological data for Flanders have been, and still are, collected by a national Belgian institute, so the figures used in this chapter are those used by the Belgian Government because separate data are not available. All figures used are collected by the Institute for Hygiene and Epidemiology. The data on HIV/AIDS in Belgium come from two sources: on the one hand from the registration of AIDS patients by doctors, and on the other hand from the registration of the HIV cases by the reference centres which confirm the positive screening tests.

The epidemiological data are described from two standpoints. Firstly, we take a look at the HIV cases in Belgium (those which have not yet developed AIDS). In this part, we deal with all people who are registered as seropositive in Belgium, which means Belgians as well as non-Belgians. In the second part, we handle the AIDS cases which have been diagnosed in Belgium. Here, a distinction is made between residents (persons who have lived in Belgium for at least five years at the time of diagnosis) and non-residents (people who had probably become infected beyond the Belgian borders).

1.3.1 Infected Persons

At the end of December 1993, there were a registered 8,420 HIV cases in Belgium.
This means that between the start of the epidemic (1981) and 1994, at least 8,420
persons had been infected with HIV. For 974 of the cases, there is not enough information to exclude "double counting", so they are not taken up in the analysis.
The AIDS phase has already set in among 1,555 of the cases during that period,
which means that 5,891 persons are seropositive but do not yet have AIDS.

Since 1987, an average of 72 new HIV infections have been counted in Belgium
per month, which means two to three a day. This situation did not vary very much
with time. We see a slight increase in 1992, but if the figures for 1993 are complete
(this might not be the case as some persons infected in 1993 could only have been
diagnosed in 1994, which would mean that these figures are missing), this increase
has stopped.

The age and sex are known for 94.7% (7,051) of all recorded HIV patients. If
we compare the number of infected men and women, we find that there are two
times more seropositive men than women. The age groups most represented are
25-29 (for women) and 30-34 (for men). For adults, the mean age at which one
is infected is 35.6 for men and 31.4 for women, which means that women are, on
average, younger at the time of infection than men.

Figure 5.1: The Development of New HIV Cases per Three-monthly Term

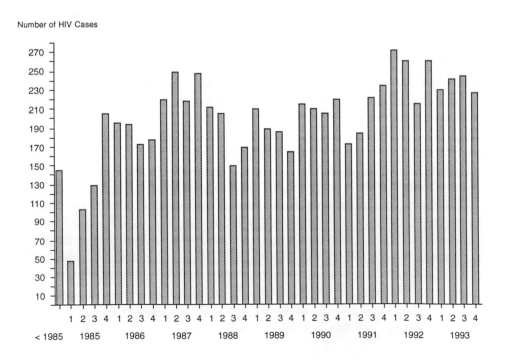

Figure 5.2: Number of Registered HIV Cases by Gender and Age (1993)

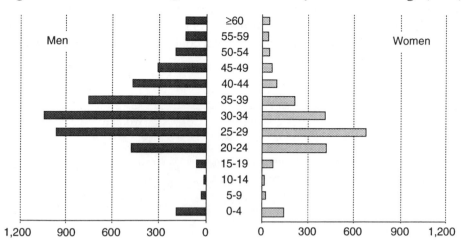

Source: Instituut voor Hygiëne en Epidemiologie / I.H.E. (Institute for Hygiene and Epidemiology), *Three-monthly Report* No. 34.

Table 5.2 gives the number of infected persons, according to their gender and probable route of transmission. These figures are known for 56.3% of all cases (4,193 persons). Table 5.2A shows the results of the Belgian population, Table 5.2B those of the HIV infections of non-Belgians in Belgium. Table 5.2C combines the two preceding tables.

Table 5.2:   Number of Registered HIV Cases by Gender and Route of Transmission (March 1994)

A. Belgians

	Men		Women		Total
	N	%	N	%	
Homosexual Contact	945	(56.6%)	–	–	945
Bisexual Contact	172	(10.3%)	–	–	172
IV-Drug Use	74	(4.4%)	44	(11.9%)	118
Homo-/bisexual IV-Drug Use	18	(1.1%)	–	–	18
Haemophilia	23	(1.4%)	–	–	23
Blood Transfusions	47	(2.8%)	40	(10.8%)	87
Heterosexual Contact	366	(21.9%)	258	(69.9%)	624
Mother to Child	26	(1.6%)	27	(7.3%)	53
Total	1,671	(100%)	369	(100%)	2,040

Source: I.H.E., *Three-monthly Report* No. 35.

From the Belgian men whose way of transmission is known, 68.5% have had sexual contact with other men. Some 5.3% have taken drugs intravenously. Transmission by way of heterosexual contact occurred in 338 cases (or 21.2%) of the male population. On the women's side, heterosexual contact is the biggest factor (68% of all female cases) for transmission of HIV.

B. Other Nationalities

	Men		Women		Total
	N	%	N	%	
Homosexual Contact	292	(18.4%)	–	–	292
Bisexual Contact	70	(4.4%)	–	–	70
IV-Drug Use	195	(12.3%)	44	(0.4%)	239
Homo-/bisexual IV-Drug Use	20	(1.3%)	–	–	20
Haemophilia	12	(0.8%)	–	–	12
Blood Transfusions	45	(28.3%)	72	(6.6%)	117
Heterosexual Contact	882	(55.4%)	900	(82.8%)	1,782
Mother to Child	75	(4.7%)	71	(6.5%)	146
Total	1,591	(100%)	1,087	(100%)	2,678

Source: I.H.E., *Three-monthly Report* No. 35.

If we look at the risk factors within the population of infected non-Belgian people, another pattern appears. Heterosexual HIV transmission dominates for both sexes: 59.7% of the men and 84% of the women have been infected in this way.

C. Total

	Men		Women		Total
	N	%	N	%	
Homosexual Contact	1,237	(37.9%)	–	–	1,237
Bisexual Contact	242	(7.4%)	–	–	242
IV Drug Use	269	(8.2%)	88	(6.0%)	357
Homo-/Bisexual IV Drug Use	38	(1.2%)	–	–	38
Haemophilia	35	(1.1%)	–	–	35
Blood Transfusions	92	(2.8%)	112	(7.7%)	204
Heterosexual Contact	1,248	(38.3%)	1,158	(79.5%)	2,406
Mother to Child	101	(3.1%)	98	(6.7%)	199
Total	3,262	(100%)	1,456	(100%)	4,718

Source: I.H.E., *Three-monthly Report* No. 35.

The total figures concerning the way of transmission show us the two biggest risk factors in Belgium. These are homosexual contact (for men) and heterosexual contact for both sexes.

Figure 5.3: Number of Registered HIV-infected Persons by Region (1994)

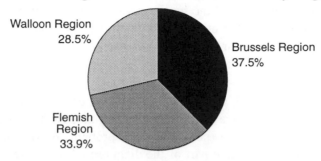

Source: *Epidemiology of AIDS and HIV in Belgium*, 1994.

Figure 5.4: Number of Registered HIV-infected Persons by Province (1993)

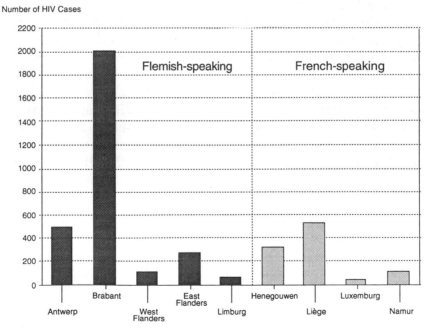

Note: The division between the Dutch-speaking and the French-speaking provinces is not completely correct. The province of Brabant is composed of two Dutch-speaking districts, one bilingual district and one French-speaking district. We made the division, however, to give an idea of which provinces belong fully or partly to the Flemish Community.

Source: I.H.E., *Three-monthly Report* No. 34.

Almost half (42%) of the infected people, whose place of residence is known, live in the Brussels region. This region is the smallest in Belgium. The other two regions, Flanders and Wallonia, contain the rest of the cases, each of them contain some 29% of the population.

There is no uniform distribution of HIV/AIDS cases between the nine Belgian provinces. More than half of the seropositive persons live in Brabant, especially in and around Brussels. The other patients mainly come from big cities (Antwerp, Ghent and Liège) and their surrounding areas.

1.3.2 AIDS Patients

As previously mentioned, we can divide the AIDS cases into two groups of residents, i.e. persons who have lived in Belgium for at least five years at the time of diagnosis, and non-residents (people who had probably become infected abroad). The former represent a large part of the diagnosed AIDS cases (63.2%), which indicates that the HIV-infected Belgian citizens had probably been infected in Belgium. Table 5.3 illustrates the number of AIDS cases according to the citizen's residential status and nationality.

If we look at the development of the AIDS cases in Belgium, we can distinguish three stadia. Until 1984, we saw a quick increase of the disease in the population of non-residents, but a rather slow one among residents. As many residents as non-residents were diagnosed as HIV-positive between 1985 and the first part of 1987. From that moment on, residents surpassed non-residents and there is an increase in the total number of AIDS patients. The decrease in 1992, and especially in 1993, has to be scrutinized due to the period prior to a certain AIDS diagnosis. As it takes several weeks to know if someone has developed full-blown AIDS or not, the complete number of diagnoses is not available; such cases are not part of any statistics. This means that the AIDS figures were not definitive at the time of recording.

Table 5.3:   Number of AIDS Cases by Residential Status and Nationality (1994)

	Belgian Nationality	Other Nationality	Total
Residents	780	231	1,011
Non-Residents	86	502	588
Total	866	733	1,599

Source: *Epidemiology of AIDS and HIV in Belgium*, November 1994.

Figure 5.5: Development of AIDS Cases per Semester (1993)

Number of AIDS Cases

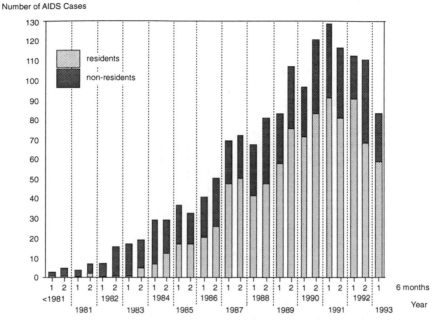

Source: I.H.E., *Three-monthly Report* No. 34.

The figures used in Figure 5.6 date from September 1993. The nationality was known for 1,486 AIDS cases at that time. Belgians count for 54.5% (808 patients) of the cases whereas the rest of the patients are of another nationality.

Considering the variable "gender", we see that 76.3% of the AIDS patients are men. For the Belgian population, this percentage is even higher: 86% of the AIDS patients of Belgian nationality are men. However, only 65% of the non-Belgian AIDS cases are male. The ratio of adult men to women is for all age groups larger than 2, except for the age group 20-29.

Relatively seen, there are more women who develop AIDS at a younger age. The age group 25-29 is the biggest among women. For men, on the other hand, 20% of the AIDS patients belong to the age group 35-39. When taking into account the variable "nationality", then the age group 30-35 is the biggest among women. Finally, it is in fact remarkable that 50.8% of the men and 62% of the women belong to the age group 25-39.

Looking at the distribution of AIDS patients between the different regions, we can see the same pattern as with HIV. Most of the AIDS patients (50.8%) live in the Brussels region, 26.9% of them in Flanders and 22.3% in Wallonia. These figures date from September 1993 and amount to 859 AIDS patients. The residence of 80 persons is unknown.

Figure 5.6:   Number of AIDS Cases according to Gender, Age Group and Nationality (September 1993)

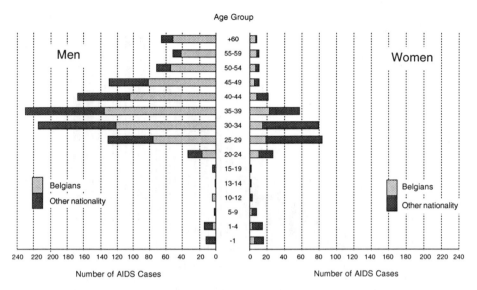

Source: I.H.E., *Three-monthly Report* No. 34.

Figure 5.7:   Number of AIDS Cases by Region (September 1993)

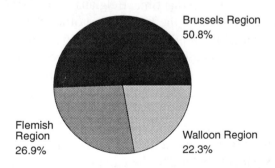

Source: I.H.E., *Three-monthly Report* No. 34.

In December 1993 the province was known for 947 of the 983 residential AIDS patients. A strong concentration of AIDS cases is to be found in Brabant (almost 60%) and another 13% of the AIDS patients live in the province of Antwerp (most of them around the city of Antwerp). The other Flemish provinces house less than 5% of the AIDS patients.

Figure 5.8: Number of AIDS Cases by Province (1993)

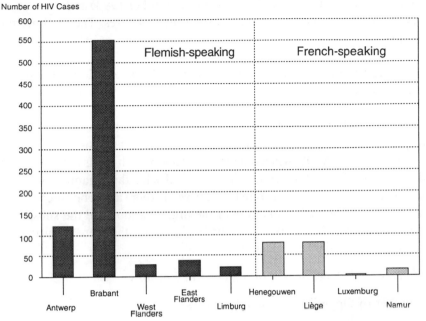

Number of HIV Cases

Note: The division between the Dutch-speaking provinces and the French-speaking provinces is not completely correct. The province of Brabant is composed of two Dutch-speaking districts, one bilingual district and one French-speaking district. We made the division, however, to give an idea of which provinces belong fully or partly to the Flemish Community.

Source: I.H.E., *Three-monthly Report* No. 34.

Table 5.4: Mortality by Year of Diagnosis and by the Duration of Observation (December 1993)

Year of Diagnosis	N	Cumulative Percentage of Deaths in AIDS Patients after x Years						
		1	2	3	4	5	6	7
<1985	18	51	58	75	83	83	92	100
1985	30	66	78	78	85	85	92	92
1986	38	59	74	84	87	90	90	94
1987	76	41	65	77	85	87	89	
1988	93	28	55	74	77	86		
1989	106	37	57	68	72			
1990	148	36	58	80				
1991	176	25	54					
1992	178	30						

Source: *Epidemiology of AIDS and HIV in Belgium*, November 1994.

Table 5.4 shows us information about the mortality of AIDS patients in Belgium. We were informed of a total of 424 deaths (by September 1993) and one lost track of 28 persons due to some physicians not reporting all cases. The total mortality rate amounts to 54%.

2   Mapping the Services and Development of Organizational Responses to HIV/AIDS

We will firstly analyse the volume and development of the overall response in section 2.1. Questions are treated such as: How many organizations have reacted to the phenomenon of AIDS, when did they react and which kinds of organizations reacted? Section 2.2 goes further into the subject of what the organizations are actually doing. In which subsector(s) are they active? Is there a link between the legal status or the organizational orientation of the organizations and the subsector in which they are active? In section 2.3 we try to find out if there are specific activities offered by particular organizations.

2.1   Volume and Development of the Overall Response

2.1.1 Number of Organizations and Activities

According to the criteria of the *Managing AIDS* project (see Chapter 1), a total of 51 organizations were identified in the field of HIV/AIDS in Flanders. These organizations provide about 224 activities – an average of some 4.4 activities per organization.

We can relate the number of organizations to the number of AIDS cases in Flanders. When doing so, one has to bear in mind that there are no figures available on the number of AIDS cases in the Flemish Community.[22] Here, we used the number of AIDS cases in the Flemish region (231) augmented by an estimated figure of the number of AIDS cases in the Dutch-speaking part of Brussels[23] (87 persons).

Table 5.5: Organizational Response in the Field of HIV/AIDS

	Number of Organizations	Number of Activities	Organizations per 100 AIDS Cases
Flanders	51	224	19.2

2.1.2 Organizational Development

In what is to follow, we take a look at the development of the different AIDS organizations. Generally speaking, the AIDS phenomenon is dealt with by rather new organizations in Flanders. However, a few older ones are also active in the field. As can be seen in Table 5.6, it was during the 1970s when 20.5% of the organizations were founded. However, another 25 organizations (51%) were set up in the 1980s and 1990s.

In the context of our chapter, it is more interesting to consider the year when HIV/AIDS activities were provided by the organizations for the first time. Table 5.7 shows the year when HIV/AIDS activities began in the different Flemish organizations. The first wave of HIV/AIDS activities was apparent in 1985; 75% of all organizations started their activities between 1985 and 1988 – reaching a peak in 1987.

The boom in 1987 might be explained by the increasing interest of the media in the phenomenon of AIDS. The first Belgian AIDS information campaigns began during this period. At the same time, the government took other different initiatives: Four AIDS reference centres were set up, as well as the IPAC and two PACCs – all in all seven organizations which explicitly dealt with AIDS. The AIDS team, which targets homosexuals (founded in a period when AIDS was seen as a homosexual disease), the STAG (Stichting AIDS Gezondheidszorg)[24], The Foundation

Table 5.6: Organizations in the Field of HIV/AIDS by Year of Foundation

Founding Year	Frequency	Percentage	Cumulative Frequency	Cumulative Percentage
< 1900	1	2.0	1	2.0
1900-1909	1	2.0	2	4.1
1910-1919	0	0.0	2	4.1
1920-1929	0	0.0	2	4.1
1930-1939	1	2.0	3	6.1
1940-1949	0	0.0	3	6.1
1950-1959	3	6.0	6	12.2
1960-1969	8	16.2	14	28.6
1970-1979	10	20.4	24	49.0
1980-1989	18	36.8	42	85.7
1990-1994	7	14.2	49	100.0
Total	49	100.0		

Frequency missing = 2

Table 5.7:   Organizations by the Year in which HIV/AIDS Activities Started

Founding Year	Frequency	Percentage	Cumulative Frequency	Cumulative Percentage
1980	1	2.1	1	2.1
1981	0	0.0	1	2.1
1982	0	0.0	1	2.1
1983	1	2.1	2	4.2
1984	1	2.1	3	6.2
1985	6	12.5	9	18.8
1986	9	18.8	18	37.5
1987	12	25.0	30	62.5
1988	9	18.8	39	81.2
1989	1	2.1	40	83.3
1990	4	8.3	44	91.7
1991	2	4.2	46	95.8
1992	1	2.1	47	97.9
1993	0	0.0	46	97.9
1994	1	2.1	48	100.0
	48	100.0		

Frequency missing = 3

and two other exclusive organizations were all new and started their activities during the above-mentioned period. Beside the foundation of these exclusive organizations, there were a lot of inclusives which started projects concerning HIV/AIDS. Figure 5.9 illustrates the start of activities according to the exclusive or inclusive orientation of the organizations. The cumulative frequency is also illustrated in the figure to show the increase in organizations which offer any kind of HIV/AIDS activity at all.

After an enthusiastic start, there was a decrease in new activities. It is, however, remarkable that four new exclusives were set up in 1990. This can probably be explained by the functions the new organizations fulfilled. Whereas the first exclusive organizations focus on more medical problems, general information and prevention; the later ones perform functions of care (e.g. self-help groups), interest representation and integration.

Looking at Figure 5.9, we can generally conclude that the first reactions concerning HIV/AIDS came from the inclusive organizations which started their activities immediately after the AIDS virus was discovered. From 1985 to 1988 the

**Figure 5.9: Start of the First HIV/AIDS Activities
by Organizational Orientation**

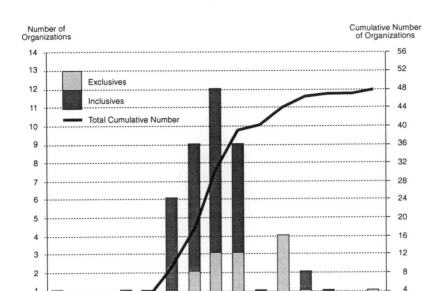

number of inclusives increased significantly. Some exclusives began activities at around the same time as the new inclusives and, thus, followed suit in the field of HIV/AIDS.

Another way to analyse the pattern in the emergence of HIV/AIDS activities is to compare them with the number of new HIV/AIDS cases during the same period. Figures 5.10 A to D illustrate these variables.[25]

On first glance, Figures 5.10 A, B, C and D show that the numbers of AIDS cases have been on a constant increase whereas the new numbers of HIV cases have been fluctuating from year to year. It was not until 1992 that the number of AIDS cases saw its first period of stabilization (even seeing a slight decrease in numbers).

From 1984 onwards, the number of new organizations starting AIDS programmes follows relatively closely to the pattern of the amount of new HIV cases. We can see the halt in 1989 as a momentary saturation of activities in the field. Looking at the cumulative figures, we can conclude that at the start, the activities increased faster than the new HIV/AIDS cases, but in 1992 there was a stabilization of activities.

**Figure 5.10: Start of New Activities Compared to the Development of New
             HIV/AIDS Cases**

A.   Number of New Activities and New HIV Cases

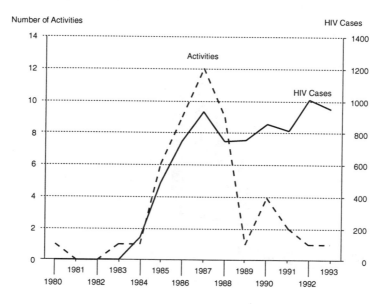

B.   Number of New Activities and New AIDS Cases

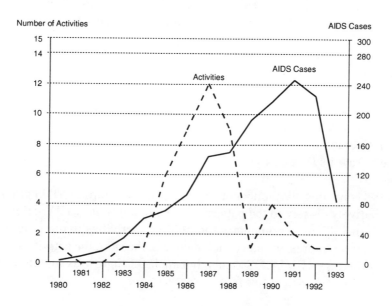

C.   Cumulative Number of New Activities and New HIV Cases

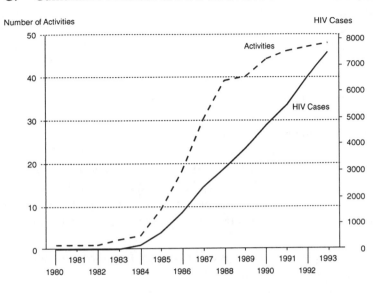

D.   Cumulative Number of New Activities and New AIDS Cases

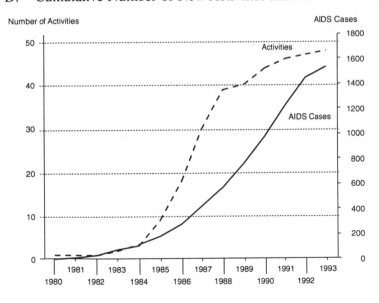

2.1.3 Organizational Responsiveness by Legal Status[25] and Organizational Orientation

Table 5.8.1 shows that most of the Flemish organizations (84%) are non-profit organizations. Most of these non-profit organizations (73.8%) are inclusives. The

private sector has no long tradition in the Belgian health care system. There are
only two active, private organizations in the field of HIV/AIDS. Strangely enough,
the public sector is neither very much represented (12% of the organizations).

Concerning the organizational orientation, 30% of the organizations are
exclusives, which means that they exclusively provide HIV/AIDS-related programmes. Among the exclusive organizations, 73.4% are non-profit organizations,
while 20% are public bodies. Among the inclusive ones, only 8.6% are public and
88.6% of the organizations belong to the non-profit sector.

Table 5.8.2 gives the figures on the organizational orientation according to the
new classification, namely Legal Status (2), which includes the categories governmental status/private and non-profit status. Governmental organizations considered here are organizations which have been established by the government.

In Tables 5.8.1 and 5.8.2 we see a change in the data, which supports the trend
that non-profit organizations are strongly represented in inclusive organizations,

**Table 5.8.1: Organizational Responsiveness by Legal Status and
Organizational Orientation**

Organizational Orientation	Exclusives	Inclusives	Total
Legal Status of the Organization			
Public Organization	3	3	6
Overall Percentage	6%	6%	12%
Column Percentage	20%	8.6%	
Row Percentage	50%	50%	
Private Organization	1	1	2
Overall Percentage	2%	2%	4%
Column Percentage	6.7%	2.8%	
Row Percentage	50%	50%	
Non-Profit Organization	11	31	42
Overall Percentage	22%	62%	84%
Column Percentage	73.3%	88.6%	
Row Percentage	26.2%	73.8%	
Total	15	35	50
	30%	70%	100%

Frequency missing = 1

Table 5.8.2: Organizational Responsiveness by Legal Status (2) and Organizational Orientation

Organizational Orientation	Exclusives	Inclusives	Total
Legal Status (2) of the Organization			
Governmental Organization	6	2	8
Overall Percentage	11.8%	3.9%	15.7%
Column Percentage	40%	5.6%	
Row Percentage	75%	25%	
Private Organization	1	1	2
Overall Percentage	1.9%	1.9%	3.9%
Column Percentage	6.7%	2.8%	
Row Percentage	50%	50%	
Non-Profit Organization	8	33	41
Overall Percentage	15.7%	64.7%	80.4%
Column Percentage	53.3%	91.7%	
Row Percentage	19.5%	80.5%	
Total	15	36	51
	29.4%	70.6%	100%

i.e. 91.7% of all inclusives are non-profit organizations. There is not such a strong majority of non-profits to be found among organizations which deal with HIV/ AIDS exclusively. The proportion of governmental exclusive organizations to non-profit ones is almost equal (40% governmental/53.3% non-profit). This also means that the government founded almost half of the exclusive organizations.

Looking at Legal Status (2) as an independent variable, 80.5% of the non-profit organizations are inclusives. A remarkable fact is that 75% of the so-called governmental organizations are exclusives.

2.1.4 Organizational Responsiveness by Region across the Different Subsectors

In this section, we examine the differences in the concentration of HIV/AIDS organizations in certain areas of Flanders (see Table 5.9).

Table 5.9: Organizational Responsiveness by Province

Province	Public Exclusives/Inclusives			Private Exclusives/Inclusives		Non-profit Exclusives/Inclusives		Total Exclusives/Inclusives	
Antwerp (province)		*(x)**						6	14
								(40%)	
Antwerp (city)	1	*(3)*	2	–	–	4	7		
Berchem	–	*(1)*	–	–	–	–	2		
Borgerhout	–		–	–	1	–	–		
Lier	–		–	–	–	–	1		
Mechlin	–		–	–	–	–	1		
Mortsel	–		–	–	–	1	–		
Brabant								6	9
								(30%)	
Brussels	1	*(1)*	1	1	–	2	5		
Leuven	–	*(1)*	–	–	–	2	2		
Tienen	–		–	–	–	–	1		
Limburg								1	2
								(6%)	
Genk	–	*(1)*	–	–	–	–	1		
Hasselt	–		–	–	–	1	1		
East Flanders								2	5
								(14%)	
Aalst	–		–	–	–	–	1		
Ghent	1	*(1)*	–	–	–	1	3		
St-Niklaas	–		–	–	–	–	1		
West Flanders								0	5
								(10%)	
Bruges	–		–	–	–	–	1		
Izegem	–		–	–	–	–	1		
Courtrai	–		–	–	–	–	1		
Ostend	–		–	–	–	–	2		

Missing Values = 1

* *(x)* = Number of organizations belonging to the category "Governmental Organizations" as a variable of Legal Status (2).

As one can see, HIV/AIDS organizations are mainly concentrated in two provinces: Antwerp and Brabant. The province of Antwerp contains 40% of all Flemish AIDS organizations. Most of these are situated in and around the city. Half of the governmental organizations are also situated in and around the city of Antwerp. Two of them are coordinating organs – the IPAC and the SOAA (LD Stedelijk Overleg AIDS Antwerpen / Municipal Deliberation AIDS Antwerp).

In Brabant, where 30% of all Flemish HIV/AIDS organizations are situated, a large proportion of them are located near Brussels. Two of the reference centres which the Government set up operate in Brabant, i.e. one at the University of Brussels and one at the University of Louvain. A possible reason for the concentration of organizations in these two provinces could be the relatively high number of AIDS cases apparent in these areas. However, it could also be due to the existence of universities and other important institutes like I.H.E. (Institute for Hygiene and Epidemiology) and ITG (Institute of Tropical Medicine).

One can discover the same pattern of concentration of organizations located in and around the bigger cities in the other provinces.

2.1.5 Organizational Responsiveness by Target Group and by Those Groups Most Affected

Most of the Flemish HIV/AIDS organizations (29) do not target a specific group; in fact, only 12 organizations specify a particular target group. These organizations are open to all those in need of their help, including foreigners (although one must add that five organizations only serve Belgian citizens). There are also five organizations that have no target group at all, but which coordinate other bodies in the field (Table 5.10).

Most of the organizations which serve a specific target group are inclusives and had already worked with that group before they integrated the aspect of AIDS into their work. Specific target groups are: youth groups, drug users, prostitutes, homosexuals, sailors, haemophiliacs and the medical profession.

While looking more closely at the organizations and their organizational orientation, we discovered a particular structure concerning the organizations and their target groups (Figure 5.11).

Table 5.10: Organizations and their Target Groups

Everybody (including Foreigners)	Citizens	Specific Target Group
29 (63%)	5 (10.9%)	12 (26.1%)

Frequency Missing = 5

Figure 5.11: Structure of the Flemish Organizations by Target Group

	Exclusives		Inclusives		
	Founded by the Government (1)	Others (2)	Founded by the Government (3)	Others General Organizations (4)	Target-group Oriented Organizations (5)
Target Groups addressed	No Specific Target Group (General Public)	Specific Target Group	No Specific Target Group (General Public)	Specific Target Group	Specific Target Group

The first group of organizations which we will consider is the exclusives established by the government. Here, we find the reference centres (three in total), the IPAC and the PACCs. These organizations do not target a specific group, but act in the so-called "interests of the general public". They offer some services for which the government is mainly responsible (screening, coordination, testing of research methods, etc.). A second group of exclusive organizations (nine in total) works for specific risk groups in the field of HIV/AIDS. Five of them explicitly target persons with HIV/AIDS, the other four aim to assist prostitutes, homosexuals, drug users or members of the armed forces.

The situation is similar for the inclusive organizations. There is a small group of governmental organizations (Group 3) and they also act in the interests of the public and are more or less connected to the first group.

Group 4 targets a large section of the public in the health care sector. Here, we find big organizations like the Health Insurance (Ziekteverzekeringen) and the CLGs (Centra voor Levens- en Gezinsvragen).[26] These organizations are involved with the AIDS problem because of their original interest in health promotion and education. The government obliges them to integrate some activities concerning AIDS into their programmes.

Finally, Group 5 consists of those organizations which target a specific population and have become involved with HIV/AIDS because of their target group. Here, we find organizations for the younger generation, homosexual men, drug users, sailors, prostitutes and organizations for people confronted with AIDS in their daily work (e.g. physicians). The big difference between Group 2 and Group 5 is the motivation behind these activities. The latter targets some risk groups and integrates the HIV/AIDS problems into its other activities relating to its specific target group. The former, however, works primarily with the problem of HIV/AIDS and only then addresses a particular risk group.

It will be interesting to look at sections 2.2 and 2.3.2 and at Figure 5.12 for differences between these five groups concerning the sort of activities they offer.

It is quite remarkable that not one organization is known which explicitly targets foreign people. However, one should in fact expect such an organization, in respect of the epidemiological figures as treated in section 1.3 (Epidemiological Development). There we saw very high figures of infection through heterosexual contact, especially in persons of non-Belgian nationality.[27] There are proposals to target this risk group in every policy note; but until today, no specific projects or organizations in the field of HIV/AIDS exist for these persons.

The groups most affected with AIDS (drug users, homosexuals and haemophiliacs) are, however, served by very specific organizations. Clearly, it is interesting to look at them in closer detail.

The haemophilia organization (see Table 5.11) is the oldest one. The AHVH (Vereniging van hemofilielijders en Von Willebrand-zieken)[28] has been in existence for more than 36 years and started its activities concerning HIV/AIDS in 1985 and, unlike many other organizations, has already had a relatively long hall of experience with HIV/AIDS since then. It targets a group of patients which have already

Table 5.11: Organizations which Target Those Groups Most Affected with AIDS

Target Group	Organization*	Founding Year of the Organization	Year when HIV/AIDS Programmes Started
Haemophiliacs	AHVH	1958	1985
Drug Users	ACT-UP	1990	1990
	ADIC	1986	1987
	VAD	1982	1988
	Katarsis vzw	1985	1985
Homosexuals	AIDS team	1987	1987
	GOC	1969	1980
	De Roze Drempel vzw	1969	1986
	WG H&G	1980	1985

* For a list of the organizations mentioned in this table with their full names and translations, see Appendix.

been accepted by society as "non-outcasts". The confrontation with a problem such as AIDS within that risk group was immediately treated by the already existing structure.

A few organizations had homosexuals as their target group. Two of them were founded in 1969 (GOC and De Roze Drempel vzw), a third one in 1980 and the AIDS Team in 1987.[29] Homosexuals have not yet been totally accepted by society and this does not seem to have changed very much over the years. Homosexuality came out into the open in the late 1960s, in the aftermath of the sexual revolution. At that time, the first organizations which focused on homosexuals started activities in the field of HIV/AIDS. During the first years after the discovery of AIDS, the disease was seen as a homosexual disease. The societal acceptance of homosexuals consequently slightly declined, and new activities in the field of HIV/AIDS began. It is clear that, generally speaking, the homosexual tradition is not as old as the haemophilian one, but this group could also lean on existing structures within its field.

The last risk group focused on here, is the one of the intravenous drug users. Compared to the other two groups, relatively new organizations are apparent which deal with HIV/AIDS, which means that activities in the field of drug use are rather new. This population is accepted by a very small proportion of society and is consequently still discriminated against. The first ever HIV/AIDS activities almost coincided with the foundation of these organizations in 1985. Perhaps AIDS and the importance of controlling this disease can push this group out of marginality.

2.2   Volume of Subsectoral Response

2.2.1 Numbers of Organizations and Activities across the Different Subsectors

Five different subsectors of activities were defined in the *Managing AIDS* project (see Chapter 1). The following table gives us the number of organizations and activities across these subsectors.

In Flanders, a lot of attention is given to prevention, education and information activities. More than 86% of the organizations provide one or more of these activities – 87 activities in total. This means that every organization which offers activities in that sector attends to two activities, on average. The power of this Prevention subsector is not surprising, judging by the methods needed to curb the AIDS virus, seeing as there is still no efficient medical solution to AIDS.

A second important subsector is Care. The 74 activities presented here focus on psychological care and individual counselling, free HIV-testing and referral services. Organizations which are active in this subsector have the highest average of activities per organization. Each organization provides a mean of 2.3 activities.

The subsectors "Control and Monitoring" and "Interest Representation" are not as popular. Nevertheless, they are offered by some 30% of the organizations. The average number of activities is 1.4 in the subsector.

Table 5.12: Organizations and Activities across the Different Subsectors

Subsector	Number of Organizations (N=51)		Activities (N=224)	Ratio Activities/ Organizations
	N	%	N	
Prevention	44	86.2	87	2
Care	32	62.7	74	2.3
Control and Monitoring	14	27.5	20	1.4
Interest Representation	17	33.3	32	1.8
Fund-raising	1	1.9	1	1
Other Activities	10	19.6	10	1

And finally, Fund-raising is not very prevalent in Flanders. As we mentioned before, most of the organizations are funded by the government and there is no large tradition of fund-raising.

Regarding the other activities, most of them come into other subsectors. Some such activities are: an HIV "talkcafé" (3 times), the coordination of an AIDS policy within the Belgian army, the selling of condoms, homosexual-specific consultations by a homo-physician (*Homo-arts* – a physician who is himself a homosexual) and the inspection of physician consultations.

2.2.2 Organizational Responsiveness by Legal Status across the Different Subsectors

In what is to follow, we look for a difference in the offer of activities between organizations with a different legal status.

If we consider the public and non-profit organizations, then the subsector of Prevention is quoted most in both cases. Care is also a popular choice for organizations.

If we look at the percentages given in Table 5.13, we find some differences between the public and the non-profit sector with respect to the subsectors of their activities. In the field of Control and Monitoring, we see a significant difference: 66.7% of the public organizations have some responsibilities in these fields whereas only 23.8% of the non-profit organizations do.

Another difference lies in the sector of Interest Representation. Half of the public organizations provide activities in this area whereas only 30.9% of the non-profit organizations do so. These figures are not in line with what one would expect. It is, in fact, unusual that public organizations are involved in interest representation. Which activities cause these results, is to be analysed in section 2.3.

If we look at the figures derived from our new classification, i.e. legal status (2), there are some shifting changes. Table 5.14 only shows the data for the governmental and non-profit organizations because nothing has changed within the private sector.

The figures according to the new legal status (2) show us two interesting facts. Within the sector of Prevention, 92.7% of all non-profit organizations provide activities in this area. This figure is very high; so this first subsector can be seen as very important to the non-profit organizations.

A second striking issue is the high number of governmental organizations which provide activities in the area of Control and Monitoring. Only 17% of the non-profit organizations have responsibilities in this field.

Another conclusion made on the basis of Table 5.13 must be moderated. There is only one governmental organization which offers activities in the subsector of Interest Representation. It is the non-profit organizations which prevail in this subsector.

While studying the subsectoral division of activities, we were also looking for differences between the organizations and their target groups. We again used the

Table 5.13: Organizations by Legal Status across the Different Subsectors

Subsector	Legal Status		
	Public (N=6)	Private (N=2)	Non-Profit (N=42)
Prevention	5 83.3%	1 50%	37 88.1%
Care	4 66.7%	1 50%	27 64.3%
Control and Monitoring	4 66.7%	0 0%	10 23.8%
Interest Representation	3 50%	1 50%	13 30.9%
Fund-raising	0 0%	0 0%	1 2.3%
Other Activities	1 16.7%	2 100%	7 16.7%

Frequency Missing = 1

four categories applied in section 2.1.5, namely the governmental organizations, the target group-oriented exclusives, the general organizations and the target group-oriented inclusives (see Figure 5.12).

In this figure, we present the percentages of organizations within a certain category[30] which provide one or more activities within the subsector[31] in question.

We can conclude that all types of organizations provide activities in the sector of Prevention. For the governmental organizations (the AIDS reference centres, the IPAC which is responsible for the coordination of the Flemish AIDS policy, the PACCs, etc), the most important activities are situated in the field of Coordination of the AIDS Policy (subsector Supervision). The target group-oriented exclusives are more or less active in all subsectors, but have an important task in the field of Interest Representation (here, we find organizations like ACT-UP, De Witte Raven [The White Ravens], The Foundation, the HIV Integration Center). The general organizations like the health insurance organizations concentrate on both the sectors of Prevention and Care.

Finally, the target group-oriented inclusives supply the most different number of activities. More then 30% of these organizations are present in each sector.

Table 5.14: Organizations by Legal Status (2) across the Different Subsectors

Subsector	Legal Status (2)	
	Governmental (N=8)	Non-Profit (N=41)
Prevention	5 62.5%	38 92.7%
Care	5 62.5%	26 63.4%
Control and Monitoring	7 87.5%	7 17.1%
Interest Representation	1 12.5%	15 36.6%
Fund-raising	0 0%	1 2.4%
Other Activities	0 0%	8 19.5%

Figure 5.12: Organizations by Target Group across the Different Subsectors

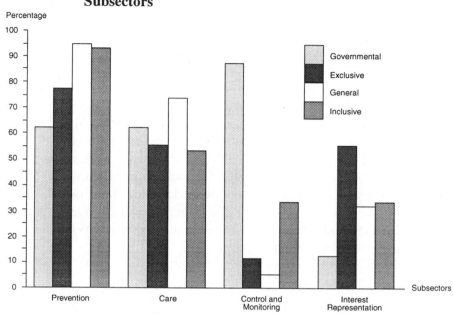

2.2.3 Organizational Responsiveness of Exclusives and Inclusives across the Different Subsectors

The most striking figure in Table 5.15 is the number of activities provided by the inclusive organizations in the subsector of Prevention. Almost all inclusives have one or more activities in this field; however, exclusives have much fewer, i.e. only 66.7%.

Another remarkable figure is found in the subsector of Control and Monitoring. We find that 46.7% of all exclusives offer such activities whereas only 20% of the inclusives do so.

2.2.4 Organizational Responsiveness by Region across the Different Subsectors

Table 5.16 gives us information on the geographical dispersal of the different subsectors. In general, the spread of the different activities is apparent in all provinces; it is only in Western Flanders that there is no regulating or controlling body. Most of the organizations are situated in the two provinces with high rates of HIV/AIDS cases, with a large expanse of activities at their disposal.

A striking figure in the table is the large number of organizations in the subsector of Interest Representation in Brabant. The province of Limburg has fewer than other areas. Even in the field of Prevention, there are only three organizations in the whole province which are involved in this subsector.

Table 5.15: Organizations by Organizational Orientation across the Different Subsectors

Subsector	Exclusive (N=15)		Inclusive (N=35)	
	N	%	N	%
Prevention	10	66.7%	33	94.3%
Care	9	60%	23	65.7%
Control and Monitoring	7	46.7%	7	20%
Interest Representation	5	33.3%	12	34.3%
Fund-raising	1	6.7%	0	0%
Other Activities	4	26.7%	6	17.1%

Frequency Missing = 1

Table 5.16: Organizations by Region across the Different Subsectors

Subsector	Antwerp	Brabant	Limburg	East Flanders	West Flanders
Prevention	18	11	3	6	5
Care	11	9	2	6	4
Control and Monitoring	5	5	2	2	0
Interest Representation	4	8	1	2	2
Fund-raising	1	0	0	0	0
Other Activities	4	4	0	1	1

2.3   Analysis of Activities – Who Does What and Why?

2.3.1 Distribution of Activities

What are the Flemish HIV/AIDS organizations exactly doing in the field? Table 5.17 enumerates all the different activities which figured in the inventory sheets and it shows the number of Flemish organizations which provide them.

Prevention is the most used subsector – 64.7% of all organizations offer education and information, and two other linked activities: AIDS Information Cam-

Table 5.17: Number of HIV/AIDS Activities Offered

	Number of activities offered	Percentage of organizations offering these activities
Prevention		
Hotline	3	5.9
Production of information material	15	29.4
AIDS information campaigns	17	33.3
Educational and information work	33	64.7
Drug-related prevention	8	15.7
Training of volunteers and health care professionals	11	21.6
Care		
Primary health care/medical services	9	17.6
Care/psychological support to people with HIV/AIDS	21	41.2
Face-to-face counselling	17	33.3
Home care services	1	2.0
Hospices, shelters, housing facilities	1	2.0
Voluntary HIV-testing and counselling	13	25.5
Buddy system	1	2.0
Referral services	10	19.6
Food bank	1	2.0
Control and Monitoring		
Epidemiological/social research	7	13.7
AIDS policy co-ordination and implementation	5	9.8
Control of blood/plasma product safety	2	3.9
HIV screening, testing, identification (contact tracing)	6	11.8
Interest Representation		
Self-help groups of people with HIV/AIDS	8	15.7
Counselling for insurance/welfare entitlements	6	11.8
Civil and human rights/protection against discrimination	9	17.6
Political lobbying	4	7.8
Legal advice	5	9.8
Fund-raising	1	2.0
Other activities	10	19.6
HIV talk-café	3	5.9
Condom distribution	1	2.0
Homosexual consultation by a homo-physician	1	2.0

paigns (33.3%) and the Production of Information Material (29.4%) are both widely mentioned.

People involved with the group: Care and Psychological Support of People with HIV/AIDS (and most of the time also of their direct environment) are more specifically dedicated to the people affected by HIV/AIDS. Of the Flemish organizations, 41.2% offer this kind of support and another 33.3% provide face-to-face counselling. This kind of psychological care is much more apparent than the more "practical" activities, e.g. a buddy system is only provided by one organization just as home care services, housing facilities and food banks are.

In line with tradition, medical activities score high with 25.5% of all organizations offering voluntary HIV-testing and counselling and 17.6%, primary health care/medical services.

2.3.2 Number and Type of Organizations across Selected Activities

It is also interesting to look at what kinds of organizations provide which types of activities. Some differences between the organizations and their activities and their legal status and organizational orientation were found, although somewhat unclear. We searched for some other factors within the classical division between public and private non-profit organizations to explain these differences. We also applied the structure presented before, based on target groups.

A few things are unusual in the subsector of Prevention. If we look at the figures concerning the Production of Information Material, we see that half of the governmental and half of the target group-oriented exclusive organizations provide these activities. The work done in the areas of education and information is provided by 94.7% of all general organizations (clearly the highest figure in the former table). The other types of organizations also score high in this activity. Drug-related prevention must, by law, be one of the tasks of the inclusive drug organizations. Training is provided by 44.4% of the target group-oriented exclusive organizations.

The two activities mentioned in the second subsector are carried out by all types of organizations. Care of and psychological support to people with HIV/AIDS is mostly provided by the inclusive general organizations. It is rather uncommon, however, in the category of the target group-oriented inclusives.

The most significant results concern the subsector of Control and Monitoring. It is almost only the governmental organizations which provide activities in this area. They concentrate on epidemiological research and AIDS policy coordination and implementation.

These governmental organizations are, on the other hand, completely absent in the sector of Interest Representation. Here, the target group-oriented exclusives are the most prevalent in these subsectors – especially concerning the activity of civil and human rights and protection against discrimination. A total of 26% of the inclusive target group-oriented organizations provide this activity.

Table 5.18: Activities Provided by the Organizations by Target Group

Organizations by Target Group Activities	Governmental Organizations (Inclusives & Exclusives) (N=8)		Target group-oriented Exclusives (N=9)		General Organizations (N=19)		Target group-oriented Inclusives (N=15)	
Prevention								
Hotline	–	–	1	11,1%	1	5.2%	1	6.6%
Production of information material	4	50%	5	55.5%	2	10.5%	4	26.6%
AIDS information campaigns	3	37.5%	3	33,3%	6	31.5%	5	33.3%
Educational and information work	4	50%	5	55.5%	18	94.7%	6	40%
Drug-related prevention	1	12.5%	–	–	1	5.2%	6	40%
Training of volunteers and health care professionals	2	25%	4	44.4%	5	26.3%	–	–
Care								
Primary health care/ medical services	2	25%	1	11.1%	5	26.3%	1	6.6%
Care/psychological support to people with HIV/AIDS	4	50%	4	44.4%	11	57.9%	2	13.3%
Face-to-face counselling	2	25%	3	33.3%	7	36.8%	5	33.3%
Home care services	–	–	–	–	1	5.2%	–	–
Hospices, shelters, housing facilities	–	–	1	11.1%	–	–	–	–
Voluntary HIV-testing and counselling	2	25%	1	11.1%	6	31.5%	4	26.6%
Buddy system	–	–	1	11.1%	–	–	–	–
Referral services	1	12.5%	3	33.3%	3	15.8%	3	20%
Food bank	1	12.5%	–	–	–	–	–	–

(Continued)

Organizations by Target Group Activities	Governmental Organizations (Inclusives & Exclusives) (N=8)		Target Group with Exclusive Orientation (N=9)		General Organizations (N=19)		Target Group with Inclusive Orientation (N=15)	
Control and Monitoring								
Epidemiological/ social research	4	50%	–	–	–	–	3	20%
AIDS policy coordination and implementation	5	62.5%	–	–	–	–	–	–
Control of blood/plasma product safety	1	12.5%	–	–	–	–	–	–
HIV screening, testing, identification (contact tracing)	3	37.5%	1	11.1%	1	5.2%	1	6.6%
Interest Representation								
Self-help groups of people with HIV/AIDS	–	–	3	33,3%	2	10,5%	3	20%
Counselling for insurance/ welfare Eentitlements	1	12.5%	2	22.2%	1	5.2%	2	13.3%
Civil and human rights/ protection against discrimination	–	–	4	44.4%	1	5.2%	4	26.6%
Political lobbying	–	–	1	11.1%	1	5.2%	2	13.3%
Legal advice	–	–	1	11.1%	3	15.8%	1	6.6%
Fund-raising	–	–	1	11.1%	–	–	–	–
Other Activities	–	–	4	44.4%	2	10.5%	4	26.6%

3 Summary and Policy Implications

3.1 Epidemiology

By the end of December 1993, at least 8,420 persons had become infected with HIV and by that time, 1,555 of them had already developed AIDS. Every day, two to three new HIV cases are registered. There are two times more men infected, but women are younger (as a rule) when they become infected. The most frequent ways of HIV transmission are through homo- and bisexual contact for Belgian men and heterosexual contact for Belgian women. For persons with another nationality, HIV/AIDS infection through heterosexual contact dominates for both sexes. Most of the infected persons live in the Brussels region, or in Brabant. The province of Antwerp also counts for a lot of the HIV cases.

In analysing the epidemiological evolution of the AIDS cases, we can divide our population into two groups. The largest one is the group of the residents (people probably infected in Belgium), the smallest one is the non-residents. The ratio between these groups has changed over time.

By the end of September 1993, 76% of the AIDS cases were male. The age groups most represented were the 35-39-year-old men and the 25-29-year-old women.

The geographical distribution of AIDS patients corresponds with that of the HIV cases. Most of the infected people live in Brabant and Antwerp and are concentrated around the bigger cities.

3.2 How Did the Flemish Organizations React to the AIDS Problem?

There is a relatively high number of AIDS organizations in Flanders – 19.2 organizations per 100 AIDS cases have been counted. These organizations are rather young because 50% of them were founded during the 1980s and 1990s, and 71% between 1970-1994. A lot of organizations started AIDS activities from 1985 onwards, reaching a peak in 1987. Afterwards, there was a stabilization in the new initiatives. A remarkable fact was that four new exclusives started up in 1990. These new organizations also offered new activities; these were directed at interest representation.

Most of the organizaions belong to the non-profit sector; the public sector is not very much represented. For the analysis of the legal status of the organizations, a new variable was constructed. The organizations were divided into governmental organizations, private organizations and organizations belonging to the non-profit sector. Only 15% of our organizations were governmental organizations and 80% were non-profits. Of the governmental organizations, 75% are exclusives. Of the non-profit organizations, however, 80% are inclusives.

The organizations are concentrated in and around the bigger cities. A high concentration is found around Antwerp and Brussels – the cities with the highest number of AIDS cases in Belgium, as well as containing important institutes like universities, the Institute for Tropical Medicine, etc.

The variable "target group" shed new light upon our data. We divided the organizations into four groups. The governmental organizations which target the interests of the public, the target group-oriented exclusives, the general organizations which target the public and the target group-oriented inclusives. The first group of organizations finds its most important task in the subsector of Control and Monitoring. The general organizations provide a lot of activities in the subsectors of Prevention and Care, while Interest Representation is more popular among the target group-oriented exclusives. The last group, i.e. the inclusives, provide an even spread of activities in all subsectors.

Looking at the division between exclusives and inclusives and the activities provided by these groups, we see that the inclusives are strongly orientated towards prevention activities. One interesting fact is that the exclusive organizations are never active in one subsector alone.

Concerning the activities, the governmental organizations take care of the epidemiological and social research and the AIDS policy coordination and implementation. The production of AIDS information material is provided by the exclusives (governmental and target group-oriented organizations), while educational and information work and psychological support are done by the general ones. Finally, the activities of civil and human rights and protection against discrimination are mainly provided by the target group-oriented exclusives.

3.3   Policy Implications

Belgium (Flanders) has reacted relatively rapidly towards the problem of AIDS. At the beginning, the government mainly concentrated on the medical aspects of the disease, but some organizations also reacted, and focused their attention on other aspects of AIDS. Today, the sector of Prevention is relatively widespread. The problems of coordination have partly been solved, but there is still not enough transparency in the different organs and structures.

A clear division of labour between the different categories of organizations is apparent in Belgium. This division is very prominent in the case of the governmental organizations which coordinate the AIDS field. They also produce information material together with other exclusives. The government itself has a certain control over all organizations as it grants money to certain AIDS projects. It must therefore be possible to build up an effective network of organizations and projects, when keeping in mind the division of labour analysed.

Looking at the Flemish data, we can also detect some deficits, which are interesting for the future AIDS policy. As has already been mentioned, there is an urgent necessity to target foreigners living in Belgium. This necessity already figures in different policy notes, however, we do not have any organizations in our directory which specifically cater for this group. Prevention material (e.g. folders) does exist in various languages (including Arabic), but in respect of the high number of non-Belgians infected with HIV through heterosexual transmission, there is a great need to organize *specific* activities geared towards this group. It could well be useful to contact the organizations which target foreign people to offer them information material specifically created for these groups.

The lack of offered practical health care by the organizations is also clearly evident. Many organizations provide psychological support to HIV/AIDS patients, but there is only one organization which organizes the buddy system which is very relevant for AIDS patient support, and one organization that offers home care.

However, activities such as legal advice and counselling for insurance/welfare entitlements are also minimally represented.

Finally, we think that structures like the AIDS Panel (AIDS overleg) and the AIDS Unit (AIDS cel) are very useful and should be further supported in the future. Coordination and cooperation should result in an effective AIDS policy in Flanders.

Notes

1   We would like to thank the Flemish Minister of Employment and Social Matters, Ms. Léona Detiège. Without the useful advice on the Flemish AIDS policy from her cabinet, and her financial support, this report would not have been able to come to fruition. We would also like to thank all the organizations which reacted and cooperated thereby enabling us to carry out our research – especially the Vlaams AIDS-Coördinaat, i.e. IPAC (The Flemish AIDS Coordination Centre), for their expert information about the Flemish AIDS problems, as well as those organizations which answered our questions, despite their busy activities.

2   After the Belgian reformation, she was divided into three communities (The Dutch- , the French- and the German-speaking) and three regions (The Flemish, the Walloon and the region of the capital, Brussels). The communities are responsible for cultural matters, education and personally-linked matters, whereas the regions for the more locally connected matters (eg. area planning, the environment, economics, etc.).

3   These ministries are:
     • The Ministry for Social Integration, Public Health and the Environment (organization and control of the blood banks).
     • The Ministry for Justice and for Economic Affairs (discrimination).
     • The Ministry of Scientific Policy and Infrastructure (research programmes on AIDS).
     • The Ministry of Employment and Labour and for the Equality of Chances (labour legislation).
     • The Ministry for Social Affairs (AIDS reference centres, reimbursement of costs incurred through HIV tests).
     • The Ministry for Foreign Affairs/Secretary of State for Development Aid (cooperation with foreign countries).

4   In Belgium, it is the Red Cross that screens the blood for HIV-antibodies. The AIDS reference centres confirm these HIV tests. If a new positive blood sample is found after such a second test, the seropositive case is reported. Afterwards, there is no obligation to report the fact that an HIV patient has developed full-blown AIDS; however, most physicians register the new cases anonymously on the basis of standardized forms. These forms must be sent to the AIDS Commission which checks the cases on their conformity with the AIDS definition and analyses the epidemiological development.

5   RIZIV: Rijks Instituut voor Invaliditeits Verzekering (National Sickness and Invaliditiy Insurance Institute).

6   See IPAC vzw Vlaams AIDS-Coördinaat (1993) *De strijd tegen AIDS in Vlaanderen. Strategisch plan voor preventie en zorg,* p. 16-18.

7   Royal Decree for the Foundation of a Supreme Council for the Coordination of the Combat against AIDS.

8   De Ryckel (1989) *Het AIDS-beleid: Een Sociologische Analyse.* Eindverhandeling (Thesis). Catholic University of Leuven: Faculty of Social Sciences, Department of Sociology, p. 82.

9   Four of them in the Flemish part of Belgium, and four in the french-speaking part.

10 Two other ministers have some significant say in the AIDS policy:
    • Minister of the Government of Flanders for Finance and the Budget, Health Institutions, Social Welfare and the Family (home health care, decisions in clinics, some inclusive AIDS organizations).
    • Minister of the Government of Flanders for Education and the Civil Service (prevention at school).

11 IPAC: Vlaams AIDS-Coördinaat (Flemish AIDS Co-ordinate).
    VIG: Vlaams Instituut voor de Gezondheidspromotie (The Flemish Health Promotion Institute).

12 IPAC vzw, *Naar een globale aanpak van de AIDSproblematiek in Vlaanderen?*, p. 3.

13 Detiège L., *AIDS in Vlaanderen. Beleidsnota 1993 van de Vlaamse Minister van Tewerkstelling en Sociale Aangelegenheden* (Minister of the Government of Flanders for Employment and Social Affairs).

14 Detiège L., *Beleidsnota 1993*, p. 51. Detiège L., *Beleidsnota 1993* (revised version, February 1993), p. 21.

15 ITG: Institute of Tropical Medicine.

16 PACC: Provincial AIDS Coordination Committee.

17 Only the Limburg PACC (nowadays called Limburgs Overleg AIDS) functioned. In Antwerp, the PACC was founded as the Stedelijk Overleg AIDS Antwerpen or SOAA (Municipal AIDS Consultation of Antwerp), because the field of work was concentrated on the town of Antwerp.

18 NFWO: National Fund for Scientific Research.

19 The most remarkable point is the increase in the budget for the target group of AIDS patients and seropositive people. There is also a higher amount of money foreseen for the education of intermediaries and for coordination.

20 Including the 25,000,000 for scientific research.

21 IPAC vzw, *Naar een globale aanpak van de AIDSproblematiek in Vlaanderen?*, p. 4.

22 cf. Part 1.3 on the epidemiological figures ('Number of AIDS cases by region').

23 The ratio of Dutch-speaking persons to French-speaking persons in the Brussels Region differs according to different sources. We took the cabinet of the Minister President of the Brussels Metropolitan Region as our source of information, which uses a ratio between 15 and 30%. So we estimate that 20% of the AIDS patients in the Brussels Region belong to the Flemish Community, i.e. 87 persons.

24 STAG: Foundation AIDS Health Care

25 While studying the Belgian (Flemish) data, it became clear that the variable "Legal Status", which contains the categories "public", "private" and "non-profit" sectors, was not useful. The difference between the public and the other sectors is not that strict anymore. There is no clear definition of what a public organization actually is. We analyse such problems in the first part of this chapter.
    As mentioned previously, the IPAC was founded by the government to coordinate and execute the AIDS policy in Flanders. One could, therefore, consider the IPAC to be

a public organization or a governmental organization at least. However, the IPAC defines itself as legal status "vzw" (vereniging zonder winstoogmerk: Association without Purpose or Gain). Many organizations have the status of vzw – even the reference centres founded by the national government have this status. This makes it very difficult to agree on a relevant difference between the public and the non-profit sector. We also found some inconsistencies in the inventory sheets which had been filled in by the organizations: e.g. three out of the four reference centres said they were non-profit organizations whereas the fourth said it was a public organization.

A second problem lies in the fact that almost all Flemish (AIDS) organizations have to be approved by the government. As we have seen earlier (see the explanation of the VIG), the VIG can support projects or organizations. The IPAC is an example of such an organization, but almost all other inclusive and exclusive organizations also receive an organization subsidy from the government or extra funding due to a project they have presented. So every organization is at least partly dependent on the government and, thus, can be seen as a kind of semi-governmental organization.

To solve this problem we defined a new variable, namely "Legal Status (2)", which distinguishes, instead of the public organizations, those organizations founded by the government (within the framework of the AIDS policy) from the private organizations and the rest of the non-profit organizations. We will call the newly-created category "governmental organizations".

26 CLG: a family planning centre.
27 See the epidemiological figures in section 1.3 relating to infections by route of transmission.
28 AHVH: The Belgian Haemophilia Society.
29 This targets not only homosexual people but it is an exclusive AIDS organization which offers a special programme for homosexual men.
30 Governmental organization, target group-orientated exclusives, general organizations or target group-orientated inclusives.
31 Prevention, Education and Information; Health Care and Social Services; Control, Intelligence, Surveillance and Monitoring; Policy Advocacy, Interest Representation, Civil and Human Rights, etc.

References

Brankaerts, J. (1987) 'Beleids- en hulpverleningsstructuren t.a.v. de AIDS-problematiek', in Baro F. e.a., *AIDS: Een multidisciplinaire aanpak.* Brussels: F.C.L.G. (Federatie Centra voor Levens- en Gezinsvragen).

De Rycke, L. (1989) *Het AIDS-beleid: Een Sociologische Analyse.* Thesis, Catholic University of Leuven, Faculty of Social Sciences, Department of Sociology.

Detiège, L. (1993) *AIDS in Vlaanderen.* Beleidsnota 1993 of the Minister for Employment and Social Affairs of the Government of Flanders.

Detiège, L. (1993) *AIDS in Vlaanderen.* Beleidsnota 1993 of the Minister for Employment and Social Affairs of the Government of Flanders (revised version, February 1993). Brussels.

I.H.E. (1992) *De epidemiologie van AIDS en HIV-infectie in België.*

I.H.E. (1993) *Trimesteriële rapporten over de toestand van AIDS in België* no. 33-34.

IPAC (1993) *De strijd tegen AIDS in Vlaanderen, strategisch plan voor preventie en zorg.* Antwerp.

IPAC (1993) *Naar een globale aanpak van de aidsproblematiek in Vlaanderen?* Antwerp. Unpublished.

Peeters, H. (1991) *Het AIDS-beleid in Vlaanderen. Een organisatiesociologische doorlichting.* Leuven: Sociological Research Institute, Catholic University of Leuven.

VIG, *Informatiemap.* Brussels: Flemish Institute for Health Promotion.

Vlaamse Executieve (1993) 'Besluit van de Vlaamse Executieve inzake Gezondheidspromotie', 31 July 1991, *Belgisch Staatsblad 28/11/1991: 26714-26719.*

Vlaamse Raad (1993) *Beleidsbrief Preventieve gezondheidszorg 1993-1997.* Flemish Ministry.

Appendix

AHVU	Association des hémophiles / Vereniging van Hemofilielijders (The Belgian Haemophilia Society)
ADIC	Antwerps Drug Interventie Centrum (Antwerp Drug Intervention Centre)
VAD	Vereniging voor Alcohol- en andere Drugproblemen (Association for Alcohol and other Drug-related Problems)
AIDS Team	The AIDS-Team
GOC	Gespreks- en Onthaalcentrum (Centre for Discussion and Reception)
De Roze Drempel	The Pink Barrier
WG H&G	Werkgroepen Homoseksualiteit en Geloof (Working Groups: Homosexuality and Belief)

CHAPTER 6

Managing AIDS. Organizational Responses to HIV/AIDS in Austria

Patrick Kenis
Christiana Nöstlinger

Introduction

Austria is generally speaking a country with a well-developed and rather comprehensive health and welfare system. The core of it, however, was developed prior to 1980, i.e. before the HIV/AIDS crisis became apparent. In this chapter we aim to evaluate how, on the one hand, the existing Austrian health and welfare system has reacted to this new and particular phenomenon by analysing its organizations, and, on the other hand, how other organizations outside the established health and welfare system have dealt with the new problem. We also enquire into the fact whether, as well as which and how new organizations have been created in order to effectively deal with the epidemic.

In the first section of the chapter we will present the institutional and epidemiological context in which HIV/AIDS activities have developed in Austria: Austria's public policy, the existing health and welfare structure, the situation of specific groups regarding HIV/AIDS and the HIV/AIDS case-load and its development. In the second section an overview will be given of the organizational response to HIV/AIDS as it developed within the specific contexts described in section 1. The overall organizational responsiveness, the development of specific areas of activities (prevention, care, etc.) as well as the development of specific single activities (condom distribution, buddy systems, needle exchange, etc.) will be discussed and related to the types of organizations which provide them. In a final part, policy implications will be formulated, indicating how the overall organizational responsiveness and effectiveness of specific types of organizations as well as the distribution of these activities could be stimulated through public policy interventions.

1   Policy Conditions: The Institutional, Social and Epidemiological Context

1.1   AIDS Policy in Austria

In Austria, the Federal Ministry of Health, Sports and Consumer Protection is the main public authority responsible for AIDS policy. Other ministries such as the Ministry for Youth and Family Affairs, the Ministry for Labour and Social Affairs or the Ministry of Justice are only marginally involved in any AIDS policies. The implementation of the policies formulated by the Federal Ministry of Health, Sports and Consumer Protection is the responsibility of the regional and local authorities, i.e. the *Länder* – since Austria is based on a federal constitution.

Before discussing the general social and health care structure as it is available to persons with HIV or AIDS, we will discuss the main cornerstones of the specific Austrian HIV/AIDS policy in short, i.e. the policy which has been developed on a federal level within the Ministry of Health.

The first initiatives were implemented rather early on in Austria in comparison to the rest of Europe. It was already in 1983 (when the first AIDS cases amongst homosexual men were diagnosed) when the reporting of AIDS cases was made obligatory. By then, the Supreme Health Council's AIDS Commission was founded as an advisory body to the Ministry of Health. Apart from the AIDS Commission, three other significant public policy initiatives regarding HIV/AIDS have been realized since then: The AIDS Law, national information campaigns and the constitution and support of the *AIDS-Hilfen*.

In 1993 the Ministry of Health issued the "AIDS Information and Prevention Concept" (Bundesministerium für Gesundheit und Konsumentenschutz, 1993). Interestingly enough it has not been published, serving only as an internal working document. By choosing this strategy, a public debate on the content and goals of this concept has been avoided, although this is exactly what has already been requested by the community for quite some time. In the concept, prevention goals are formulated as well as suggestions on how to reach them.

The document recommends a division of labour with respect to the provision of information on HIV/AIDS: The ministry considers itself responsible for conceptualizing, printing and providing materials for the general population, whereas the regional *AIDS-Hilfen* and the *AIDS-Informationszentrale Austria* (the clearinghouse and documentation centre for the AIDS-Hilfen) and other organizations active in the field of HIV/AIDS should produce information material for specific target groups, such as drug users or homosexual persons. On a practical level, this division of labour has been in place for many years now. As a result of this concept, the last brochure which targeted women was produced in 1985 by the former national Austrian AIDS-Hilfe; the most current brochure which targets young people was produced in 1987. The most current brochures by the Ministry of Health address health-care workers and sex tourists.

1.1.1 The AIDS Commission

In 1983 the *Austrian AIDS Commission* was set up by the Ministry of Health as one of the first health policy measures for HIV/AIDS. The commission is made up of experts from the areas of dermatology, epidemiology, hygiene, internal medicine, immunology, social medicine, virology and blood-bank experts. The AIDS Commission is expected to meet regularly and give suggestions as to health policy measures; it acts as the advisory body to the Ministry of Health regarding AIDS and is primarily directed towards the prevention of the further spread of HIV/AIDS.

This advisory board has been criticized by many non-profit organizations active in the field of HIV/AIDS. Representatives of the most affected communities were excluded from the board, and so were professional health care or social workers with expertise in this field. Social scientists were neither heard. Thus, the Austrian AIDS Commission did not abide to WHO-standards, which clearly recommend close cooperation with communities directly or indirectly affected by HIV/AIDS. Although a representative of the regional *AIDS-Hilfen* has been sitting on the commission since 1985, it's agenda is still very biased towards technical questions and deals primarily with the medical aspects of HIV/AIDS.

1.1.2 AIDS Regulations and the AIDS Law

An important public policy measure was enforced in 1986 – the Austrian AIDS Law. It was considered necessary because the then-existing regulations referring to epidemics and STDs were not considered to be generally applicable to the case of HIV infection and AIDS (i.e. the *Epidemiegesetz* [The Law of Epidemics] and the *Geschlechtskrankheitengesetz* [The Law of Sexually Transmitted Diseases]). The *Maßnahmen gegen die Verbreitung des erworbenen Immundefektsyndroms* (Measures against the Spread of the Acquired Immune Deficiency Syndrome), as the law was called, was amended in 1989, 1991 and 1993 and is now called the *Aids Gesetz 1993* (The 1993 AIDS Law). It points out the following:

- The conditions for an AIDS diagnosis (i.e. a positive HIV-antibody test and at least one AIDS-related disease).
- The mandatory anonymous reporting of AIDS cases (not of HIV) and deaths caused by AIDS by general practitioners, hospitals and pathologists.
- The prohibition of HIV-positive sex-workers from working and the obligatory regular three-monthly compulsory HIV test for sex-workers.
- The requirement of mandatory pre-test counselling and the passing on of information to HIV-positive diagnosed persons by physicians.[1]
- The regulation of the quality control of HIV-antibody tests and blood screening.

- The instruction to the Ministry of Health to monitor and fund studies on the epidemiological development of HIV/AIDS.
- The requirement of a comprehensive information concept issued by the Ministry of Health regarding the HIV routes of infection and prevention measures.
- The stipulation that activities concerning the counselling and care of persons with AIDS provided by institutions and associations can be funded on a federal level. Such institutions can only be funded in relation to their case-load and on the condition that they have a physician at their disposal.

In addition to this law, there are several decrees and recommendations as to the measures of hygiene in hospitals, the undertaking of an HIV-antibody test within the bounds of hospital treatment, drug-rehabilitation programmes, research on sources of infection, etc.

The AIDS Law and other regulations reflect the main philosophy behind the AIDS policy of the Ministry of Health in Austria fairly well: a combination of rigorous rules on regulating and administrating the disease (on HIV tests, sex-workers, reporting, etc.) and some half-hearted and weakened WHO standards (advocating HIV-test counselling to only a limited degree; a commitment to a comprehensive AIDS information campaign which is poorly specified with respect to its implementation; a rather weak statement on funding non-profit organizations with, at the same time, strong rules on the conditions for financing – WHO, 1990).

1.1.3 National Information Campaigns

As has been mentioned above, the AIDS Law specifies that the Ministry of Health is responsible for the preparation and implementation of comprehensive information campaigns. The ministry's goal is to inform the public about HIV/AIDS, especially regarding the ways of transmission and preventive measures. The most important features of these public campaigns can be summarized as follows: on average, such campaigns are implemented once a year and last for about one month (on the radio, television and billboards). Generally, they have not been directed towards any particular target group; they carry very general preventive messages, and only sometimes anti-discrimination messages, and up until now, only once have the campaigns been explicit enough to show a condom on billboards. This may explain why only 75% of the Austrians perceive condoms to be a useful tool in preventing HIV, while condom acceptance in the population still seems to be very low. In 1992 only 45% of all people aged 14 to 49 years of age showed positive attitudes towards condoms (Bundesministerium für Gesundheit und Konsumentenschutz, 1993).

The public information campaigns are regularly evaluated by large polls: they concentrate on the awareness of the population of the campaigns, their effects, as well as the behaviour of the population. Interestingly enough, however, these polls hardly seem to have an influence or an impact on the prevention policy. Political considerations seem to exert more of an influence however. The substantial messages to be communicated by the 1994 prevention campaign were changed because of a fear of negative results in the approaching elections (*Falter* 30/1994: 8). Instead of dealing with sexuality in an explicit but humorous way it was decided to target young people via role models and pop-culture celebrities. However, this particular campaign constituted the first effort ever to target young people via a special TV-campaign. It was well received by young people: Of 3318 interviewed adolescents, 90% remembered the information that condoms provide an effective protection against HIV, 64% remembered social integration of HIV-infected persons as an additional aim of the campaign. A third of those young people who do not use condoms on a regular basis intend to do so in the future after having seen the video-clips of the 1994 public AIDS campaign (Wimmer-Puchinger, 1995).

One of the main problems of the Austrian prevention campaigns, however, is that they are poorly funded. As far as funding is concerned, in 1992 for example, Austria spent about US$ 400,000 on public prevention campaigns (compared to $ 2,000,000 in Germany and $ 1,000,000 in Switzerland). In 1993 this budget was increased to $ 800,000 (Kenis/Marin/Nöstlinger, 1994).

1.1.4 Supporting the AIDS-Hilfen

In 1985, the *Österreichische AIDS-Hilfe* (ÖAH) was founded as a service organization for people directly and indirectly affected by HIV/AIDS. Besides primary prevention, its main task was to assist infected people by combining self-help programmes with professional assistance. The ÖAH had its roots in community-based organizations which targeted homosexual men – the group most affected by the epidemic at that time. Also, thanks to some committed and open-minded civil servants at the Ministry of Health, the ÖAH, being financed by the Ministry, could develop a broad range of activities to deal with the spread of HIV/AIDS and its social consequences. This Austrian model – a national organization financed by the state, with its roots in the community affected – was also considered by WHO as a good model to deal with the problem. WHO tried to convince other countries to follow it. The creation of the ÖAH – originating in a collaboration between the community, a highly committed physician and civil servants – could not guarantee a conflict-free cooperation in the years after 1985. The ÖAH, as an independent non-profit organization – though exclusively financed by the state – developed new initiatives which were not always approved by the funding Ministry of Health. An additional conflict developed between the regional outlets in the federal provinces and the national "headquarter". Seeking more autonomy, some of the regional AIDS-Hilfen opposed the centralized management. As a result of ongoing conflicts the ÖAH was closed down in 1990 and totally restructured. Since 1991, regional Austrian AIDS-Hilfen, each independent organizations, have been operating in seven of the nine Austrian federal provinces. Although the regional AIDS-Hilfen are now expected to raise funds mainly on the regional level (where they are successful only to limited and varying degrees), the Ministry of Health is still the main funding agency of the regional AIDS-Hilfen with about $ 3,400,000 annually.

This turn of events in 1990 led to the virtual disappearance of the national AIDS community. Whereas this community was politically very active and visible between 1985 and 1990, now, organizations seem to be struggling along more individual paths without raising much public awareness.

On summarizing the Austrian HIV/AIDS policy one can conclude that the current approach reaffirms a tradition of centrally integrated policy-making, i.e. mainly formulating and implementing regulations from above with little participation by those affected, and by providing very general messages of information.

1.2   The General Health and Welfare System

As described in more detail in Chapter 1 of this volume, the country studies presented concentrate on the HIV/AIDS activities which have developed in a specific and specialized way. The analysis therefore excludes those activities which are provided by the health and welfare structure in a general way (the so-called inclusive inclusive organizations[2]). However, in order to compare countries regarding the situation of people affected, it is also important to have a knowledge of the general context, i.e. of those structures which are generally, and not exclusively available to HIV/AIDS-affected persons. As far as the availability of such general offers is concerned, there are two possibilities. Firstly, generally available services (such as medication, care, social security, etc.) are often also available to HIV/AIDS-affected persons. Secondly, however, it can be that services which are generally available to everybody are – in the case of HIV/AIDS – not so generally accessible or offered. These we call "silent resources" since they keep "silent", or, in other words, are less available and accessible to HIV/AIDS-affected persons. Instances of such silent resources will be identified and described in somewhat more detail in section 2.1.2.

1.2.1   Primary Health Care and the Insurance System

Structures for primary health care are not fully developed in Austria. As effective primary health care should combine medical, psychosocial and social services, this lack has significant consequences for both the prevention of HIV and the treatment of persons living with AIDS. Although Austria accepted the WHO guidelines "Health for All 2000" in 1978 as one of its primary goals in health and social policies, the coordination of social and medical services has not yet been achieved. Relating the existing situation of primary health care in Austria to the WHO standards, the following can be concluded: Diagnostic and curative services are widely offered, too few prevention and rehabilitation services have been implemented so far, and existing welfare and social services do not relate to the health care system. In general, training for health care professionals does not include concepts of primary health care. Health care is mainly financed by the compulsory insurance system, aiming at the treatment of acute diseases and hardly considering prevention activities. The data which will be presented later will reflect these observations to a significant degree.

With respect to the insurance system, however, it is crucial to look at its accessibility first. The Austrian social insurance system (i.e. health insurance, pension insurance and accident insurance) is a compulsory one, which currently covers 99% of the population. Compulsory health insurance covers medicine (with a prescription charge to be paid), medical treatment, therapeutic substances (with a share of 10-20% to be paid by the insured person), general dental treatment and dentures (with a relatively large share to be paid by the patient for high-quality technical items), and in-patient treatment and hospital costs (with an index-linked daily charge to be paid by the patients not exceeding a maximum of 28 days). Roughly a third of the population (e.g. 38% in 1990) have an additional private health insurance. The benefits of additional private health insurance are better hospital accommodation, reduction of waiting time for examinations and the treatment by a physician of one's choice (Rack, 1992).

In the next paragraphs we will briefly examine how these general conditions affect people with HIV/AIDS and how the health care system actually responds to their particular needs.

1.2.2 Hospital Care and Medication

People affected directly by the epidemic, such as PWAs (people living with AIDS) or HIV-infected people who become ill, are mostly treated in the AIDS wards of departments of internal medicine or dermatology in public hospitals. General access to these facilities is granted and so is medication. AZT, as an example of drugs available for the treatment of HIV infection, like any other anti-viral drug, is covered by health insurance and given if prescribed. Currently, three drugs are approved for prescription in Austria, Zidovudine (AZT), DDI and DDC.

With respect to the care of AIDS patients, the integration between hospital facilities and other forms of formal and informal care is somewhat underdeveloped. Some hospitals have already started to closely cooperate with out-patient clinics, day clinics, or networks of home care services. A barrier to these efforts is that home care services are generally not very active in the field of HIV/AIDS. A new legislation covering the expenses for home care services has not existed long enough to be evaluated in terms of its effectiveness for AIDS patients.

Compared to other countries, AIDS patients in Austria seem to have a relatively low life expectancy, particularly when the long-term prognoses of people living with AIDS are compared with those of other European countries (Zangerle/ Klein, 1994). Moreover, it seems that the rate of people dying of AIDS within the first three months after diagnosis is extremely high in the metropolitan area of Vienna. The relative risk of people diagnosed and of dying within this three-month period appears to be three times higher than for patients living elsewhere in Austria (OR=3.2; revealed by multiple logistic regression). This is a particularly unexpected result taking into account that everyone is generally covered with health insurance and that the overall accessibility to the medical system is granted – even to anti-viral therapies. Thus, possible reasons for this worrisome fact may go beyond medical explanations: In many cases a significant delay in the HIV diagnosis seems to exist and, consequently, the same is true for the reporting of AIDS. For the affected individual, a late diagnosis leads to a delay in treatment, which then has a significantly reduced efficacy. Particularly, if patients do not belong to what still many physicians perceive as the typical "AIDS risk group", diagnoses are delayed. This not only occurs due to a lack of medical training, but has to be understood in a societal context where AIDS is still considered to a large extent as a self-inflicted disease of certain groups. In addition, such a societal climate also influences the affected individual's health behaviour. While feelings of rejection may also play a role, the realistic fear of discrimination might further aggravate the reluctance to consult the medical system. Given the geographical differences in survival times, substantial differences in the access to and the quality of the AIDS-specific medical and psychosocial treatment seem to exist throughout the country. This issue still requires further scientific investigation, however.

1.2.3 Care Allowances

A care allowance legislation regulates the financial allowances for people in need of care services, giving them the option to choose between all different types of care services available – and to pay for them. The degree of care allowance received depends on the hours of care needed; this is decided on by expert approval usually by physicians (in rare cases it can also be performed by social workers and other qualified professionals). It remains to be seen if this type of financing will actually result in a better provision of home care services due to a broadened and improved offer of services. It might depend on the general social situation of the people affected, whether they can afford to spend the money received on home care services and other support mechanisms in the end or whether they will use the money received just to cover their daily living expenses. First experiences show that this indeed seems the case for many people living with AIDS since the disease leads to a significant reduction in their income.

1.2.4 Psychosocial Support Structures

The emotional and psychosocial well-being of somebody being infected with HIV clearly affects his/her ability to cope with the disease. This may directly or indirectly influence the progression of the HIV disease, and indeed growing evidence of psychoneuroimmunological AIDS research suggests that psychosocial factors eventually play a potential role in delaying its progression. Moreover, the provision of psychosocial support increases the subjective living quality of people with HIV/ AIDS (Franke, 1990). Consequently, psychosocial and psychological support must be considered crucial activities in HIV/AIDS-related service provision.

Counselling and the various forms of psychosocial support in general are either delivered by statutory or non-profit organizations. A network of decentralized psychosocial services (*Psychosozialer Dienst*) has been partially implemented to function as a provider of basic mental health care (covering psychiatric out-patient care and rehabilitation from psychiatric disorders, illicit drug use and other forms of dependencies, as well as individual counselling for a broad range of critical life events). Besides this basic network, a number of organizations provide psychological counselling, ranging from church-affiliated to feminist organizations. Psychotherapy, as an intensive form of counselling and psychological introspection, is partly covered by health insurance. Although being HIV-infected is not necessarily a sufficient precondition for the indication of psychotherapeutic treatment, this coverage could potentially improve the psychosocial situation of people affected with HIV/AIDS. It would, however, require a sufficient number of psychotherapists on the "free market" being willing to treat clients with HIV/AIDS-related problems. But so far even psychotherapists – as most professional groups in psychosocial services – have been reluctant to integrate these clients.

1.3 The Situation of Specific Groups in Austria

More than a decade into the AIDS epidemic, it has also become clear that certain social groups have been more affected by the epidemic than others. Among these groups are: homo- and bisexual men, intravenous drug users (IV-drug users), ethnic minorities and young people. Women in general, but in particular those who belong to the latter three groups, are even more affected than their male counterparts. Haemophiliacs are a group that were extremely at risk of HIV infection in the first years of the epidemic, today still constituting a considerable portion of AIDS patients. In what is to follow we will briefly describe the social and health context of these groups most affected by HIV/AIDS in Austria.

1.3.1 Homo- and Bisexual Men

Within the Austrian gay community, as in most Western countries, the threatening existence of HIV has transformed the norms and attitudes towards unprotected sex to a certain extent. Available evidence suggests that men who label themselves as gay perceive condom use as a normative and effective means of preventing infections (Bochow, 1994). While this is true for certain groups of gay men, it is by no means true for all people with homosexual practices. Accepting safer sex norms obviously has much more to do with social norms than with sexual practices. Here it has to be noted, however, that some significant barriers to homosexual self-identification still exist in Austria. For years now there has been pressure from the community to abolish the specific laws that discriminate against and criminalize homosexual persons. This legislation (§209, 220 and 221 of the Austrian Penalty Law) contains three major points which are all relevant to aspects of HIV prevention: first, the age of consent for homosexual acts is not equal to the age of consent for heterosexual acts; second, the law prevents the setting-up of organizations which aim at the promotion of homosexuality; and third, the promotion of homosexual lifestyles (e.g. via brochures, billboards and any other media) is illegal.

Contrary to this existing situation, it is generally known that a social atmosphere which accepts homosexuality constitutes an essential part of structural prevention. The legal framework would be one of the most important prerequisites to combat both the subtle discrimination and the structural violence to which persons with a homosexual lifestyle are exposed in everyday life.

The social situation of people with a homosexual lifestyle varies a lot across different regions. While the gay community in urban areas has created some structures (social meeting places, counselling centres, activist groups, etc.), it is still difficult to set up similar support mechanisms in the rural regions. Some efforts have been made in this respect, but with fairly limited success due to the existing homophobia in Austrian society.

1.3.2 IV-Drug Users

Epidemiological figures on illicit drug use in Austria are scarce. Estimations are hard to give and range around the figure of 23,000 for so-called "hard-drug users". In Vienna alone, 103 drug deaths were reported in 1993 ("Wiener Drogenbericht 1992/1993", 1994: 15).

It is often argued that due to the political and economic changes in the neighbouring states, i.e. in the countries of Central and Eastern Europe, more and higher-concentrated heroine is being supplied, which would explain the increase in the drug problem. It is difficult to either falsify or verify this "anecdotal" knowledge since detailed studies neither exist on the drug market nor on the drug consumer.

However, in their effort to tackle the drug problem, policy-makers mainly follow a medical and regulative approach (Pfersmann/Presslich, 1994: 26; 145). In 1985 a harsh narcotics law was introduced. According to this law, exemption from punishment for consumers is only possible if the accused undergoes an obligatory therapy. The Methadone Act of 1987 – the other important legal measure with respect to illicit drug use – represents, to a certain extent, a deviation from abstinence as the aim of treatment. Methadone programmes, however, are limited and strongly regulated. Other measures such as a more liberal law with respect to the possession of drugs or a distinction between soft and hard drugs are not considered to be politically feasible.

In evaluating the approach used so far, one could conclude that the medical solution has not proven to be successful in solving the drug problem.

Most of the institutions which deal with drug patients have waiting lists between three and six months for detoxification and therapy; this poses a major barrier for the motivation of patients willing to undergo such treatment. The situation for methadone treatment is similar: Not everybody who is to go on a rehabilitation programme can get treatment right away. The policy that HIV infection is a prerequisite in order to qualify for a methadone programme is highly controversial.

The general supply of substitution drugs (e.g. methadone) also varies considerably, that is, across regions. Consequently, drug users are generally dependent on the access to illegal drugs. As a result, they may have to turn to crime, are at risk of HIV or hepatitis infection and perhaps may die of a drugs overdose.

Recently, the number of young adolescents dependent on various types of drugs has also increased. There is no particular institution which provides adequate services for this group. Young people are either dealt with in drug institutions, setting the grounds for "typical drug careers", or in departments for child and adolescent psychiatry, where no specialized drug-related services are provided.

While in other areas of professional medicine active participation by patients is seen as a useful tool for treatment, efforts of drug users to organize themselves are hardly tolerated by the medical establishment. Drug user self-help groups have tried to get started (e.g. the Junkie Bond in Vienna), but have failed so far. None of them, however, have ever received any public support.

1.3.3 Prisons

The number of HIV-infected persons in Austrian prisons has reached 56 cases in 1992[3] (Pont/Kahl/Salzner, 1994: 168). A quarter of these persons can be accounted to the CDC-stage IV, meaning that they have already developed manifest symptoms of severe immunodeficiency. The HIV seroprevalence in Austrian prisons is estimated to be five times higher than in the general population (approximately 1% and 0.18% respectively; Kunz, 1992). Most of them are reported to be IV-drug users. It is estimated that 5% of the prison-population have been using IV-drugs. Since sterile needles and condoms are generally not available in prisons and drug-related and sexual risk behaviour is evident, prisoners are at a particularly high risk of HIV transmission.

Prison inmates who suffer from AIDS are treated in special hospital units or discharged once they fall seriously ill. Substitution treatment for drug users in prison is possible, but is actually only implemented to a limited extent.

1.3.4 Haemophiliacs

Currently, approximately 700 persons are suffering from haemophilia in Austria; 21% of this group are HIV-infected. The annual routine screening of all factor VIII products was introduced in Austria in 1985; however, almost all haemophiliacs became infected before this time. All those persons who have been infected with HIV through infected blood have received compensation. It was negotiated that people had to refrain from suing the pharmaceutical industries when accepting such a financial compensation. However, when it turned out in 1993 that patients had become infected by life-saving drugs even after 1985, the medical companies were sued nevertheless. These trials are still going on and pensions for the patients affected are under discussion. In general, haemophiliacs feel that they are not adequately represented and that their situation is not fully understood in society. Even most interest organizations for haemophiliacs tend to primarily deal with issues of financial compensation; the psychosocial needs of persons suffering from haemophilia – be they infected with HIV or not – are hardly met.

1.3.5 Women

Compared to other Western European countries, the theoretical equality of both sexes in Austria has been put into practice to a somewhat lesser degree than elsewhere (e.g. labour market participation, political and social decision-making, participation in leading positions, etc.). This clearly influences the woman's control over her social situation.

With respect to the woman's health status, fewer women than men describe their state of health as excellent (28% as compared to 36%). Fifty-five per cent of women (as compared to 47% of men) think that they suffer from ill health – complaints which have been labelled by a male-dominated medical science as "the female syndrome" (fatigue, headaches, insomnia, etc.). However, the reason for this fact might have much more to do with the woman's lower social status in society than with a "typical female proneness to psychosomatic disorders".

Women as an affected group are less visible, service offers targeting women are scarce. However, recently a trend towards more women-specific or women-friendly services has been observed, which could be interpreted as an acknowledgement of the above-mentioned gender differences. But although the number of women's self-help groups, for instance, has increased during the last decade, initiatives are still few: the existing ones range from prenatal treatment to women's self-help after cancer treatment. The main objective of these self-help initiatives is to offer an alternative to the patriarchal health system. Existing women's projects and democratic grass-roots initiatives (e.g. the recent initiatives to combat violence against women) organized by and for women can be understood as one way to respond to the hierarchical and anti-women structures of male-dominated political institutions. With a constantly growing number of HIV-infected women, Austria faces similar patterns with respect to the epidemiological development as observed in many other European countries. Women in Austria want to participate more in social decision-making without a doubt, but the more these interests lie in socially marginalized spheres, the more it is difficult to become visible and get support.

1.3.6 Young People

HIV prevention for young people can only be effective when embedded in the context of an overall sexual health education; this concept emphasizes not only the biological but also the psychological and social components, such as attitudes towards HIV/AIDS, aspects of adolescent sexual relationships and social and communicative skills in this context. While it is true that sexual behaviour has undergone some changes during the last two or three decades, many of the taboos related to human sexuality in general, and to adolescent sexuality in particular, still exist. The public debate in Austria is first and foremost concerned with the issue as to who should provide sex education, the parents or the schools? Studies have shown that many parents experience difficulties in talking to their children about sexual matters, and if they do, the information provided often does not suffice. Parents have been seen to consider comprehensive sex education in schools as an additional support to this sensitive educational task (Wimmer-Puchinger/Schmitz, 1994). Furthermore, sex education would have to react to the reality that adolescents are sexually active: 43% of all Austrian adolescents have their first experience of heterosexual intercourse at the mean age of 15.5 years. More than a third of all adolescents do not use any form of contraception at this "psychosexual milestone" (Nöstlinger/Wimmer-Puchinger, 1994). A recent evaluation of the effectiveness of sexual education programmes in Austrian schools revealed that only 47% of adolescents aged 14 to 18 had received any form of sex education.

Information on how to avoid the unwanted consequences of sexual behaviour should not be withheld from adolescents, if we are to reduce teenage pregnancy, abortion rates and HIV transmissions in this age group. In this light, however, it is striking that in particular conservative catholic pressure groups still oppose sex education in schools as well as the abortion law.

Some groups of young people are of particular concern with respect to health promotion and sex education, mostly because they are out of school or are part of psychologically or socially marginalized groups: unemployed youths, homosexual adolescents, drug-using adolescents, young girls who have experienced sexual violence, and adolescents from ethnic minorities.

1.4   The Epidemiological Development in Austria

The development of new AIDS cases in Austria has been increasing not only in absolute numbers (see Figure 6.1), but also each year compared to the previous year (see Figure A2, Annex I). By the end of 1994, 1,340 AIDS cases were reported, of which 994 have died.

Figure A1 in Annex I compares AIDS cases and AIDS ratios in Austria to other countries. Two different groups can be determined with respect to the AIDS ratio: Countries with an AIDS ratio above 250 cases per 1 million inhabitants (France, Italy, Spain and Switzerland) and countries with an AIDS ratio less than 250 cases per 1 million inhabitants (Austria, Belgium, Germany, Hungary, the Netherlands, Portugal, Sweden and the United Kingdom).

Since there is no mandatory reporting of HIV in Austria, no exact figures on HIV infections can be given. Approximately 4,500 persons are aware of their HIV infection, whereas it is estimated that in addition to this number, between 4,500 and 10,500 persons are HIV-infected without knowing about their immune status.

As Figure 6.2 shows, the regional comparison in Austria reveals some strong differences between the Austrian federal provinces. Vienna and Upper Austria have the highest number of reported AIDS cases. The highest number of female AIDS cases is reported in Vienna, followed by Upper Austria and Styria which is due to the distribution of routes of transmission regarding AIDS, which also differs from region to region.

Figure 6.3 shows that in Austria the transmission of AIDS is most prevalent from homo- or bisexual contact. AIDS cases due to intravenous drug use rank second, but are on the rapid increase. For women, intravenous drug use and heterosexual contact are the two predominant routes of transmission. Here, the gender dimension is important since more women with AIDS have been infected by way of heterosexual contact than men. The figure shows that the transmission category "unknown/other" ranks third. In terms of prevention it would be worth-while to hypothesize about how infections could have arisen in this group. This is not simple and two clues should be noted (which are shown in Figure 6.4): the age distribution and the development of new infections in this group corre-spond with those in the group of heterosexual transmissions. Therefore, hetero-sexual transmission in Austria could have contributed to many more AIDS cases than the official AIDS statistics reveal at first sight. This must still remain specu-lative, however.

Due to the relatively high overall number of AIDS cases related to heterosexual transmission, Austria has a particularly individual character when it comes to the epidemiological pattern of European countries: the main route of transmission for countries in the north of Europe is still homosexual contact, whereas for countries in Southern Europe it is intravenous drug use.

In terms of routes of AIDS transmission, regional differences can be observed: Most of the AIDS cases in Vienna, Styria, Salzburg and Lower Austria have occurred through homo- or bisexual contact, whereas regions more to the west report most of their AIDS cases coming from IV-drug users.

Figure 6.4 shows the age distribution at the time of diagnosis of people living with AIDS. The difference between the two main routes of transmission (homo- and bisexual contact, intravenous drug use) is salient. Both groups show typical

Figure 6.1:   Cumulative Numbers of PWAs and AIDS Deaths (1983-1994)

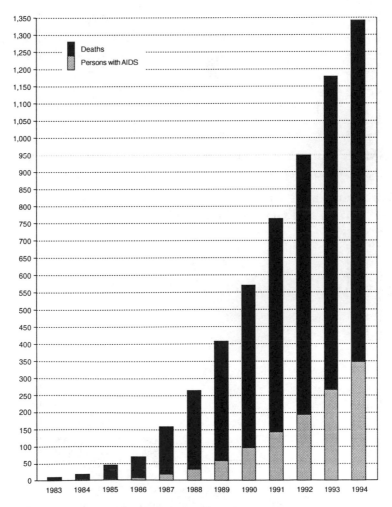

Source: Bundesministerium für Gesundheit und Konsumentenschutz, Sektion Gesundheitswesen, *Österreichische AIDS-Statistik, Periodische Berichte.*

**Figure 6.2:   Regional Distribution of AIDS Cases in Austria
by Gender (1983-1993)**

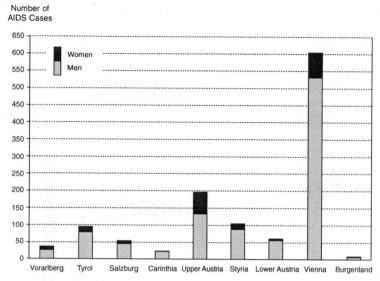

Source: BM für Gesundheit und Konsumentenschutz, Sektion Gesundheitswesen, *Österreichische AIDS-Statistik, Periodische Berichte.*

**Figure 6.3:   Cumulative Numbers of PWAs by Transmission
Group and Gender (1983-1993)**

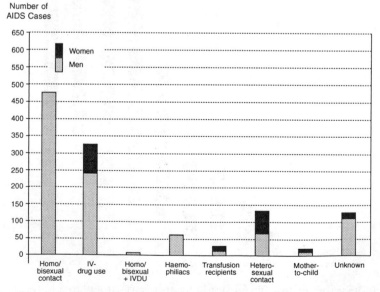

Source: BM für Gesundheit und Konsumentenschutz, Sektion Gesundheitswesen, *Österreichische AIDS-Statistik, Periodische Berichte.*

Figure 6.4: Age Structure of Austrian AIDS Cases (1993)

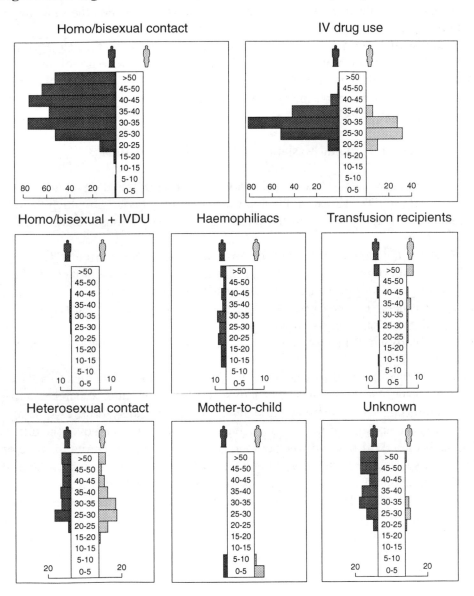

Source: Bundesministerium für Gesundheit und Konsumentenschutz

patterns: Among IV-drug users with AIDS, persons aged 30-35 are most affected. However, among homo- or bisexual men two age groups are most affected: persons aged between 30-35 and 40-45. This indicates that there are two different age cohorts, which probably differ also socially. Such differences would have to be considered in terms of prevention strategies even within one and the same target group.

Heterosexual transmission is relatively evenly distributed among all age groups. Most affected are men and women aged between 25 and 30 years of age. This indicates that – given the incubation period between HIV infection and the onset of the disease – many people in Austria had probably already become infected during their adolescent years.

2   The Organizational Response to HIV/AIDS in Austria

In this section we will describe and analyse the organizational development regarding HIV/AIDS in Austria. First, we will give an overview in which the different types of responses are all analysed together. The questions to answer in this first part are:

- How can the degree of this overall Austrian response be interpreted?
- Do types of organization (legal status, inclusive and exclusive, function of organization) differ in their degree of organizational response?
- To what degree is the overall organizational response distributed across geographical regions and social groups?
- And, finally, how did the organizational response as it exists today develop over time?

In a second part we will give a similar analysis to the one above, this time however, analysing each different area of activities (prevention, care, research, control and monitoring, interest representation, fund-raising) separately. From this, we aim to answer the question as to what the overall response distributed over the different areas of activities is and whether there are certain types of activities more or less predisposed to be offered by certain types of organizations. Finally, in a third part, certain single and most relevant activities (e.g. condom distribution, information work, self-help, etc.) will be presented and discussed in more detail. The main questions to be answered in this part are twofold: on the one hand, the sheer quantitative distribution of these activities and, on the other hand, the question as to how the provision of these activities is related to certain types of organizations.

2.1   The Overall Organizational Response

2.1.1 Number of Organizations in the Field of HIV/AIDS

According to the selection criteria outlined in Chapter 1, a total of 105 organizations are active in the field of HIV/AIDS in Austria. On average, about 6 different types of activities are provided per organization; in total 645 activities are provided by all organizations.

Table 6.1: Organizational Response to HIV/AIDS in Austria

Number of Organizations	Organizations/ 100 AIDS Cases	Organizations/ Rate per Million Citizens	Number of Activities
105	7.5	14.6	648

The general question as to whether this organizational response is major or minor, or whether it is "sufficient" or not, is difficult to answer. Table 6.1 relates the number of organizations to the number of AIDS cases and the number of citizens. It is, however, difficult to effectively analyse these figures for a single country. It is fully indeterminate how many organizations should be active for how many citizens or persons with HIV/AIDS. An alternative way to interpret this figure is, first, to compare it to the figure of other countries. This helps to relate the organizational response to the size of the country as well as to the country's case-load. A second approach which would make sense of these data is to analyse the ratio of organizations dealing with HIV/AIDS in a specific country to what would theoretically be possible if all organizations were active that potentially could be involved in HIV/AIDS-related activities (this pertains to what will later be referred to as "silent resources"). Thirdly, one can analyse the degree to which the organizations are distributed across geographical areas, target groups and organizational types. This last analysis, which will give indications as to the structural causes leading to the organizational responses other than the AIDS case-load, will be extensively dealt with later.

When we compare the number of organizations in Austria to that of the other participating countries in the "Managing AIDS" project, Austria belongs to the middle group regarding the total number of organizations per country (see Chapter 1). From the same data, it also becomes clear that a relationship between the AIDS case-load or number of citizens and the degree of organizational response in the field of HIV/AIDS does not exist. The reason why Austria does not figure at the lower end regarding its overall organizational response is probably, first, because Austria is a well-developed welfare state in which many organizations already existed in the field of health and welfare long before the problem of HIV/AIDS was recognized; secondly, because Austria has a federal structure with many separate provincial competencies in the field of health and welfare. Given these institutional factors, the question arises, however, as to why Austria is not at the higher end when compared to other countries. Here, the reason may be that the state is considered to be the appropriate centre of response to HIV/AIDS in Austria. This implies that the problem is defined above all as a medical and administrative one which can best be dealt with by the medical sector as well as by the administrative regulations. Thus, the development of a broad and varied range of organizations in the field of HIV/AIDS has not been promoted.

2.1.2 Overall Organizational Responsiveness by Type of Organization

I.   LEGAL STATUS

Table 6.2 indicates that, as everywhere in Europe, it is also in Austria that private businesses play next to no role in coping with the social dimension of AIDS (i.e. with respect to prevention, care, research, control and monitoring and fund-raising activities).

Austria seems to display a relatively high degree of *etatization* due to the country's relatively high proportion of public organizations in the field of HIV/AIDS (38%) from an international perspective. The overall European distribution is about 1/3 public to 2/3 voluntary non-profits – about 1/4 to 3/4 in the USA.

However, compared to other sectors in health and welfare within Austria, the fact that more than half of all organizations are private non-profit institutions makes them cross-sectorally a rather exceptional example of *associationalism*. Consequently, cross-national comparison leads to opposing conclusions in comparison to those of comparing sectors: AIDS policies seem to be more state-centred in Austria than elsewhere in Western Europe, but more private non-profit oriented than most other health and welfare policy fields in Austria today. At this point it is too early to explain this discrepancy. It will become more clear when we discuss the division of labour which exists between the non-profit and public sector regarding the provision of specific activities in sections 2.2 and 2.3.

II.   ORGANIZATIONAL ORIENTATION

With respect to organizational orientation, about 1/5 of all organizations exclusively deal with HIV/AIDS (see Table 6.2). The significance of this rate is difficult to interpret as such. To make sense of this data, it should again (1) be compared with data from other countries in this volume, (2) be related to how this rate influences the provision of specific activities (which is done in sections 2.2 and 2.3) or (3) it should be related to an analysis of silent resources, i.e. an analysis of what is and what is not generally done by inclusive organizations in the health and welfare sector. Conclusions on this will be formulated in the last part of this chapter after having presented the data on the different levels of analysis.

When analysing the cross-tabulations in Table 6.2, it becomes obvious that public organizations generally tend to provide HIV/AIDS activities beside other activities (only one state organization is exclusive). While 2/3 of private non-profit organizations also deal with HIV/AIDS inclusively (65% inclusives vs. 35% exclusives), exclusive organizations tend to choose the legal form of private non-profits: 96% of all exclusives are non-profit associations (Table 6.2). This phenomenon will also be more closely analysed and explained below.

Table 6.2: **Organizational Responsiveness by Legal Status and Organizational Orientation**

Organizational Orientation	Exclusives	Inclusives	Total
Legal Status of the Organization			
Public Organization	1	39	40
Overall Percentage	1%	37%	38%
Column Percentage	4.3%	47.6%	
Row Percentage	2.5%	97.5%	
Private Organization	0	2	2
Overall Percentage	2%	2%	2%
Column Percentage	0%	2.4%	
Row Percentage	0%	100%	
Non-Profit Organization	22	41	63
Overall Percentage	21%	39%	60%
Column Percentage	95.6%	50%	
Row Percentage	35%	65%	
Total	23	82	105
	22%	78%	100%

III. ORGANIZATIONAL FUNCTION

What kind of organizations are active in the field of HIV/AIDS in Austria? According to Table 6.3, those dealing exclusively with HIV/AIDS, or the so-called AIDS service organizations (ASOs), are the second-largest group of organizations. Among the organizations dealing with HIV/AIDS inclusively, those who offer HIV/AIDS programmes in drug treatment institutions are the largest group, but even in terms of absolute numbers, they come up slightly more frequently than ASOs. The number of different activities provided by the group of ASOs is, however, significantly higher than activities provided by drug service organizations. Health authorities rank third before interest groups and hospitals.

An interesting polarization can be observed among the inclusives: on the one hand, a large group of medically-oriented institutions (which can be interpreted as another confirmation of the observation that the medical approach is very prominent in Austria), and on the other hand, a relatively outspoken, large group of organizations which represents the social interests of those communities affected.

Table 6.3:   Types of Organizations

	Number of Organizations	Percentage excluding ASOs	Percentage
AIDS Service Organization (ASO)	19	18.1	–
Drug Treatment Centre	23	21.9	26.7
Health Authority	15	14.2	17.4
Self-help and Interest Group	14	13.3	16.3
Hospital	10	9.5	11.6
General Welfare Organization	9	7.7	10.5
Research Centre	6	5.7	7.0
Family Planning Centre	4	3.8	4.6
University	4	3.8	4.6
Legal Authority, Prison	1	1.0	1.2
Total	105	100	100

Organizations other than medical institutions and community organizations are very poorly represented in Austria, i.e. general welfare organizations, youth organizations, women's organizations, prisons, etc. This phenomenon will also be more closely analysed and explained below.

IV.   "Silent Resources" in the Field of HIV/AIDS in Austria

The organizational responsiveness in a country can also be evaluated by comparing the actual organizational response to what would theoretically be possible, if all or almost all potential organizations were involved. Table 6.3 has shown us that most of the organizations involved in HIV/AIDS-related activities in Austria are actually either AIDS service organizations (exclusive organizations), drug organizations or health authorities, all of which are very closely linked to HIV/AIDS. However, it is rather impossible to define the potential of all possible actors with regard to HIV/AIDS in a particular country. In order to come closer to its *accurate estimation*, we looked at the area of prevention and information related to HIV/AIDS in more detail. In an additional survey, we addressed 1,210 organizations from the overall health and social sector, which we considered to be possible providers of HIV/AIDS prevention activities. The survey unravelled some interesting facts: We could not only confirm that there were indeed no other organizations active apart from the 105 we had already identified, but could analyse the type of organizations which keep silent when it comes to HIV/AIDS. Organizations which target women, young people or families, which could use their resources to reach their target groups by adding HIV/AIDS to their agenda, are generally not involved in any AIDS-related prevention activities. The same is true for companies and private firms or the various branches of the trade unions.

2.1.3 Distribution of Organizational Responsiveness

When evaluating the organizational response on an overall level, it must obviously be considered how these organizational responses are distributed along different dimensions. The questions then are: Whether or not and why the organizational response is distributed evenly among the different social groups affected or whether it is distributed evenly or not between the different geographical areas, etc. Is an uneven distribution across social groups, for example, an indication for group-specific services, case-loads or does it indicate that some groups get more resources allocated than others? These are important questions not only for a better understanding of the organizational responsiveness but also for the evaluation of the situation of those affected.

I.   DISTRIBUTION ACROSS SOCIAL GROUPS

To some extent, an analysis of the target groups of the organizations active in the field of HIV/AIDS runs parallel to what has been said on the types of organization. One of the most important lessons learned from more than a decade of HIV/AIDS-related prevention experiences is the greater effectiveness of group-specific programmes. Prevention activities which address specific target groups allow for a

Table 6.4:   Organizations by Target Group*

	Number of Organizations	Percentage of Organizations
No Specific Target Groups	29	27.5
PWAs/ HIV+ Persons	18	17.1
Drug Users	24	22.8
Homo-/Bisexual Persons	10	9.5
Young People	8	7.6
Health Workers	3	2.8
Haemophiliacs	2	1.9
No Personal Services	7	6.7
Other	4	3.8
Total	105	100

*   "target group" refers to an organization's *primary* target group more direct response to the needs of certain groups rather than the vague, general messages which go out to the masses through very general campaigns.

Given this, it is interesting to observe that 27.5% of all organizations active in the field of HIV/AIDS in Austria do not address any specific primary target group. Our data show that some groups of people who have specific needs with respect to HIV/AIDS, e.g. young people or women, are only targeted by organizations to a minor extent. This again has to do with the minimal involvement of inclusive organizations.

Finally, 7% of the organizations active in the field of HIV/AIDS do not offer any services to persons at all, but coordinate other bodies' policies, e.g. the *AIDS Commission* as a case in point of a purely consultative and coordinating body.

II. DISTRIBUTION ACROSS GEOGRAPHICAL AREAS

In what follows, an analysis will be made as to what extent the federal provinces differ in how they promote HIV/AIDS-related activities. The next table gives us an overview of this analysis by showing the number of organizations in each of the nine federal provinces.

Forty-four per cent of all organizations are to be found in Vienna, which, as the capital and at the same time one of the nine federal provinces, is located in the east of the country. More than 50% of all AIDS cases have been reported in Vienna; therefore the demand for specific activities will doubtlessly be higher there than in any other region. The reason for this could be that the anonymous atmosphere of a big city attracts persons falling ill with AIDS or that the political and societal

Table 6.5:   Organizations by Region and Number of AIDS Cases

Federal Province	Number of Organizations	Percentage of Organizations	Percentage of all AIDS Cases
Vienna	46	43.8	51.0
Lower Austria	2	1.9	4.6
Burgenland	1	0.9	0.9
Upper Austria	14	13.3	16.6
Salzburg	7	6.6	4.4
Tyrol	8	7.6	8.8
Vorarlberg	13	12.4	2.9
Styria	10	9.5	8.8
Carinthia	4	3.8	1.8
Total	105	100	100

context of most of the provinces does not favour activities in the field of HIV/AIDS as much as would be needed. Finally, the high number of organizations in Vienna can also be explained by the fact that almost all organizations operating with a national geographical scope are also located in Vienna.

While it is clear that an organization's location only indicates its scope of activities to a minor extent, it should also be mentioned at this point that the decentralization of the Austrian *AIDS-Hilfe* (ÖAH) was also encouraged to stimulate more activities within the single provinces, especially through subsidies by the provinces. So far, neither a substantial increase in the financial contributions by the provinces nor a substantial increase in the level of activity of most AIDS-Hilfen could be observed. The decentralization of the AIDS-Hilfen has obviously not (yet) resulted in the hoped-for push for innovations on an organizational level.

2.1.4 The Development of Organizational Response, 1981-1993

Table 6.6 shows that the majority of organizations were founded during the last decade, i.e. since the time when AIDS became acknowledged as a health problem. The foundation of these organizations between 1981 and 1993 is, however, not solely due to the creation of organizations only dealing with HIV/AIDS. Interestingly enough, of the 46 organizations founded in or after 1981, 27 (i.e. 55%) are organizations which deal with HIV/AIDS among other activities. In comparison, 22 exclusives were founded in the same period. Of all the inclusive organizations, however, 24 organizations (47%) were founded before 1981, and 27 organizations (53%) were founded thereafter. This indicates that those organizations founded before 1981 have stayed relatively absent from the new problem HIV/AIDS.

More relevant than age is the year when HIV/AIDS activities were first provided when analysing organizational responses. Just over a quarter of all organizations, including the ÖAH, started their activities in 1985 and 1986, instigating a great surge towards institutionalization, accompanied by corresponding attention from the media. Apart from 1991, in which 14 new organizations were founded in the course of the regionalization of the Austrian AIDS-Hilfe, this 1985/1986

Table 6.6: Organizations in the Field of HIV/AIDS by Year of Foundation

Year of Foundation	Number of Organizations	%
< 1981	27	37
≥ 1981	46	63

(Missing values: 32)

Figure 6.5: Year HIV/AIDS Activities Started

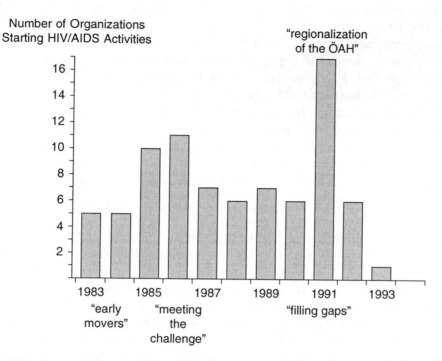

(missing data: 24)

starting boom has come down to a number of four new organizations on average per year since 1987.

If we now relate the year of the first HIV/AIDS activities to the type of organization, a widespread assumption in the literature on non-profit organizations would lead us to expect that exclusive organizations tend to precede inclusive organizations and non-profit organizations to come before public agencies; the theory being that communities affected start organizations as a reaction to state failure and to the failure of existing inclusive health and welfare organizations. In Austria we find just the opposite, exclusives *follow* inclusives (Figure 6.6) and voluntary non-profits follow state organizations (Figure 6.7).

In general, Austrian organizations dealing with HIV/AIDS among other things became active before the foundation of exclusive organizations. An exception to this rule is the *AIDS Commission,* which was initiated by the Ministry of Health and which is almost exclusively composed of medical experts. This again lucidly illustrates the emphasis on the medical and administrative response in Austria.

Even more remarkable than the atypical sequencing of organizational forms is the fact that the foundation of new organizations dealing exclusively with HIV/

Figure 6.6:   Year HIV/AIDS Programmes Started by Inclusive/Exclusive Orientation and Reported Number of AIDS Cases

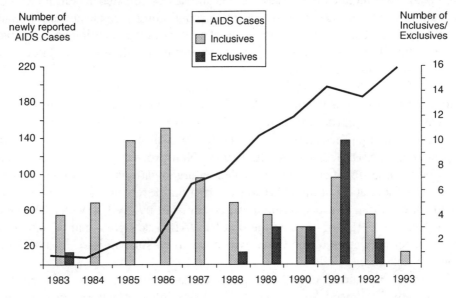

(missing data: 34)

Figure 6.7:   Year HIV/AIDS Programmes Started by Legal Status and Number of Reported AIDS Cases

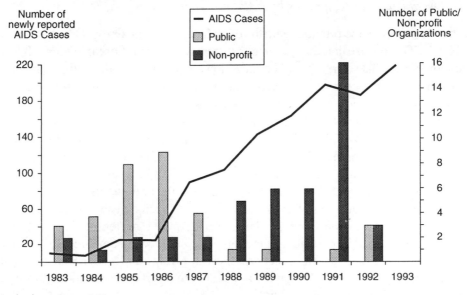

(missing data: 32)

AIDS has been continuing throughout the last years: in many countries HIV/AIDS has started to be "normalized" since about 1989, in the sense that states have attempted to reintegrate relevant services into already established health and welfare institutions by absorbing exclusives rather than continuing to create new ones. Apart from the fact that such a public policy is not evident in the Austrian case, the fact also remains that traditional inclusive organizations still do not seem to become active in the field of HIV/AIDS.

Prima facie, a "state failure" cannot be concluded from the Austrian data. State actors reacted to the problem of HIV/AIDS already at a point in time when only one case was known (compared to the 32,000 cases it took the USA to come up with any form of public action). Moreover, Austria was the first country in Europe to pass special AIDS legislations (July 1983). Non-profit organizations started in 1983 with some single activities (provided by organizations for homosexual persons). The foundation of the ÖAH was the first major reaction from a non-profit organization, though also sponsored and co-initiated by civil servants. The peak one notices in 1991 – in terms of the first HIV/AIDS activity – can be explained by the decentralization of the ÖAH, which was then split up into seven autonomous organizations.

In general, non-profit organizations reacted later than the state, constituting a "second wave" of responses to HIV/AIDS. A possible explanation for this could be that, in principal, in Austria expectations are that in a situation of crisis the state should become active. Only in the second phase, once the limits of state activity had become apparent, did the non-profit organizations try to fill the gaps.

2.2   Organizational Responses by Area of Activity

As has been seen in the previous part, the overall organizational response in the field of HIV/AIDS in Austria is composed of a differentiated set of organizations. It has been illustrated that some types of organization are more active than others and that social groups and regions are covered to different degrees by organizational activity. It is of course important not only to evaluate the overall degree of organizational response to HIV/AIDS but also to look to the areas of activities where the organizational responses take place. It obviously makes a difference whether the organizational responses mainly consist of prevention activities or whether research or policy coordination are the primary activities provided in a particular country.

Consequently, in what is to follow we will describe and analyse the following aspects for each of the areas of activities which have been considered in this study (prevention, care, research, control and monitoring, interest representation and fundraising): their overall importance; their relative importance as compared to the other areas of activity; their distribution across social groups and geographical areas; their composition by type of organization; and their degree of integration through policies and other forms of cooperation.

Table 6.7:   Number of Organizations Active in Different Areas of Activities

Activities	Prevention	Care	Research	Control & Monitoring	Interest Representation	Fund-raising
Overall						
n	82	81	23	22	39	11
%	78.1	77.1	21.9	21.0	37.1	10.5
Legal Status						
Public	33	28	14	17	8	2
Non-Profit	47	51	9	5	30	9
Private	2	2	0	0	1	0
Orientation						
Exclusive	19	63	4	4	14	7
Inclusive	63	18	19	18	25	4
Region						
Vienna	29	32	11	14	21	6
Lower Austria	2	2	0	0	0	0
Burgenland	1	1	0	0	0	0
Upper Austria	14	13	2	1	5	0
Salzburg	6	6	4	1	2	2
Tyrol	6	7	1	2	3	1
Vorarlberg	12	10	1	2	4	0
Styria	9	7	3	1	3	2
Carinthia	3	3	1	1	1	0
Regions with a High AIDS Prevalence	58	59	17	18	32	9
Regions with a Low AIDS Prevalence	24	22	6	4	7	2

I.   PREVENTION ACTIVITIES

Eighty-two organizations, or 78% of all organizations active in the field of HIV/ AIDS, provide some type of prevention and information activity in Austria. Activities related to either prevention or care are the ones most often provided in

Austria. A possible explanation for this high rate might be that prevention is a type of activity which can be provided *ad hoc* and eventually by almost every organization, e.g. only once a year and without any specific commitment (e.g. only distributing some brochures). At the same time, prevention may be a type of activity organizations are eager to report because of the important status it has received in the general HIV/AIDS debate. This would imply that the high absolute and relative numbers of prevention activities do not necessarily mean that Austrian regions and social groups are in fact well-covered by such activities. It could equally point to the fact that an organization whose primary activity in the field of HIV/AIDS is not prevention also tends to report prevention activities.

To test the above theses on the basis of the data available, four types of evidence can be assessed, i.e. (1) by verifying how many organizations have prevention as one of their primary tasks or at least define it as a permanent one; (2) by analysing how prevention activities are distributed across geographical areas and social groups; (3) by analysing the distribution of the types of organization which report prevention activities compared to those who do not provide prevention, but would be in a good situation to do so; and finally, (4) by analysing existing public prevention policies with respect to their goals, scope and resources made available.

(1)   Primary prevention as the organization's main task
How many organizations actually have prevention as a permanent and primary activity in Austria? This is not only a matter of definition but has more and further important implications. It is well known that prevention initiatives are most effective when they are provided on a permanent basis and are embedded in the social context which they aim to address. Although this is difficult to evaluate in the national context, the criterion of prevention as a permanent and primary task applies to approximately only one fourth of the organizations which report any such activities.

Thus, prevention activities, as reported by the organizations, do not seem to require a high degree of specialization. Prevention activities were reported by 82% of the organizations which provide care-related activities, by 87% of the organizations which carry out research, by 86% of the organizations involved in policy coordination, by 80% of the organizations involved in interest representation and by 82% of those which organize fund-raising. Thus, prevention seems to be provided no matter what the primary task of an organization is.

(2)   Distribution of prevention activities over geographical areas and social groups
Although regions with a higher prevalence of AIDS cases are generally better covered with prevention activities, no significant correlation between the AIDS prevalence and the number of HIV prevention activities is apparent. Some geographical regions, however, are extremely poorly covered with prevention activities, as can easily be seen in Table 6.7 (e.g. Burgenland, Lower Austria, Carinthia, etc.).

Some social groups are generally better reached than others: homosexual persons, for instance, are better provided with prevention activities than other groups, and in some areas, prevention activities for drug users are more often provided (which is the case in Vorarlberg for example).

(3) Types of organizations involved in prevention activities
Public and non-profit organizations provide prevention activities just as much as the inclusive and exclusive organizations do. No significant correlation was found with respect to both legal status and organizational type. Such an undifferentiated response is contrary to what has been found to be effective in terms of HIV/AIDS prevention: An EC-concerted action on the assessment of HIV/AIDS prevention strategies between 1989 and 1992 in various population groups has described group-specific prevention activities delivered by non-profit organizations as specific directives for effective future work (Dubois-Arber/Paccaud, 1994). The Austrian data show that there is little organizational development with respect to HIV/AIDS in the area of inclusive inclusive organizations.

(4) The degree of integration through public policies and other forms
     of cooperation
Although the formal regulation through the AIDS Law has aimed at establishing a certain division of labour between the national and the federal level, this has so far not been achieved successfully. On a national level some general prevention campaigns have been launched (as has been described above), while on the federal level the development of only a few independent HIV/AIDS-related activities were observed.

   This poor development might be partly explained by the fact that the AIDS Law defines the Ministry of Health as the main actor in this area, which consequently has led to the passive attitude of other actors such as health authorities on the federal level. This could be seen as an even counterproduvtive effect of this specific law. National HIV/AIDS prevention, as it is framed in the national AIDS prevention concept, should, however, aim at flexible, non-coercive strategies to be carried out by public (both national and federal) and non-profit organizations. While it is true that this division of labour can be considered useful, political suggestions would be required as to the integration of these different actors. Thus, it is not surprising that almost no activities concerning coordination (such as umbrella organizations, national platforms or networking activities on national, federal or local levels) have been developed.

   On the basis of the above, the thesis formulated earlier can be affirmed: The high absolute and relative number of prevention activities must be cautiously interpreted. It certainly does not reflect a comprehensive and differentiated set of prevention activities, which could eventually cover all social groups in all geographical areas.

II.   CARE

(1)   Medical and psychosocial care activities as the organization's main task
Although activities related to the area of care are reported to be provided by almost
as many organizations as prevention (77% of all organizations), this figure should
be interpreted differently. Contrary to prevention, care is a type of activity which
is probably only reported when provided rather substantially.

The fact, however, that so many organizations are active in the field of care
confirms the general pattern of dealing with diseases in Austria, favouring a purely
medical approach over an integrative one. By the same token, this does not automatically imply that a comprehensive coverage is given. With respect to care, some
significant problems, which became visible on the basis of our data, must be
mentioned. Although a general accessible and technologically highly-developed
system of medical care is given, in the field of HIV/AIDS – as in many other areas
of health care (e.g. chronic disease, care for the elderly, etc.) – problems on the
consumer's side must not be overlooked. In some areas, no hospitals exist at all
for the treatment of AIDS patients and there seem to be some important differences
between hospitals in terms of the quality of care.

With respect to extramural care, we have to consider the reluctance of many
general practitioners to treat HIV-infected persons. Patients are consequently forced
to seek specialized hospital departments, even if their condition would not require
them to do so.

The cooperation with non-medical services is significantly underdeveloped in
Austria, a system of primary health care has not yet been established. Thus, not
only the provision of non-medical care services is hindered, but also the financial
coverage of this type of service is complicated compared to purely medical treatment.

(2)   Types of organizations involved in care activities
The missing integration of medical and non-medical services in Austria has further disadvantages for the case of HIV/AIDS. The existing medical infrastructure is only poorly equipped to deal with the psychosocial consequences of the
problem. Thus, the development of a whole series of new exclusive organizations – all involved in care-related activities – can be explained by the failure
of the existing medical infrastructure to adequately deal with HIV/AIDS. This
also explains the under-representation of inclusive organizations. Most of those
involved in care are public hospital departments ("AIDS wards"), which, by
definition, have been counted as inclusives. Again, also for care-related activities, we have to conclude that the normalization of HIV/AIDS has not yet been
established.

*(3)   The degree of integration through public policies and other forms
       of cooperation*
For the care sector, no AIDS-specific policy has been discussed since it has been
assumed that the general health care system had been responding sufficiently to
HIV/AIDS and the corresponding needs of people affected. That this has not
happened, however, can also be concluded from the fact that the development of
a number of specialized AIDS wards has never provoked general discussions, neither
on the justification nor on the effects of such wards. Interdisciplinary working groups
or any other form of communication networks have not yet been established, neither
on the national nor on the federal level. Some initiatives to set up a network and
cooperate between hospitals were started by highly motivated and committed health
care workers on the community level in Vienna. The AIDS ward at the University
Hospital of Innsbruck also regularly organizes a special AIDS training day for its
health care personnel.

III.   RESEARCH

(1)   The overall importance of research activities
Research as an area of activities related to HIV/AIDS is generally not very prominent in Austria. Activities in four areas have been assessed (social, clinical, epidemiological, and virological research). In order to interpret the data, however, it
is important to note that some very active pharmaceutical companies involved in
vaccine and genetic research have not been included in the data set since they did
not provide any other HIV-related activity. Social research as an activity is reported
more often than research in other areas. This does not mean, however, that this
number equals the social science research projects carried out in the field of HIV/
AIDS. It can be explained by the fact that some organizations from the non-profit
sector reported client statistics as a research activity since they consider research
as an important additional task for evaluation or conceptualization of their work.

(2)   Types of organizations involved in research activities
Research in the field of HIV/AIDS is bound to the "classical" research institutions
(e.g. universities, hospitals, etc.). The tendency of non-profit organizations to
contribute to research, although they often lack the resources to do so, should be
noted. However, research activities are significantly more often undertaken by
public organizations (chi square p-value=0.0014).[4]

*(3)   The degree of integration through public policies and other forms
       of cooperation*
The degree of integration through policies and other forms of cooperation in the
area of research is mainly framed by the Ministry of Science and Research, which
is the main public body for financing research. It has implemented a research

emphasis with specific grants for social research in the field of HIV/AIDS. Research is also being commissioned by the Ministry of Health. The integration of the sector seen as a whole is relatively low since a research community is virtually non-existent. Some exceptions have been reported, however, e.g. two newsletters for medical professionals communicating research results, or the annual Austrian AIDS Congress which addresses medical-clinical professions almost exclusively. Once a year the Austrian World AIDS Day event is organized in cooperation with some research institutions and public organizations.

IV.   CONTROL AND MONITORING

(1)   The overall importance of control and monitoring activities
Some tasks related to this sector (blood screening/plasma/product safety, quality control of HIV test kits, medication, etc.) are covered by well-established, mainly public institutions. Compared to other areas of activities one could even conclude that this is the most developed sector in Austria. With respect to the overall importance of this area of activities, one must differentiate between the above-mentioned control activities and those activities which are related to policy coordination.

(2)   Type of organizations involved in control and monitoring activities
The provision of control and monitoring, which also includes policy coordination, is strongly linked to public organizations (chi-square p-value=0.0001). This might be regarded as a rather obvious finding, were it not that private interest government is an otherwise widespread phenomenon – especially in Austria. Private interest governments are arrangements under which an attempt is made to make associative, self-interested collective action contribute to the achievement of public policy objectives; in other words to provide public goods, such as policy coordination and control, by non-profit organizations. This phenomenon, which in Austria – compared to other European countries – is particularly prominent in the industry and social security sector, is absent in the case of HIV/AIDS. This is puzzling since many reasons could be named for why such a form of governance would be very effective. Further research will have to determine whether this is because private interest government requires well-established, old organizations or whether this has something to do with the specific case of HIV/AIDS.

(3)   The degree of integration through public policies and other forms
of cooperation
This area of activities, seen as a whole, is regulated and integrated through the AIDS Law and a series of other regulations. The first organization active in this sector was the *AIDS Kommission*, the advisory body to the Ministry of Health. Policy coordination, however, does not only function by means of laws and regulations:

Some significant problems of competence, commitment and funding have developed between the federal provinces and the national authorities – as the ministry itself has pointed out in the national AIDS prevention concept. Some interesting efforts have been reported on the federal level as well, e.g. a clearing-house for AIDS initiatives and self-help groups, which has been set up by the regional health authority in Vorarlberg.

v.   INTEREST REPRESENTATION

(1)   Overall importance of activities related to interest representation
Both the quantitative significance in itself, as well as its importance related to other areas of activities, seem to be low. Interest representation is not very visible, although many cases of discrimination against persons with HIV/AIDS have been reported in previous years. Interest representation, so it seems, is thus not provided on a regular basis, but more on an individual level when single incidents have been followed up. Given the social and societal context in which HIV/AIDS is embedded, many organizations obviously have the feeling that this is an important activity, but resources are missing to provide interest representation effectively. In general, interest representation is mostly linked to large membership organizations which have financial resources other than subsidies from the state. This type of organization is, however, almost totally absent in the social field in Austria.

(2)   Distribution across social groups and geographical areas
Many organizations only provide interest representation once they are confronted with specific incidents of discrimination. Very few organizations define this as their primary task. As a result, some social groups are better provided with interest representation with a tradition in being politically active in other fields (e.g. organizations for homosexuals).

(3)   Types of organizations involved in interest representation
By definition, interest representation is provided by non-profit organizations. The fact that the role of non-profit organizations in general is rather underdeveloped in Austria, provides an additional explanation for the low occurrence of these activities. A significant relationship has been found between the exclusive/inclusive orientation of the organization and interest representation (chi square p-value=0.008 for exclusive organizations). Not surprisingly, exclusive organizations are significantly more often active when it comes to interest representation. The reason for this finding can be multiform: Specific and new interests and problems which are linked to HIV/AIDS can only be covered by general interest organizations to a certain extent; therefore, specific organizations had to be created to deal

with these problems, i.e. exclusive HIV/AIDS organizations. Another reason could be that the specific problems related to HIV/AIDS provoke conflicts of interest in inclusive organizations (on how to deal sensitively with issues such as sexuality, drug abuse, etc.); this could prevent them from taking a clear standing. Still another hypothesis could be that interest intermediation can only concentrate on a single issue. In this respect, it would be interesting to analyse whether interest organizations from other fields also tend to be exclusive in character.

(4)   The degree of integration through public policies and other forms
      of cooperation
The degree of integration can be described in general as low. No peak organizations have developed in this area, which would primarily focus and coordinate interest representation of different organizations in the field. Equally, interest representation is not only invisible on the sectoral level, but also somewhat non-existent in public life: Activism is in general rather uncommon in Austria.

VI.   FUND-RAISING

(1) The overall importance of fund-raising
Fund-raising in the general welfare sector hardly exists in Austria, but seems to be slowly emerging in relation to HIV/AIDS. However, very few activities were identified in this field. This can be explained by the fact that organizations active in the field of HIV/AIDS mainly rely on public funding and cannot afford to invest time in the allocation of private funding since this is a very time-consuming activity. Those few organizations tending to engage in such activities are exclusive ones (chi square p-value=0.0004 for exclusives).

(2) The distribution across social groups and geographical areas
Only a few scant activities were reported by special organizations (e.g. the "Life AIDS Ball" which is organized once a year). These few organizations which are involved in fund-raising are mainly exclusives. But whether an organization in Austria engages in fund-raising or not seems to depend to a certain extent on the knowledge of the situation of people directly affected by HIV/AIDS. Exclusive organizations are more knowledgeable in this respect than any other type of organization. Thus, one can conclude that there is a trend of exclusive organizations being more active in fund-raising than inclusive organizations. The benefits of this activity are primarily directed towards AIDS patients, although some activities have been directed to prevention efforts as well (e.g. the 1993 World AIDS Day rock concert).

2.3 Analysis of Selected Single Activities: Who Does What and Why?

2.3.1 Distribution of Selected Single Activities

The rate at which selected activities develop in Austria will now be explained in more detail. The ten selected single activities chosen for this analysis are those which we consider crucial in dealing with HIV/AIDS. In Table 6.8, it is illustrated how many organizations provide these activities in Austria, how many organizations compared to the total number of organizations provide them (%), what types of organizations provide them (legal status, orientation, region) and how many organizations provide them in regions with a low AIDS prevalence compared to regions with a high one.

The objective of the present part is to analyse and explain the frequency of these different activities. This can be done by analysing each single activity by answering three questions: (1) Why can the activity be considered crucial when it comes to dealing with HIV/AIDS? (2) What is the frequency and distribution of the activity in Austria? (3) How can one explain the frequency of the activity?

Information work is crucial when it comes to general prevention. More than ten years of behavioural research in the field of HIV/AIDS have shown that the provision of basic information constitutes a necessary prerequisite for any attempted behavioural change.

Although many questions referring to how to provide the relevant information most effectively are still unsolved, people clearly need to know the basic facts about HIV/AIDS and understand them as necessary prerequisites before they can make their choice regarding any behaviour that poses a risk for HIV infection.

General educational and information work as a single offered activity ranks highest among all organizations. Since this does not say much about the specifics of the prevention activity itself, we also looked at the production of information material. Fifty-eight per cent of all organizations (61 organizations) provide both of these activities.

Information material such as prevention booklets are generally produced by governmental agencies and health authorities; information for specific target groups is largely missing (even for young people or women, not to mention information for marginalized groups such as prison inmates, prostitutes, or young bisexual or homosexual persons who seem to constitute a specific and "hard-to-reach" subgroup within the bisexual or homosexual population). Another gap has been observed in the provision of information for ethnic minorities: no information material is produced in foreign languages.

Virtually all types of organizations are involved in the basic provision of HIV-related information. This explains why no significant relationship between this activity and an organization's legal status was found. One would expect particular

Table 6.8:   Ten Selected Single HIV/AIDS Activities Offered

Activities	Information Work	Condom Distribution	Needle Exchange	Face-to-Face Counselling	HIV-Testing	Medical Care	Terminal Care	Buddy Systems	Blood-Screening	Self-help Groups
Overall										
N	61	28	13	48	24	18	10	6	2	16
%	58.1	26.7	12.4	45.7	22.9	17.1	19.5	5.7	1.9	15.2
Legal Status										
Public	23	4	1	16	12	12	2	0	2	1
Non-Profit	37	23	12	30	12	6	8	6	0	15
Private	1	1	0	2	0	0	0	0	0	0
Orientation										
Exclusive	16	6	5	10	7	5	4	5	1	10
Inclusive	45	22	8	38	17	13	6	1	1	6
Province										
Vienna	22	9	3	16	7	9	4	3	2	9
Lower Austria	1	1	0	2	2	0	1	0	0	0
Burgenland	1	0	0	1	0	0	0	0	0	0
Upper Austria	13	1	0	9	3	3	0	0	0	2
Salzburg	5	3	2	3	1	2	0	1	0	1
Tyrol	2	3	2	4	3	1	2	0	0	0
Vorarlberg	7	5	4	7	5	2	1	0	0	2
Styria	9	5	0	5	2	1	1	1	0	2
Carinthia	1	1	2	1	1	0	1	1	0	0
Regions with a High AIDS Prevalence	46	18	5	34	15	14	7	4	2	13
Regions with a Low AIDS Prevalence	15	10	8	14	9	4	3	2	0	3

inclusive organizations to be more active in this respect since the overall number of inclusive organizations is much higher. With the exception of interest organizations for homosexual persons which are very active in printing and providing their group-specific HIV-related information material, the lack of information material could be interpreted as the failure of inclusive organizations to use their resources in the field of HIV/AIDS. In general, however, exclusive organizations are much more active in terms of producing their own HIV-related information material: a significant relationship was found between this variable and exclusive organizations (chi square p-value=0.0007).

Condom distribution is considered an important prevention activity. Making condoms available to people at a low cost and low threshold is an important prevention activity. For many people, the adoption of safer sex practices is controversial, and psychological barriers still exist around the issue of condom use in particular. Giving away condoms can be a useful strategy to facilitate a change in the negative attitudes towards condoms. This may ultimately help to make the condom a socially and psychologically better accepted method of contraception and HIV prevention. This would be particularly important with respect to the heterosexual man's present attitude towards condom use.

One would expect to see that most of the organizations that provide any kind of AIDS prevention would also give away condoms; however, Table 6.8 shows that this activity is provided by 27% of all organizations (or 28 organizations). Given the fact that 58% of all organizations engage in information activities, it is puzzling that only less than half of them distribute condoms. Many organizations are obviously teaching safer sex but expect their clients to get condoms from elsewhere. Hence it could be argued that such prevention strategies will not effectively reduce the existing gap between knowledge and attitudes on the one hand, and personal behaviour on the other.

With respect to the organizations' legal status, a significant relationship (chi square p-value=0.003) has been found with significantly more private non-profit organizations distributing condoms. This is a surprising result as condoms could be distributed in many public places, such as schools, the military, in hospitals, and other statutory organizations. The organizational orientation, however, does not have an influence on whether or not an organization provides condoms free of charge. No significant statistical relationships have been found with respect to this variable.

The availability of **needle and syringe exchange** activities is particularly relevant in reducing the further spread of HIV transmissions in the drug-using population. For drug organizations, one could say that providing this activity already constitutes a choice for a very specific approach to the drug problem (i.e. harm reduction); it can mean, for example, that drug workers accept the clients' drug-taking lifestyle and that, as professionals, they not necessarily stick to the therapeutic goal of a drug-free life.

Most of the drug organizations in Austria, however, still opt for the paradigm of therapy and abstinence and only very few low-threshold organizations work in the context of harm reduction. Only 13 organizations (or 12%) reported this activity. This is not only a small portion of all organizations active in the field of HIV/AIDS, it also constitutes a fairly small portion of the overall number of drug service organizations. Moreover, with respect to the 13 organizations enormous regional differences can be observed. This reflects that drug policies are shaped by regional and local authorities.

As an outcome of these different policies, the smallest federal province in Austria, Vorarlberg, actually has the highest number of needle-exchange programmes and is most active in this type of drug-related HIV prevention (4 organizations provide their clients with clean needles in Vorarlberg).

The legal status of an organization involved in drug-related work seems to matter a lot when looking at whether or not an organization gives away clean needles or exchanges used ones. Private non-profit organizations provide these types of services more often than public organizations (chi square p-value=0.013). It is important to notice here, however, that drug organizations in Austria are mainly public. Due to binding policies connected to their legal status, it may be difficult to be effectively involved in this type of drug-related HIV prevention.

No significant relationship has been found with respect to the organizational orientation. The assumption, however, that more inclusive organizations (i.e. drug service organizations) would be expected to provide this activity (8 inclusive organizations as compared to 5 exclusive ones) is being questioned by our data. It are mainly the *AIDS-Hilfen*, which are exclusives by definition, that provide needle-exchange facilities. Thus, our data show that exclusive organizations play a major role in drug-related HIV prevention in Austria. Taking the target group specifics into account, the question remains, however, as to whether or not prevention related to the issue of drug use should be part of the services provided by the *AIDS-Hilfen* or whether it should be related more directly to drug service organizations. This, however, would mean that drug service organizations would need to become more active in the field of HIV/AIDS.

Face-to-face counselling and psychotherapy are considered supportive for people living with HIV or AIDS in coping with their critical life events. The counsellor may accompany clients through the different stages of the HIV infection and support him/her in dealing with the various resulting problems. This can not only lead to an increased quality of life; research on psycho-immune reactions has shown that emotional well-being may result in an extended time of asymptotic HIV infection (an actual delay in the onset of AIDS) and eventually in an increase in the survival time with AIDS.

Face-to-face counselling is a generally widely distributed activity provided by many organizations with direct client contacts (48 organizations or 46% of all organizations engage in face-to-face counselling). Since the number of organizations providing this activity does not tell us much about either the continuity nor the quality of this service, we also looked at psychotherapy available for HIV-infected persons or AIDS patients. This specific type of continuous counselling could be considered a more substantial service requiring certain training standards on the counsellors'/therapists' side as well as a deeper commitment on both the clients' and the therapists' side. While an overall of 45 organizations provide different types of face-to-face counselling, only 12 organizations reported offering psychotherapy. Thus, psychotherapeutic counselling constitutes only 1.8% of all HIV-related activities. The absence of a wide range of inclusive organizations, such as the well-established psychotherapeutic institutions or counselling centres, can be considered as extremely problematic. Again, here the data point to the fact that these institutions have somehow failed to integrate HIV/AIDS into their services. They tend to refer people affected with HIV/AIDS to specific organizations (such as the *AIDS-Hilfen*), rather than to counsel or treat them within the organization. One can only speculate as to why HIV/AIDS is dealt in such a way: a lack of training or a reluctance to deal with the typical patient groups could be possible reasons.

All types of organizations active in the field of HIV/AIDS, however, try to bridge this gap in the provision of psychosocial support. Thus, neither the organizations' legal status nor their organizational orientation, however, can explain the absence of these two important activities. No significant relationships have been found related to these variables. All different types of organizations are involved in the provision of these activities.

Voluntary HIV-testing and counselling are crucial in terms of HIV/AIDS prevention for a number of reasons. Although HIV-testing can be considered a preventive measure, the issue of HIV-testing is still highly controversial when applied as a screening method: Normative reasons stress the importance of the concept of informed consent but testing at a very early stage of HIV infection is considered important for adequate treatment. On analysing this particular activity in more detail, we have to look critically at how Austrian organizations deal with the term "counselling": Clearly, adequate pre- and post-test counselling is not provided in all places where HIV-testing is offered.

Here, the most salient example for the misuse of the concept of informed consent is the testing policy of public hospitals in Vienna. HIV tests are being performed on a routine basis with all in-patients in the city's hospitals. This kind of misuse of a patient's informed consent, which is clearly not in line with any of the WHO or national government recommendations, is seriously criticized by many organizations. Given this background, it is difficult to interpret the overall number of 24 organizations involved in voluntary HIV-testing. It was impossible to evaluate the pre- and post-test counselling procedure applied by the organizations within the given research design. Some of the regional AIDS-Hilfen, however, reported that pre-test counselling was being performed and that only on the basis of its outcome was it decided whether or not to carry out the HIV antibody test.

In the case of voluntary HIV-testing and counselling, neither the organizations' legal status nor their organizational orientation explain the absence or presence of this activity. No significant relationships have been found related to these two variables. This finding is due to the fact that mainly two specific types of organizations provide this activity: regional AIDS-Hilfen and the AIDS departments of public hospitals.

AIDS-specialized medical care plays a role in secondary prevention, but it is first and foremost essential to people who are suffering from AIDS. In Austria, AIDS-specialized medical care is mainly provided in AIDS wards, which have developed as the response to HIV/AIDS by the medical system.

Interestingly enough, private practitioners play next to no role in the care for people with HIV/AIDS. While it is true that AIDS-specialized medical care requires complex treatment and expensive medication, adequate training, and sensitivity for the particular emotional and social situation that the people affected find themselves in, the question is whether it is really only the structure of the separated AIDS wards that is capable of providing these qualities. In Austria, however, there has been no public debate about this issue. Its possible negative "side-effects" have hardly been discussed.

Our data show that AIDS-specialized medical care is offered almost exclusively by hospitals with an AIDS ward and in only few other hospital departments. Organizations offering AIDS-specialized medical care constitute 17% of all organizations which provide any HIV/AIDS-related activities. Only very few private practitioners are known to be involved in the provision of AIDS-specialized medical care (Fazekas, 1991).

As a consequence of this specific development, people affected tend to rather seek these specialized hospital departments since it is there where they expect to get the best care available. In turn, the medical system outside these structures does not consider itself liable for HIV/AIDS treatment. While we cannot answer the question as to whether separating AIDS from other diseases has been the best way to deal with the virus (from a medical point of view), it has certainly hindered a broader commitment of the medical community. Practically speaking, HIV-infected persons are trapped in a situation where they have to consult an

AIDS-specialized department even when they have a medical condition that has nothing to do with their immune status whatsoever (a broken bone or toothache, for example).

All of the hospitals which provide AIDS-specialized medical care are public institutions. Considering a useful division of labour, it makes sense that this activity is in the Austrian context mainly provided by public organizations (e.g. hospitals). Thus, a significant relationship was found between public organizations and this activity (chi square p-value=0.008 for public organizations). But it should also be considered that if a system of primary health care is to be established which would have positive effects (for HIV/AIDS patients in particular, but not for this patient group alone), a stronger commitment on the part of private practitioners would be needed.

The importance of **terminal care**, which is usually provided in hospices as well as on an individual basis, has also been recognized for other deadly diseases, such as cancer for example. HIV/AIDS is directly and indirectly closely linked to highly ambiguous issues such as dying and death, which most people are not prepared to deal with. Issues related to dying often evoke conflicts and uncertainties not only for volunteers, but also for professional health care workers. Consequently, such issues do not have enough room in the professional routine of the established health care system, although, from a humanitarian point of view, they stand for the respect with which the patients are treated.

Some of the hospital departments with a specialized AIDS department offer terminal care facilities, as do some other organizations (e.g. home care services). An overall of 10 organizations were identified nationwide where palliative care was reported. This is mostly performed as a client-oriented service, e.g. by a social worker or a nurse who has received additional training in palliative care. Although there are a few hospices in Austria, they do not accept AIDS patients but rather concentrate on cancer and the like.

With respect to the relationship between terminal care and both the organizations' legal status and their organizational orientation, the chi-square tests did not reveal any significant correlations. As can be seen in Table 6.8, however, there is a trend that more non-profit organizations are involved in this activity (eight non-profit organizations compared to only two public organizations). Since most AIDS patients actually die in public hospitals, one should reflect on how the daily hospital routine would allow to integrate terminal care more effectively.

Buddy systems – as a very different means of emotional support – have proven to be very successful in caring for people living with HIV/AIDS, helping out with their daily needs and by just being there to have somebody to talk to. Buddy systems work exclusively with volunteers and provide the necessary services, which most traditional home care services experience difficulties in providing due to their organizational structures.

In Austria, buddy systems have developed almost exclusively within the context of the AIDS-Hilfen; therefore they are only offered by six organizations throughout the country. By the same token, this means that not all AIDS-Hilfen can actually offer buddy systems. Buddy systems also require a lot of training and ongoing supervisory activities, which is difficult to offer for smaller organizations.

Funding problems seem to be the most important reason for this shortage. In many cases, the AIDS-Hilfen have more requests for buddies than they can actually provide patients with. For organizations not linked to the AIDS-Hilfen trying to establish a buddy system, it is very difficult to get funding outside of the context and network of the regional AIDS-Hilfen. The *Buddy Verein* in Vienna is the organization that seems to work most effectively in this respect, given the number of buddies trained and the number of patients that are taken care of, and also given the range of additional practical services offered (such as repairs, cleaning, etc.).

With respect to the buddy system, an organization's legal status does have a significant influence on whether or not a buddy system is being provided. As expected, more non-profit organizations reported this activity. This result is not very surprising since a buddy system provides services that could be defined as best provided by volunteers and people affected directly or indirectly by HIV/AIDS themselves.

Buddy systems are almost only run by exclusive organizations; this can be explained by the fact that buddy systems are mostly provided within the context of the regional AIDS-Hilfen. Only one inclusive organization (a church-affiliated organization with a very active and autonomous HIV/AIDS unit) reported the provision of a buddy system. Interestingly enough, no other inclusive organizations, such as home care service organizations or drug service organizations, have so far ever tried to establish a buddy system for their clients. Thus, the data support the idea that very specific HIV/AIDS-related services are best provided by very specific types of HIV/AIDS organizations.

Blood-screening, plasma and product safety are of utmost importance in the general prevention of further HIV transmissions, but they are of extreme concern for persons suffering from haemophilia in particular. Suffering from this blood defect means dependence on a drug that potentially could pose a severe risk of HIV infection. It has turned out that these drugs did in fact pose a danger even after safe screening methods were in place. However, reliable techniques of safety control are generally used now, and consequently this issue has more or less faded away in the general AIDS debate.

Inclusive inclusive organizations (which refers to HIV-testing labs and diagnostic centres) were not part of the data analyses. Thus, only two public organizations were found with respect to this particular activity – the monitoring of all blood products is done by these specific public organizations. This still constitutes an important and basic preventive activity in terms of avoiding further HIV infection through the contamination of blood products.

Self-help groups are in many ways important. Self-help is based on the idea that people become experts due to a certain relevant experience that they have in common; this is believed to be an important source as compared to professional training. This approach has proven to be particularly successful in the case of HIV/ AIDS. For people affected by HIV/AIDS, learning that one is not alone can mean a significant step towards the acceptance of the HIV infection. Self-help groups are also means of fighting the social isolation which accompanies the HIV infection. And finally, such organizations often provide interest representation which helps in expressing and demanding basic human rights and fighting discrimination.

Self-help groups of people with HIV/AIDS were only identified in 16 cases (constituting 15% of all organizations), and have been founded mainly in the context of the AIDS-Hilfen or interest groups of homosexual persons. Given the importance of preventing self-isolation for HIV-infected people, organized self-help should be further promoted. While the people have to be motivated to organize themselves, they also need some supportive structures to be successful with this. Drug users, for example, have not succeeded in organizing themselves, although various groups have launched efforts several times (e.g. the Austrian Junkie Bond, which only existed for a limited time).

After interpreting these results in more detail, it must also be mentioned, though, that the overall number of 16 reported activities rather exceeds the actual offer of self-help groups. Some of the organizations also reported "potential" offers for self-help, which at the time of data assessment were not active but could be reactivated on request. Although this is difficult to estimate, supposedly a total number of ten active self-help groups were active at one specific point in time (operating on a constant basis, with regular meetings, a certain number of clients, certain activities, etc.).

Self-help in Austria seems to be strongly correlated to an organization's legal status. Similar to the case of buddy systems, self-help is reported significantly more often by exclusive organizations (chi-square p-value=0.0001). This is not a surprising result since these activities can be considered to be typical for the profile of AIDS service organizations. It could be argued, though, that if people affected by the disease only organize themselves within the context of AIDS service organizations, their social isolation and stigmatization might be further aggravated. This could be particularly true for two main reasons for the regional AIDS-Hilfen in the federal provinces: First of all, social discrimination seems to be much stronger in the rural areas than in big cities, and secondly, the public image of the AIDS-Hilfen in these regions seems to be very much associated with the interests of homosexual men. Therefore, a self-help group within the context of the AIDS-Hilfen might not be acceptable to HIV-positive women or to haemophiliacs for example. Again, the regional disparities support this explanation: 9 out of 16 self-help groups were found in Vienna, 3 federal provinces reported 2 self-help groups each, and 1 reported only 1 self-help group in the entire province. This leaves us with an overall of 4 federal provinces in Austria where no such offer exists (see Table 6.8).

In summary, from the above results pertaining to the 10 most relevant activities, we can say that activities related to education and information work are provided most frequently. Very specific activities, however, such as condom distribution or needle exchange programmes, which have proven to be at the core of successful HIV/AIDS prevention, are not provided sufficiently and frequently enough to really have an impact. Secondary prevention strategies such as buddy systems or self-help groups are not being promoted enough to really make a difference for the people affected. They are not available in all parts of the country and are not accessible to all affected groups.

3   Conclusions and Policy Implications

The organizational response will now be evaluated on the basis of the afore-mentioned results. The main findings will be summarized and evaluated in such a way that relevant policy implications can be drawn from them. In what is to follow, three dimensions should be considered when evaluating the organizational respon-siveness in the field of HIV/AIDS in Austria: the rate of organizational response, the types of organizations involved in the organizational response and the distri-bution of the organizational response across social groups and geographical areas.

3.1   Degree of Organizational Response

3.1.1 Overall Organizational Response

The Managing AIDS project has identified 105 organizations which are active in the field of HIV/AIDS in Austria. Although the extent to which these organiza-tions are actually involved in HIV/AIDS-related activities differs a lot, an overall of 648 activities have been reported by these organizations.

The major response towards HIV/AIDS in Austria lies first and foremost with the regional AIDS-Hilfen and statutory agencies. Compared to most other Euro-pean countries, the public sector in Austria is more active with respect to HIV/AIDS. And it is in Austria where compared to other countries the public sector is rela-tively speaking more active than the general non-profit sector.

In Austria, public health policies pertaining to HIV/AIDS are centrally directed, "top-down" approaches – as is generally the case with publicly recognized health problems. The national AIDS policy comprises legal measures, general information campaigns, funding of the AIDS-Hilfen and other regional AIDS service organizations. With respect to the latter, however, there seems to be a significant lack of both recognition and funding from statutory agencies.

Our results show that the epidemiological situation in Austria does not correspond with the development of HIV/AIDS-related activities. The presence or absence of certain HIV/AIDS-related activities can be better explained by an organi-zation's legal status and by whether an organization is inclusive or exclusive. Specific activities which can be considered as being at the core of effective HIV/AIDS prevention and care (e.g. condom distribution, needle exchange programmes, self-help groups, and buddy systems, to name only some of them) are significantly more often provided by exclusive and non-profit organizations. With respect to the overall involvement of inclusive organizations, our data confirm that there are significant gaps in using silent resources, i.e. involving a wider range of inclusive organizations in HIV/AIDS-related work. This can be interpreted as a further effect of the "AIDS exceptionalism", that still hinders a normalization of HIV/AIDS in this country. Many actors, be they involved in HIV-related areas or in the general health and welfare sector, still hold the view that AIDS is an extremely particular disease and hence has to be treated differently. This runs parallel to the marginalization of people affected, and can be found on all levels: that of the single organization, the overall related health and welfare scctor, and society as a whole.

3.1.2 Organizational Response by Areas of Activity

On the basis of the results – when analysed along the lines of the different areas of activities – it is quite difficult to draw definite conclusions regarding the factors which explain the different number of organizations active in these areas. It can, however, be implicitly concluded that this distribution does not reflect the problem-load, the epidemiological case-loads nor the needs of the people directly and indirectly affected by HIV/AIDS. It seems to relate, to some extent at least, to the public versus non-profit ratio to the distribution of organizations which are active in a specific subsector. Another influence might be exerted by the fact that organizations which are active in the less frequented areas (research, control and monitoring, interest representation and fund-raising) also tend to be significantly more often active in prevention and care. Consequently, what really can be concluded as a policy implication is that a further division of labour and better role definition is needed between the different actors. A necessary prerequisite would therefore be a better integration of the AIDS field and some structures to facilitate networking among the organizations. Provided this exchange of knowledge and information occurs, certain types of organizations will almost automatically develop. Strategies therefore must be twofold aiming at both specialization and normalization: some specific activities that have proven to be relevant should be directly promoted, whereas on the overall sectoral level, strategies should aim at involving a broader variety of organizations.

3.1.3 Frequency of the Ten Most Relevant Activities

HIV/AIDS-related activities, which can be considered as being at the core of effective prevention and care have been analysed in further detail. Among these, information activities are the most frequent ones, followed by counselling activities. By the same token, these activities are the most general ones among the ten selected ones. While it is important to recognize the significance of the work being done in this field, these data also show that activities which require a certain degree of specialization or extensive training clearly are provided less frequently. Our data have clearly demonstrated this. Here, it is obviously not so much the quantity of activities that should be increased, but rather the specialization and training which may be needed on how to provide more effective services.

Activities which aim at enhancing an infected person's quality of life (e.g. AIDS-specialized medical care, counselling, emotional support, self-help activities, etc.) are also distributed to a different degree according to the type of activity. It is these activities in particular which involve people directly and indirectly affected by HIV/AIDS that are less frequently provided. This is rather worrisome since it is exactly these activities which have been proven to make a difference for an infected person and his/her ability to cope with HIV/AIDS. Our data show that many more programmes would be needed that promote self-help and fight the isolation of HIV-infected people in Austria. In this respect, it would be extremely important that further research be carried out to determine the psychosocial needs of persons with HIV/AIDS. Next to nothing is known of how the existing service offers actually correspond to the needs of the HIV/AIDS-affected person.

3.2 *Types of Organizations Involved in HIV/AIDS*

3.2.1 Legal Status: The Role of the State versus that of the Third Sector

Although the non-profit organizations constitute 60% of all organizations (vs. 38% of statutory agencies), it is nevertheless justified to say that the major impact lies with the state. This is due to the role of the state as the general funding agency for a large portion of non-profit organizations (AIDS-Hilfen and most of the drug treatment centres are exclusively funded by the state). While this grants general access to the organizations' services from the client's point of view, issues of independence, control, and cooperation from the organization's interests should equally be considered.

When it comes to HIV/AIDS prevention, some of the activities that can only be provided by certain types of organizations are particularly effective, such as condom distribution and needle/syringe exchange in the field of primary prevention, as well as self-help groups or buddy-systems with respect to secondary prevention. Public, inclusive organizations are obviously not prepared to provide these activities to the same extent as their counterparts in the third sector. Since only 23 (22%) exclusive organizations are active, their numbers of activities have to be limited. It can therefore be concluded that it is an almost impossible expectation that the overall availability of activities could live up to the demands and needs of the HIV-affected person. While it is true that not all HIV/AIDS-related activities can be normalized, the effect of only having some organizations which try to meet the needs of those directly and indirectly affected by HIV/AIDS is twofold: Not only is it an overburdening task for these few organizations, it can consequently also aggravate the social isolation which the HIV-infected person may experience; this, in turn, can lead to a kind of "ghetto" of community-based organizations.

Other reasons for the so-called "under-development" of these activities could be the historical development of the welfare sector in Austria, which has always been strongly linked to the public sector: therefore, self-help has not had a long tradition. Since AIDS is burdened with the stigma of socially undesirable behaviour, it is even more difficult for people to organize self-help.

Since the health and social sectors are centrally and publicly regulated, voluntary work has not been in existence for very long. Working with committed and trained volunteers has been shown to be very successful in the field of HIV/AIDS (e.g. buddy systems, home care services, etc.), but the provision of this specific kind of support and care needed is widely missing in Austria. Here, a normalization of the AIDS phenomenon would be without doubt feasible and achievable, if more training and supervision were facilitated for workers and volunteers in established home care services. Efforts should be made on a policy level to integrate these services and consequently to overcome the barriers which prejudices related to HIV/AIDS still constitute.

In terms of a classical distinction between the public and non-profit organizations we find that public organizations rather provide activities such as research, control and monitoring, whereas non-profit organizations provide activities in the field of interest representation. But when it comes to client-specific services, such as prevention or social and psychosocial care, the unclear division of labour leads to overlapping activities and under-served target groups. According to the recently issued national AIDS prevention concept, general prevention should be covered by the ministry while prevention programmes targeting specific social groups should be launched by the regional AIDS-Hilfen. It remains to be seen how this concept can be effectively implemented. The experience of the last years has shown that the loopholes in national prevention campaigns have to be filled by the

AIDS-Hilfen as well. Due to passivity on the national level (in most cases), exclusive organizations have started prevention campaigns for specific target groups, even if this task had not been originally assigned to them. Some of the regional *AIDS-Hilfen* for example have been very active with respect to young people, developing prevention campaigns with specific methods such as peer-group education or issuing adequate prevention materials to be used within the teenage population.

Although it is important to leave the decision whether or not to become active in a certain field of prevention or care to the individual organization, it can nevertheless be influenced by many factors, such as personal motivation, resources, access to specific target groups, feasibility of specific programmes, etc. If we are, however, to guarantee that all groups will be covered by prevention messages, a policy aiming at a clear division of labour is needed. As an outcome of this unclear division of labour, women, for example, have almost totally been left out of primary prevention. It was also in the field of secondary prevention where we observed very little initiatives for women-specific programmes, such as counselling for birth control, prenatal or natal care, or programmes for HIV-infected mothers and their children.

We have shown that, in general, non-profit organizations have responded to HIV/AIDS to various extents, depending on the region and the different social groups. Private for-profit organizations virtually play no role in the overall picture of the organizational response in Austria. Interestingly enough, non-profit organizations reacted later than public organizations; this could indicate a state failure in early HIV/AIDS-related policies. Non-profit organizations responded in what could be described as a second wave. In the history of more than ten years of HIV/AIDS-related work, some major conflicts have arisen between these two pillars (e.g. division of labour, methods and topics of prevention, etc.). The conflict surrounding HIV-testing is an additional example: basically, this involves technical and ethical questions. The latter are still debated between the national authorities, who tend to follow WHO standards in terms of anonymity and counselling, and some federal authorities who implement more coercive policies, such as HIV-screening in public hospitals without informed consent. Here, a clear-cut centralized decision would be needed in order to achieve the nationwide implementation of WHO guidelines.

In addition, a national AIDS concept has been requested by non-profit organizations active in the field of HIV/AIDS for some time now. Such a concept, which clearly has to go beyond what has been issued so far would have to trigger off a profound nationwide debate involving all relevant actors to come to grips with their goals, strategies, and possible evaluation methods. If such a concept is worked out by the entire community, there are clearly higher chances of its implementation.

3.2.2 Organizational Orientation: Exclusives versus Inclusives

We could identify only a fairly small number of exclusive organizations active in the field of HIV/AIDS as compared to their inclusive counterparts. While inclusive organizations constitute about 87% of all organizations, it is essential to understand the significance of the exclusive organizations' predominant importance. Exclusive organizations actually provide the most relevant activities in terms of effective prevention and care for people with HIV/AIDS significantly more often than inclusives. Inclusive organizations, such as family planning centres, organizations for young people, unions, etc., are not as active as they could be, given their resources, access to target groups, and other organizational features. In this respect, as has already been pointed out above, support and training issues are crucial to achieve further organizational development.

With respect to the broad range of HIV/AIDS-related activities, which are in fact (and which could potentially be) offered by inclusive organizations, a clear-cut division of labour is missing. Since there is no public policy regarding such a division of labour (neither between inclusives, nor between exclusives and inclusives), the approach of integration and normalization of AIDS in Austria is rather suppressed than favoured.

The absence of an effective division of labour between different types of organizations results in significant gaps in the provision of certain activities, to which, in turn, some organizations have to react. Primarily exclusive organizations are overburdened due to the number of specific services that are provided only by them. As the main actor among the non-profit organizations in the field of HIV/AIDS, the regional AIDS-Hilfen play an extremely important role in the provision of virtually all relevant HIV/AIDS-related activities. Given their resources, both in terms of budget and in terms of staff, the work-load that is assigned to them is clearly more than burdensome. A division of labour would hence also be needed to relieve the AIDS-Hilfen of the burden by transferring tasks which could be performed by other organizations to them. Thus, strongly needed capacities would be free to fulfil activities the AIDS-Hilfen and other exclusives are better prepared to deal with due to their organizational characteristics.

Given the overall organizational field in the sector of health and welfare, it can be concluded that 105 organizations being active in the field of HIV/AIDS is a fairly small number. There are, however, potential silent resources that could be used for prevention and care. In order to enhance the overall organizational development, public health policy would have to give incentives to mobilize these organizations by facilitating a broader community commitment. Crucial issues in supporting inclusive organizations which could potentially become active are: training, funding, management issues, and anti-discrimination measures.

Possible barriers to integrate some of the established organizations of the health and welfare sector could be seen in their high degree of professionalization, which to some degree constitutes a certain organizational inflexibility. This actually seems to hinder the development of new activities in the field of HIV/AIDS in particular. Thus, the lessons learned from HIV/AIDS should be used as a further step towards the necessary reorganization of the health care system, which the government has basically agreed upon by accepting the WHO guidelines "Health for All by the Year 2000". Certainly, not only people affected by HIV/AIDS could benefit from achieving the specific goals of this programme: orienting the health care system towards primary health care, a further integration of health and social services, a general upgrading of psychosocial and social services and an increase in non-hospital services would contribute to the well-being of people, be they infected or not.

3.3 Distribution of the Organizational Response

3.3.1 Distribution of the Organizational Response across Social Groups

One of the most remarkable results is that more than one third of all organizations do not address any specific target groups (e.g. women, young people, bisexual or homosexual persons, etc.). With respect to HIV/AIDS-related information and educational work in particular, which is provided most often as a single activity, whether or not a prevention message will work effectively very much depends on social norms and group specifities. The whole body of scientific evidence that research on prevention has brought about so far points to the necessity of group-specific messages. Again, this is why a clear concept of "who does what and for whom" would be necessary.

In the following section we will therefore reflect on what the organizational response to HIV/AIDS in Austria means for different social groups. As in most other countries, not only the degree to which different groups are served varies a lot, but also the degree to which different social groups have been able to organize services for themselves. Consequently, strategies for the groups most affected by HIV/AIDS will be developed upon.

I.   STRATEGIES TARGETING HOMOSEXUAL AND BISEXUAL PERSONS

Homosexual men constitute the group most affected by HIV/AIDS. As in most countries, including Austria, they have succeeded to organize specific prevention activities more than any other group affected by HIV/AIDS. Relying on the already existing organizational infrastructure, homosexual men as a group have responded to the AIDS epidemic by setting up AIDS-related services, and they did so even though legal measures that discriminate against homosexual persons are still in place. The abolition of these constraints would be the most urgent policy measure to be undertaken. Furthermore, certain groups of persons with a homosexual behaviour, such as young homosexual or bisexual men, must not be excluded from prevention messages. Given the limited resources of community-based organizations for homosexual/bisexual persons, it is also doubtful whether these organizations can reach all persons at risk of HIV infection through homosexual contact. Not all persons with a homosexual behaviour identify themselves as being homosexual, in particular in areas where discrimination is high. Public prevention messages would have to react to this.

II.   STRATEGIES TARGETING DRUG USERS

Organizations in the field of drug-related work constitute a large portion among inclusive organizations. The question as to how to integrate HIV prevention into drug-related services has been shaped by the general debate on different drug treatment approaches. Low-threshold programmes provide HIV-related services such as needle exchange and condom distribution, whereas therapy institutions which follow an abstinence approach still do not integrate HIV/AIDS-related activities. Most of the drug treatment centres, however, work according to the latter approach. Only a few low-threshold programmes have developed, although programmes such as needle exchange or needle distribution have proven effective – in the short run, in the prevention of HIV transmission, and, in the long run, also in treating drug abuse. With respect to drug policies, a greater flexibility in service offers is certainly needed in Austria. Integrated drug concepts would be needed (pertaining to a division of labour between therapeutic institutions and community-based organizations), which would promote the health status of the drug user. While the psychosocial services for drug users have to be expanded upon, binding drug policies, which for example do not permit to give away clean needles in hospitals, should also be put into question. One could pose the ethical question: If we are not capable of curing society's drug problem in the long term, why further aggravate the drug user's health conditions in the short term?

III.   STRATEGIES TARGETING WOMEN

Not one single women's organization and only very few general organizations which directly target women were identified. Given the recent trends of the epidemiological patterns, targeting women should rather be a high priority in public health planning. Activities are needed on an overall level of the general population (addressing women's risks, addressing the role of heterosexual transmission and of shared responsibility in the context of heterosexual partnerships, etc.), as well as addressing women's heterogeneity: specific programmes for drug-using women, young women, pregnant women, mothers of infected children, etc. While it is true that most women become infected with HIV through sexual contact with a man, it is clearly not sufficient to only claim men to be the source of infection. Women have to be addressed specifically in order to be aware of their heightened risk since men have been excluded from these kind of messages for too long now: be it with respect to specific contraceptive methods, general sexual health, and the overall responsibilities in the area of human reproduction.

The interesting question here, however, is, why have so relatively few programmes for women developed in the field of HIV/AIDS? Given gender-specific characteristics and the existing wider female support networks in the closer personal environment, one would expect women to be more visible. It seems, however, that in the case of HIV/AIDS, the typical female support structures (e.g. traditional family ties and peer support networks) have failed to support HIV-infected women. But the effective organizational counterpart (such as support groups for homosexual men, for example) are virtually non-existent for women. So far, women's organizations have failed to integrate HIV/AIDS into their agenda, as have AIDS organizations, which have continued to ignore gender-specific issues in every respect. Effective AIDS policies would have to aim at both using and strengthening social networks for the benefit of women and stimulating a further organizational development in targeting women affected by HIV/AIDS both directly and indirectly.

IV.   STRATEGIES TARGETING YOUNG PEOPLE

To target young people is of extreme importance if the future spread of HIV/AIDS is to be limited or halted. Analyses of the recent epidemiological figures show that in Austria young people are at risk of becoming infected with HIV; prevention is clearly of utmost importance. The general dilemma with sex education programmes in this country has already been discussed. It has to be stressed, however, that political priority should be given to the implementation of such programmes. HIV/AIDS prevention should be an integrated part of these programmes. A nationwide prevention message should be granted by the school authorities, providing the necessary information and hands-on training (e.g. how to use a condom correctly) to all age groups of adolescents and to all types of schools. Equal access – independent of education – has to be assured. Additionally, innovative programmes are needed such as peer-group education for young people with specific needs, e.g. young homosexuals or young drug users, to only name two of the many groups with specific needs. Organizations that have started to develop such specific programmes should be strongly supported.

V.   STRATEGIES TARGETING PEOPLE LIVING WITH HIV OR AIDS

Comprehensive psychosocial support has been defined as a committed and understanding support through all stages of HIV infection. This would have to include a wide range of service offers: HIV-testing facilities providing adequate pre- and post-test counselling, low-threshold, non-bureaucratic and easily available counselling facilities, adequate medical treatment facilities, flexible home care services, cooperation with families, etc. Public inclusive organizations in most cases are not adequately equipped to provide such services. The lack of professional training in these organizations complicates matters further: crucial activities, such as case-management and networking, for example, are barely offered in Austria.

Promoting non-profit organizations with experience in delivering such services (buddy programmes, home services, etc.) would contribute to a reduction in costs: Hospital care often means not only additional emotional distress and isolation, it is also much more expensive. Offering more outpatient-facilities and home care services would effectively reduce the overall costs of health care.

On the organizational level, e.g. at the level of hospital departments, comprehensive care for AIDS patients could be much better reached by restructuring the inflexible work routine. A greater flexibility in working hours, the implementation of quality standards and supervision and emotional support of the staff are only some options that can help to avoid burn-out for health-care workers in the field of HIV/AIDS.

A general reorientation of the health care system is strongly advised. We have given several examples for why not only AIDS patients would benefit from re-oriented health and social policies. Compared to other health and social problems – e.g. the drug problem, care for the elderly, or cancer – HIV/AIDS is clearly a minor one. But the specifics of AIDS as a medical and social phenomenon very much illustrate the need for a change in dealing with health and disease in general.

3.3.2 Distribution of the Organizational Response across Geographical Areas

The declared political aim of the restructuring of the Austrian *AIDS-Hilfe* was to achieve a stronger involvement on the federal level in the field of HIV/AIDS. To really evaluate the organizational response in this respect, a longitudinal follow-up study would be needed. Our data show, however, that the aim of a stronger federal participation has not yet been reached. Hence, HIV/AIDS-related activities should be much more promoted on a federal level, requiring first and foremost a stronger financial commitment on the part of the federal authorities. Activities pertaining to care and psychosocial support for example, are clearly defined as federal matters and thus, it has to be assured that people with HIV/AIDS can have access to the care they need no matter where they happen to live and what disease they are affected with. This picture is reflected not only by the uneven geographical distribution of organizations and activities, but also by the total absence of certain activities in some areas. Surprisingly, this refers not only to low-threshold or self-help and voluntary activities, which would already require a certain degree of normalization as a prerequisite, but also to activities which are provided by the traditional health care system (e.g. AIDS-specialized medical care). Some regions do lack facilities for specialized medical care in the area of HIV/AIDS, which can be explained by the fact that highly-specialized departments are not affordable in regions where AIDS cases are few. This argument brings us back to what has already been questioned above: First, it remains to ask whether such a high degree of specialization is needed at all costs. Secondly, the role of physicians and their insufficient involvement in the medical care for people with HIV/AIDS has to be evaluated critically. And thirdly, with respect to the geographical distribution of services, we ought to question why people who are in need of specific services have to go to places outside their communities to be treated.

HIV/AIDS-related policies should therefore much more promote the community-based provision of services, which, in turn, would favour the normalization of HIV/AIDS in society. This would additionally help to fight discrimination and isolation, which people with HIV/AIDS are still suffering from.

3.4 General Conclusions

On the basis of the above-presented results and their discussion, some general conclusions can be formulated. Although the overall organizational response to HIV/AIDS has developed fairly well in Austria (e.g. general access to services, public funding for AIDS service organizations, an increase in the state's responsibility for general information campaigns, etc.), there is an underdeveloped integration among the existing organizations as well as a lack of division of labour. The relatively small number of non-profit organizations might explain why specific activities that have proven to be successful in responding adequately to HIV/AIDS in other countries, e.g. buddy systems, self-help groups, needle-exchange programmes, condom distribution, etc. are only provided to a limited degree in Austria. It also became clear in the Austrian case that the few existing exclusive non-profit organizations tend to deliver services no other organizational form does. Conclusively, a comprehensive HIV/AIDS policy needs, first, to pay specific attention to these types of organizations and allocate specific resources to them. Second, it has to find ways to increase the mobilization of silent resources in order to enhance the integration and normalization of the HIV/AIDS phenomenon. And third, it has to respond more adequately to the needs of specific groups of clients, such as women, IV-drug users, young homosexuals and the youth in general.

From an overall public health perspective, some of the specific conclusions which follow from the study are extremely important, not only because they could potentially improve the organizational response in the field of HIV/AIDS, but also because other areas of health and welfare problems could benefit from the innovative organizational approaches developed in the field of HIV/AIDS. Shifting the overall focus from disease treatment and cure to disease prevention and health promotion, for example, constitutes a public health approach which is gaining more and more importance. The public health field of HIV/AIDS has been one of the first to have fully implemented this approach. A further integration of medical and psychosocial services as well as a promotion of self-help approaches would hence also be necessary for people who need home care, who suffer from whatever chronic disease.

The AIDS phenomenon has shown how strongly interlinked disease, dying and social inequality is even in a generally homogeneous society such as Austria. However, the strong, passionate and innovative commitment of many persons and organizations active in the field of HIV/AIDS, which has been attempted to document here, has also brought about the chances to balance out these inequalities.

Notes

1   With respect to the regulation of HIV-antibody testing, an additonal decree to the AIDS Law (September 1994) specifies that only if risk behaviour is to be assumed should persons who have tested negative receive post-test counselling.

2   In contrast to exclusive and inclusive organizations which are covered in the present survey, "inclusive inclusives" are not. These are organizations which do not deal explicitly with HIV/AIDS in a different or differentiated way. An example of such an organization would be one providing housing facilities for people in crisis situations: such an organization might also do this for seropositive persons or those with AIDS, perhaps even without knowledge of their particular medical condition or even disregarding it. Another example would be a family planning centre which offers information on AIDS as one sexually-transmitted disease among many without offering any AIDS-specific educational activities.

3   Figures are based on Austrian prisons that test more than 80% of their inmates on HIV-antibodies.

4   Note that with respect to the organizations' "legal status", chi-square statistics were calculated only for 103 organizations; the two private organizations were excluded from the statistical analysis. Note also, that all significant relationships refer to a chi square < 0.05.

References

Bochow, M. (1994) 'Reaktionen homosexueller Männer auf HIV und AIDS', pp. 279-290 in: Heckmann, W./Koch, M. (Eds.), *Sexualverhalten in Zeiten von AIDS. Ergebnisse sozialwissenschaftlicher AIDS-Forschung*, Band 12. Berlin: Edition Sigma.

Bundesministerium für Gesundheit, Sport und Konsumentenschutz (1993) *AIDS-Informations- und Präventionskonzept.* Unpublished Document. Vienna: Ministry of Health and Consumer Protection.

Bundesministerium für Gesundheit, Sport und Konsumentenschutz (1995) *Österreichische AIDS-Statistik. Periodischer Bericht*, April 28, 1995. Vienna: Ministry of Health and Consumer Protection.

Dubois-Arber, F./Paccaud, F. (1994) 'Assessing AIDS/HIV Prevention: What Do We Know in Europe? European Community Concerted Action "Assessment of the AIDS/HIV Preventive Strategies" ', *Sozial- und Präventivmedizin* 39 (Suppl. 1): 3-13.

Falter Nr. 30 (1994) 'AIDS in Wien. 410 Tote', pp. 8-12. Vienna: Falter Verlag.

Fazekas, C. (1991) 'AIDS and Austrian Physicians', *AIDS. Education and Prevention* 3 (1).

Franke, G.H. (1990) *Die psychosoziale Situation von HIV-Positiven. Ergebnisse sozialwissenschaftlicher AIDS-Forschung*, Band 5. Berlin: Edition Sigma.

Kenis, P./Marin, B./Nöstlinger, C. (1994) *AIDS-Management in Österreich im internationalen Vergleich*, Band II. Forschungsendbericht. Studie im Auftrag des Bundesministeriums für Gesundheit und Konsumentenschutz. Vienna: European Centre for Social Welfare Policy and Research.

Kunz, C. (1992) *Virusepidemiologische Informationen* Nr. 8. Vienna: Institute of Virology, University of Vienna.

Nöstlinger, C./Wimmer-Puchinger, B. (1994) *Geschützte Liebe – Jugendsexualität und AIDS. Eine internationale Vergleichsstudie*. Vienna: Jugend und Volk.

Pfersmann, D./Presslich, O. (Eds.) (1994) *Drogensucht und Therapie*. Vienna: Verlag Wilhelm Maudrich.

Pont, J./Kahl, W./Salzner, G. (1994) 'HIV-Epidemiologie und Risikoverhalten für HIV-Transmission in Haft in Österreich', pp. 167-173 in Pfersmann, D./Presslich, O. (Eds.), *Drogensucht und Therapie*. Vienna: Verlag Wilhelm Maudrich.

Rack, H. (1992) *The Health Care System in Austria. A Survey – Reforms of the Past Decade*. Vienna: Federal Ministry of Labour and Social Affairs.

Wiener Drogenbericht 1992/1993 (1994) Vienna: Büro des Drogenkoordinators, Magistrat der Stadt Wien.

Wimmer-Puchinger, B. (1995) *Evaluationsstudie der AIDS-Kampagne 1994*. Im Auftrag des Bundesministeriums für Gesundheit und Konsumentenschutz. Vienna: Ludwig Boltzmann Institut für Gesundheitspsychologie der Frau.

World Health Organization (1990) *Guidelines for Counselling about HIV Infection and Disease*. WHO AIDS Series Nr. 8. Geneva: World Health Organization.

Zangerle, R./Klein, J.P. (1994) 'Unterschiede im Überleben von AIDS Patienten in Österreich'. Presentation at the *Vth Austrian AIDS Congress*, September 9-10, 1994, Vienna.

CHAPTER 7

Managing AIDS in Italy

Emma Fasolo

1   Institutional, Policy and Epidemiological Context

1.1   Public AIDS Policy

In 1988, AIDS was put on the list of infectious diseases which must be reported by law, however, there is no obligation to report HIV cases. Every case of AIDS is reported by the doctor who made the diagnosis to the regional government and to the *Higher Institute of Health (Istituto Superiore di Sanita, ISS)*, using a special form that includes more than 30 variables. Besides the national register of AIDS cases, there exists another one that records patients who are being treated with AZT. Blood donations are subjected to obligatory screening for HIV infection. Forty-five out-patient centres for sexually-transmitted diseases are now linked in a national system of vigilance. The results of these tests remain anonymous. The data are passed on to the Higher Institute of Health, which issues quarterly reports – thousands of copies of which are distributed throughout the country.

The national AIDS policy is thus extremely centralized at the level of health care, medical research (for which more than 100 billion lire [US$ 62 m.] have been allocated in 5 years) and monitoring. Priority with regard to policy choices is given to health care aspects.

The government has enacted a series of initiatives and financial commitments since 1990, some of which are exceptional when compared to commitments made in other public health sectors.

Law 135, of 5 June 1990, defines a "Programme of Urgent Measures for the Prevention of AIDS and the Fight against It". This law, and the subsequent decrees implementing it, constitute a systematic plan of action aimed at directing the decisions of regional governments and the non-profit sector.

On the economic side, 2.1 trillion lire ($ 1,300 m.) have annually been appropri-
ated for the construction and renovation of specialized departments in hospitals,
and more than 157 billion lire ($ 97 m.) have been allocated to hire, train, and offer
incentives to staff. Unspecified funds have also been provided for research, prevention and information, and to support volunteers. Sixty billion lire ($ 37 m.) have
been earmarked for medical treatment at home by public health agencies (*The Local
Health Units, USL*), 38 billion lire ($ 23.5 m.) to improve services for drug users
and 6 billion lire ($ 3.5 m.) for centres for sexually-transmitted diseases.

The coordination of measures to implement this plan has been entrusted to an
Interministerial Committee; this is made up of representatives of the Ministries of
Health, Social Affairs, University and Scientific Research, Public Education,
Labour, Defence, Justice, the Interior, and Public Works.

We can conclude that since approximately two years ago the central government
has made an important commitment to the fight against AIDS, involving all of those
institutions which are able to make contributions in various forms in order to
confront this epidemic. Law 135/1990 also emphasizes the "exceptional urgency"
of this measure and provides for exemptions from current regulations relating to
the hiring of staff in the public sector.

However, even earlier than that, since 1985 in particular, there has been a response on the part of the authorities concerning diagnostic testing and health
remedies. During that year, a national law urged the regional governments, who
have jurisdiction in the matter, to institute diagnostic and therapeutic services for
persons with HIV and AIDS at Local Health Units. It can be said that public agencies
and the medical profession began paying attention to AIDS before the private sector
and social welfare workers.

However, members of the non-profit sector were the first to undertake activities
aimed at education and prevention, and also to take the psychological and social
aspects of the disease into consideration. These first activities occurred within the
framework of services for drug users and, almost simultaneously, within those
organizations that defend the rights of homosexuals.

The same Law 135/1990 recognized the importance of the role played by non-
profit agencies, not only by providing them with financial assistance but by making
consultation with them a part of the planning process. The involvement of the non-
profit agencies in the plans implemented by the public sector is no longer occa-
sional but has recently been institutionalized in the form of *Forum AIDS Italia*,
and it should help to overcome the main inadequacies which exist in volunteer
activities in this area, namely, the isolated and rather unsystematic nature of their
efforts. Forum AIDS Italia brings together the main non-profit organizations which
concern themselves with AIDS. The representatives of these organizations, together
with high-level government officials and experts (above all doctors), make up the
National Commission for the Fight against AIDS, chaired by the Minister of Health.

It acts as a consultative body to the Government for the implementation of those measures provided for in the plan.

1.2 Major Issues of Conflict in Public Debate

At present, the main conflicts and the problems which remain unsolved seem to be the following (keeping in mind that the general policy picture is, in a sense, "fluctuating" and that what is true today might change in a very short period of time):

a) Educational and information campaigns are still inadequate despite the impulse given to this sector – both by the government and by single organizations – in order to sufficiently inform the population in general and young people in particular.

   The news supplied by the mass media often heightens irrational anxieties and fears – regardless of the intentions behind these campaigns; only accurate scientific information and well-planned health education might help to reduce this. Many scholars agree that the social perception of the danger of AIDS has far exceeded the actual danger, without having produced any significant changes in the behavioural patterns of those considered to be at risk.

b) The social pressures made by associations of PWAs (persons with AIDS) and by persons with HIV on the social security system to obtain anticipated retirement benefits, or at least to reduce the time necessary for getting a pension for those unable to work, have so far been unsuccessful.

c) As has already been mentioned, large funds have been assigned to the regional governments for the setting-up of social and health-related home services for AIDS patients. Yet, most regions find it difficult to put these facilities into practice. The main reason can be found in the scarcity of specialized personnel willing to take on such tasks. However, managers of health services are reluctant to use volunteers (who are too scarce in this field) because they fear the risks involved in taking on people with insufficient medical training. On the whole, the institutions regard AIDS far more as a dangerous disease than a social and psychological problem.

d) For this reason, and out of humanitarian motives, a few non-profit organizations are beginning to appeal to the public powers in order to have the organization of homes for small groups of patients approved and financed. But for the moment, only a limited number of organizations have been realized, despite the increasing need for them. This kind of service often encounters a hostile attitude from the surrounding population, among other difficulties.

e) In general it can be said that, except for ambulatory drug treatment, there is a persistent dichotomy between the treatment offered to patients within hospitals and the relative abandon they are left to during the intervals between hospital in-patient treatment.

f) The recent reform of the national health system is causing additional problems to patients: some medicines must now be paid for (at least partially) by the patient him/herself. The same is true for other serious chronic illnesses, but due to the smaller number of AIDS patients, the polemics of the reform are not focused on their particular needs.

In addition, as a result of the reform, most drugs necessary for prolonging life, which used to be part of the ambulatory treatment, can only be given to in-patients. Due to the shortage of beds in certain areas, the waiting list for some hospitals is becoming dangerously long.

A more detailed description of these and other issues can be found in relation to the analysis of the programmes offered by organizations and is summed up in the last part of this chapter.

1.3   HIV/AIDS and the General Health and Welfare System

The *National Health Service (NHS)*, which has replaced the earlier insurance system, has guaranteed all citizens, irrespective of their employment and financial circumstances, health assistance in its different forms since 1978. Although envisaged as being financed solely from tax revenues, the NHS today draws its main support from the compulsory contributions deducted from employees and their employers who are taxable under the previous insurance system (which covers over 90% of the population, including pensioners and family members). Those who do not fall into the above-mentioned groups pay an income-related contribution. The state also makes an annual financial contribution, which has been increasing considerably over the years.

Health assistance is provided through services available at public or private centres and, to a limited extent, by means of transfer in order to reimburse expenses sustained by Italian citizens.

During the 1970s, the Italian state carried out the decentralization process envisaged by the constitution. This involved the health and welfare sector to a significant extent. Consequently, the local authorities were assigned responsibility for all the administrative functions whereas the regions were responsible for planning and financing programmes and activities related to HIV/AIDS. The regional governments are also still responsible for the prophylaxis of infectious diseases and are bound by the principles set out by the state, which has the power to direct and coordinate the regional activities.

The regions also have legislative power regarding the basic regulations established by the laws of the national state, which provides the regions with the necessary funds to carry out their functions. However, unlike the health service, there is no national law which governs the welfare sector in an integrated way, setting guidelines and general principles valid for the whole country.

This might partly explain why at the time the HIV/AIDS emergency arose, the central government was able to use the provisions provided by the National Health Law (no. 833/1978) for enacting the special regulations described in section 1.1 of this chapter, while the welfare system was mostly left to the initiative of the local authorities with obvious consequences regarding their erratic development.

However, it is also within this field that the regional laws on welfare reveal the presence of common trends and of a basic philosophy which might represent an incentive to promoting better services for people with HIV/AIDS. Among the principles expressed by the regional legislation there is a need to integrate health care in all cases where the well-being of the individual cannot be achieved via the medical approach alone; favouring action which allows the subject to remain in his/her own living environment while institutionalized services should remain a last resort. The patient and the family as a whole should be considered and assisted through integrated services; there should be a mobilization and involvement of all community resources; a structured involvement of public and non-profit organizations on the territory coordinated by the public sector is also necessary.

The problem is that, in spite of the principles expressed by the regional legislation, there is a marked lack of application not only because of the scarcity of financial and technical resources and the shortage of adequate professional staff, but also, as far as people with HIV/AIDS are concerned, because of the priority given to other needs and categories that are more visible in number and are, in a sense, better "accepted" by public opinion. This will be discussed in section 2.1.

1.4 The Epidemiological Development

The first AIDS cases recorded in Italy were a few male homosexuals. In 1983, the first Ministry of Health circular letter on this subject pointed out that "so far, this Ministry is not aware of any proven cases of the Acquired Immune Deficiency Syndrome in our country" (circular letter no. 64, 3 August 1983). The same note pointed out that "the syndrome is extremely deadly", optimistically appraising the death rate at "up to 60%".

Immediately after this, however, at the beginning of 1985, there was a sharp increase in the epidemic curve with a reversal in the percentage of cases found in the largest risk groups (homosexuals and IV-drug users). Whereas in 1984 these had accounted for 70% and 30% of all known cases respectively, only two years later, in 1986, the percentage breakdown of AIDS cases stood at 28% for homosexual and bisexual males, 59% for IV-drug users, and 10% for haemophiliacs and blood transfusion patients.

On 31 December that same year, the number of recorded AIDS cases in Italy was 525, with 295 deaths. But the figure had risen to 1,704 by 31 December 1987, 5,853 as at 31 December 1989, while in 1992 the steep increase in the epidemic curve can be seen from the following figures: 12,754 as at 31 March, 13,668 as at 30 June, 14,783 as at 30 September, and 15,780 as at 31 December. On 31 March 1993 the cases reported to the Higher Institute of Health numbered 16,860. When one considers that it took about 90 days to report AIDS cases to the Ministry of Health after diagnosis, this means that an underestimation of 40% existed. The actual number of AIDS patients in Italy at the beginning of 1993 was probably nearer to 17,000. Of all the reported cases of AIDS, 9,048 had died between 1985 (when the reporting of cases became obligatory) and 1993.

Lastly, the estimated number of AIDS patients by the end of 1993 was approaching near to 20,000 – 9% of which were non drug-using heterosexuals.

There are no visible signs of the epidemic slowing down even if the curve seems to be stabilizing. Due to the long incubation period of the disease one can assume that most patients became infected in the early 1980s when the information campaigns for the general public had not yet begun on a vast scale. An exact assessment of the number of persons with HIV is not possible because it is not mandatory to report these cases. However, from epidemiological studies their number is estimated to be between 70,000 and 100,000.

Figure 7.1:   Cumulative Number of AIDS Cases and Adjustments for Reporting Delays

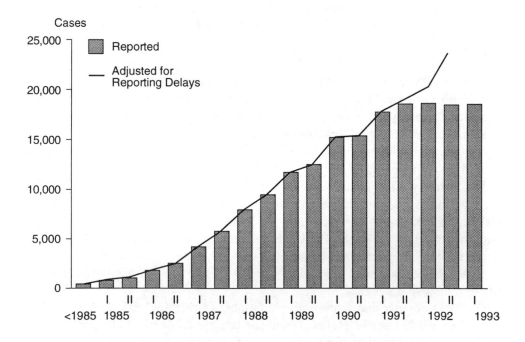

Source: Centro operativo AIDS. Istituto Superiore di Sanita.

Drug users remain the main risk group in absolute terms: the percentage of drug users has grown more than any other group. At the present time they account for 69% of the total whereas the relative number of haemophiliacs and multiple transfusion AIDS patients has declined to 2.5%. Another problem linked to drug addiction is the number of paediatric AIDS cases: with 334 cases of children under the age of 13 (in 1992), 92% of whom have been infected by their mothers. Italy (after Spain and France) has the third-largest number of indigenous cases of AIDS in Europe, i.e. children of HIV-positive, intravenous drug-using mothers.

In view of the high proportion of HIV-positive cases and the young age of the IV-drug-using population, it is likely that the number of at-risk pregnancies will also continue to increase.

Finally, whereas there seems to have been a reduction in the number of homo- and bisexuals suffering from AIDS, who now only account for 15% of the total – probably as a result of the information and prevention campaigns set in motion by organizations responsible for the members of this group – heterosexual intercourse is becoming increasingly more marked as a means of transmitting the virus.

2 Mapping the Services and the Development of Organizational Responses to HIV/AIDS

2.1 Volume of Development of the Overall Response

2.1.1 Number of Organizations and Activities

The public and non-profit organizations involved in different HIV/AIDS-related activities (as specified in section 1) number about 1,550. Of these, 1,335 (87.5%) have been analysed in this study. Those impossible to reach are mostly clinic-diagnostic centres (*centri diagnostico-clinici*) since many of them are in the process of being reorganized following a law passed in 1990. These centres are medically specialized units in charge of HIV screening, out-patient therapy, the periodic control of seropositive persons and of people at risk.

Moreover, 50 organizations have been studied in depth through detailed interviews. They have been selected according to the following criteria:

- geographical breakdown: 5 organizations were interviewed in each of the 10 major cities across the country;
- legal status: 20 organizations are public, 30 private non-profit;
- inclusive or exclusive orientation: 36 belong to the former group, 14 to the latter. Note that the exclusive ones are only 2.7% of the total, but they were preferred for the interviews since their activities and operation seemed particularly interesting for research purposes.

Table 7.1: **Number of Organizations by Legal Status and Organizational Orientation**

	Public	Private Non-Profit	Private For-Profit	No Reply[*]	Total	%
Inclusives	539	753	5	1	1,298	97.2
Exclusives	10	26	0	0	36	2.7
No Response	0	0	0	1	1	0.1
Total	549	779	5	2	1,335	100

[*] As far as the "no reply" questions are concerned, one of the inclusive organizations failed to state its legal status, and in the case of another one we do not know the sector to which it belongs (i.e. public, private non-profit or commercial), and whether it is exclusive or inclusive.

The first thing to note in this distribution is that non-profit organizations outnumber the public ones because it is among them that a high number of services for drug addicts can be found. The division of labour between private and public sectors in the care of drug users is explained in more detail in section 2 of this chapter. However, there are very few commercial organizations, and none of them offers services exclusively in the field of HIV/AIDS.

Also very limited in absolute (36 in all) and relative numbers are the exclusive organizations. An explanation for this scarcity, which might seem peculiar for a country like Italy, can be found in section 2.1.4. In any case, their number seems reliable because it is difficult for the organizations to work without being registered by the National Institute of Health which provided the data. This is because of the fact that these organizations almost completely rely on public funds.

Table 7.2: **Distribution of Organizations by Legal Status and Organizational Orientation (in %)**

	Public	Private Non-Profit	Private For-Profit
Inclusives	98.2	96.7	100
Exclusives	1.8	3.3	0
Total	100	100	100

Table 7.3: Number of Organizations by Type of Organization and Legal Status

	Public	Private Non-Profit	Private For-Profit	Total
Drug Treatment/Counselling Centres (Out-patient and Communities)	473	718	3	1,194
Health Units (Out-patient and Residential)	53	3	0	56
Social Service Organizations	3	23	1	27
Self-help and Interest Groups	0	20	0	20
Education or Information	1	13	0	14
Tests and Blood Control	12	1	0	13
Epidemiological and Social Research	4	0	0	4
Blood/Plasma Product Banks	3	0	0	3
Total	549	778	4	1,331
No response	4			

2.1.2 Organizational Development. Responsiveness by Region and Geographical Area

Diagnostic and therapeutic medical units (56 health units and 13 organizations for tests and blood control) for HIV/AIDS were set up within the public sector from 1985 onwards. The first to make a move were the regional governments of Lombardy and Latium which had the largest number of cases. The other public health and inclusive facilities subsequently equipped themselves as the epidemic curve rose; this varied considerably from one region to another. At the beginning of 1989 only two regions, one in the north, Val d'Aosta, and one in the south, Molise, still had no reported cases, and at the beginning of 1991 there were 8 cases in Val d'Aosta and 4 in Molise, compared with 2,873 in Lombardy and 1,171 in Latium.

The following table relates the global number of AIDS cases to the number of inhabitants in order to compare regions with different sizes in population.

It therefore appears that if in absolute terms three regions only (Lombardy, Latium, Emilia-Romagna) account for over half the cases recorded, as far as the

Table 7.4: Distribution of AIDS Cases by Year and Region and Rates per 100,000 Inhabitants

Regions	1982	1983	1984	1985	1986	1987	1988	1989	1990	1991	1992	1993	Total	Rate per 100,000
Piemonte	0	0	3	8	37	66	133	162	196	284	281	45	1215	27.1
Val d'Aosta	0	0	0	0	0	0	0	1	7	9	5	2	24	21.4
Lombardia	0	2	13	80	166	342	560	793	917	1,126	1,004	41	5,044	56.7
Trentino-Bolzano	0	0	0	0	1	3	6	5	7	18	24	3	67	15.6
Trentino-Trento	0	0	0	1	2	5	7	15	14	21	29	8	102	23.0
Veneto	0	0	3	11	28	56	95	153	199	210	222	25	1,002	23.1
Friuli Venezia Giulia	0	0	1	1	3	10	11	15	24	24	32	7	128	10.4
Liguria	0	0	0	8	28	64	99	143	173	206	219	21	961	53.1
Emilia Romagna	0	0	7	20	35	117	173	226	284	368	402	46	1,678	42.4
Toscana	0	0	0	12	30	54	100	164	204	209	245	30	1,048	29.3
Umbria	0	0	0	1	2	2	10	21	11	24	34	3	108	13.4
Marche	0	0	1	2	9	13	35	33	42	57	63	9	264	18.7
Lazio	1	3	3	18	48	122	233	342	404	460	514	84	2,232	44.6
Abruzzi	0	0	0	0	3	8	6	18	24	24	22	2	107	8.8
Molise	0	0	0	0	0	0	0	1	3	3	2	1	10	3.1
Campania	0	0	2	4	16	27	64	74	94	106	167	28	582	10.7
Puglia	0	1	0	5	7	36	49	60	108	139	150	18	573	14.8
Basilicata	0	0	0	0	2	1	3	4	9	10	9	3	41	6.7
Calabria	0	0	0	4	3	15	12	15	36	33	39	8	165	8.0
Sicilia	0	0	2	5	21	37	74	101	162	158	170	27	757	15.4
Sardegna	0	2	0	11	11	33	71	65	109	105	130	29	564	35.4
Estero	0	0	2	4	3	5	11	17	19	23	11	3	100	–
Ignota	0	0	0	0	0	0	2	4	16	21	38	7	88	–
Total	1	8	37	195	455	1,016	1,754	2,432	3,062	3,638	3,812	450	16,860	29.8

Source: National Institute of Health.

residential population is concerned, the disease has spread more rapidly in Liguria, putting it second after Lombardy and Sardinia. It is also obvious that there are a great many differences between north and south: namely that in the southern regions, except Sardinia, the absolute number of cases, as well as the incidence rate are clearly much lower.

Although about 88% of the organizations provide treatment and rehabilitation facilities for drug users and are of the inclusive type, very few of them are able to indicate the exact date in which their activities for HIV/AIDS got started. Their attention toward clients with HIV/AIDS developed gradually. Summing up, it can be stated that the HIV/AIDS problem was firstly dealt with as a medical issue and within the public structures. The private non-profit and exclusive organizations have started in the last four to five years.

Turning now to the way in which the organizations are distributed throughout Italy, it seems that the regions in Central Italy with the largest number of AIDS cases (after the North-West) have fewer organizations than the North-East – even than the South where there are fewer recorded cases. Finally, there are about twice as many organizations in the North (East and West), in proportion to the number of patients, than in the South and on the islands.

As far as the geographical scope of organizations is concerned, the majority are local. This is due to the fact that the National Health Service (NHS) has developed the implementation of health policy on first-level Local Boards (*USLs*) which have a population of approximately 50,000 to 400,000 people. These services are responsible for conducting the HIV screening of risk groups – particularly drug users. As far as the therapeutic communities are concerned, they are only equipped to deal with a comparatively small number of clients – with a few exceptions, namely the oldest and best established ones which treat people from all over Italy.

Table 7.5: Number of Organizations by Geographical Area and Legal Status

	Public	Private Non-Profit	Private For-Profit	No Response	Total	%
North-West	178	273	1	1	453	33.9
North-East	103	175	1	1	280	21
Centre	113	153	2	0	268	20.1
South and Islands	155	178	1	0	334	25
Total	549	779	5	2	1,335	100

Table 7.6:   Distribution of Organizations by Region

	Number	%
Piemonte	122	9.1
Val d'Aosta	4	0.3
Lombardia	277	20.7
Trentino-Alto Adige	21	1.6
Veneto	116	8.7
Friuli Venezia Giulia	25	1.9
Liguria	51	3.8
Emilia Romagna	123	9.3
Toscana	93	6.9
Umbria	37	2.8
Marche	47	3.5
Lazio	86	6.5
Abruzzi	29	2.2
Molise	5	0.4
Campania	50	3.7
Puglia	109	8.2
Basilicata	13	0.9
Calabria	23	1.7
Sicilia	66	4.9
Sardegna	39	2.9
Total	1,336	100

The social and welfare services have a narrow territorial scope. On regional, national and multinational levels, however, there are organizations whose activities are mainly to curb the spread of the disease, educate the public, carry out preventive programmes, and to lobby and promote civil rights. With regard to these latter aspects, the organizations claim that it is becoming increasingly obvious that co-operation and linkage with organizations in other countries with similar aims is necessary. This is also the case for non-profit organizations, which were originally brought in to mainly exchange information and to provide mutual support at a time when the spread of the disease was very limited and the categories affected by it were the object of social discrimination.

Table 7.7: Distribution of Organizations by Territorial Domain

	Public	Private Non-Profit	Private For-Profit	No Response	Total	%
Multinational	6	4	0	0	10	0.8
National	11	12	0	0	3	1.7
Regional	24	3	0	0	1	4.6
Local	511	727	5	1	1,244	92.8
No Response	2	0	0	1	3	0.2
Total	554	780	5	2	1,341	100

The slight difference between the number of organizations enumerated (1,336) and the number of replies is due to the fact that some organizations work on more than one geographical level and have therefore given more than one reply.

2.1.3 Organizational Responsiveness by Target Group

As far as the clientele is concerned, both public and third-sector organizations deal in the vast majority of cases with clients of specific risk groups (particularly drug users). The reason for this is that these institutions had originally been set up to deal with the drug problem before AIDS had emerged; they have neither changed their target even though they have broadened their functions.

However, the spread of the epidemic among the heterosexual population, as indicated above in section 1 of this chapter, is a clear indication that it is necessary to increase the number of services addressed to the population at large. In relation to this, one can see that 77 public and 55 private social welfare agencies stated that they did not have any specific target group. Of these, only 7 in the public sector, and 10 in the private sector, restrict their services to Italian nationals. The fact that foreign nationals are also accepted by the remaining 70 public and 45 non-profit organizations is important now that immigrants from African and Asian countries, who are sometimes affected by HIV/AIDS, are on the increase. It should be noted, however, that the public services provide the most comprehensive services (proportionally), even though they are fewer in number than in the private non-profit sector.

It should be noted that there is slightly more universal coverage of activities related to HIV/AIDS in the organizations in the North-East and Centre of Italy. But this is not due to any difference in social and health policy on the part of the organizations concerned, but simply to the fact that these are the areas with the

Table 7.8: Number of Organizations by Service Access for Clients and Legal Status

	Public	Private Non-Profit	Private For-Profit	No Response	Total
Service Access for:					
Everyone (including foreigners)	70	45	2	0	117
Italian Citizens	7	10	0	0	17
Specific Groups	470	724	3	1	1,198
No Response	2	0	0	1	3
Total	549	779	5	2	1,335
%	41.1	58.4	0.4	0.2	100

Table 7.9: Distribution of Service Access for Clients by Geographical Location of Organizations (in %)

	North-West	North-East	Centre	South and Islands
Service Access for:				
Everyone	6.2	10.0	14.9	6.3
Italian Citizens	1.6	1.1	1.5	0.9
Specific Groups	92.1	88.2	83.6	92.8
No Response	0.2	0.7	0	0
Total	100	100	100	100

largest concentration of organizations working mainly for the defence of civil rights, prevention and information rather than the provision of direct assistance to clients.

One of the conclusions that one may draw regarding the AIDS policy field is that, generally speaking, it reflects what one finds in other areas of Italian social and health care policy. As the disease has spread, the development of welfare-oriented initiatives has increased, especially in the North when compared to the South. Coordination or control is sparse and public authorities have predominantly developed structures for medical care. Neither the public nor the private sectors have a policy restricting the right of access based on the nationality of their clients or their place of residence. They are there, however, to cater for the practical needs of particular groups of clients who are not only HIV-positive or suffering from full-blown AIDS, but also from other serious problems such as drug addiction, homelessness or poverty.

2.1.4 Organizational Responsiveness by Legal Status

In order to explain why by far most services – both public and private – which have responded to HIV/AIDS are drug-specific organizations, one should consider the general social policies in Italy for the so-called "groups at risk".

Drug abuse is a problem that is worrying the authorities and public opinion a great deal, not only due to the high number of dependent young people but because it is connected with both macro- and micro-criminality and has reflections even on our migration policy.

All of the most recent Italian laws in this field show a trend towards repressive measures. Drug abuse is defined as being a criminal offence: some consequences are that immigrants selling drugs are expelled and prisons are overcrowded with drug users.

As a reaction to this rather punitive attitude, the social and health organizations for drug users – both public and private – had to take over the tasks related to the psychological and social rehabilitation of their clients with HIV/AIDS. These structures were generally ready to play that role because they were not working in isolation, but were supported with medical advice by the Local Health Units and by the courts for information about drug users affected by HIV/AIDS. Infected persons committing minor criminal offences are referred to the therapeutic communities instead of being sent to prison.

Since the discovery of AIDS, both the private and public sectors have dealt very differently with drug addiction. The private sector was originally responsible for setting up the first residential therapeutic communities; these have subsequently increased in number and have been contracted into the health care system. They were mostly run by volunteers.

However, in the public sector the problem was dealt with mainly on an out-patient basis, the most common forms of treatment being medical treatment and individual psychological counselling services. Since the residential therapeutic communities in the private non-profit sector had already acquired sufficient experience, they could be used by the public sector for individuals who did not use out-patient treatment – making it unnecessary to set up any public residential facilities in most cases. This implicit separation of areas of competence (medical/psychological out-patient treatment in public institutions; rebuilding the personality through work, community life, separation from the home and previous social environment by living in private residential facilities) still remains – though to a lesser degree. When AIDS appeared in Italy, residential facilities – where community life increased the risk of infection – wanted to know whether they were taking in HIV-positive persons.

Therefore, drug users who are referred to or who apply to therapeutic communities are nearly always tested, although an HIV test is normally not compulsory except in the case of blood transfusions. They are accepted even if infected, but the communities are informed of their condition and take the necessary precautions, i.e. they inform those people in closest contact with the patients (doctors, nurses, psychologists, instructors, group leaders, depending on the internal organization of the community).

Homo- and heterosexual persons affected with AIDS have not been given any special attention by policy-makers as yet. Homosexuals have not been regarded because they are able to organize themselves up to the point of sometimes becoming "interlocutors" of the government within Forum AIDS Italia (section 1.1) and also because they are relatively small in number. Although they are not formally discriminated, they are isolated.

Heterosexuals have not been considered by policy-makers because the problem is only now becoming evident. It has been mentioned that the local governments are trying to organize home services and are coming up against great difficulties. Again, the policy plans at the central level seem to anticipate the capacity of the local administrators to implement them.

Thus the organizational response to the social and medical aspects of the epidemics has worked for drug users because it was already prominent before the onset of AIDS, as well as the fact that drug users are a subject of major concern.

The other people without such an additional problem like drug abuse have few social organizations to refer to. This is either because they are a minority or because their condition (removed from public consciousness until recently) is seen as only a medical problem to be dealt with by the test and diagnostic centres and by the hospitals, or to be illustrated within the national prevention campaigns addressed to the whole population.

As one would expect, medical research centres, blood banks, and agencies responsible for ensuring that products are harmless and for carrying out HIV tests are all public (with one exception in the area of testing) as these are activities which relate to national health policies. The reverse applies, however, to those organizations whose main purpose is to educate and inform the public. The exception here is the AIDS help-line which has been set up at the Higher Institute of Health (ISS). This is a help-line which not only provides counselling and information but also puts people with HIV/AIDS in contact with diagnostic and treatment centres, guaranteeing anonymity. It has been in operation for several years, and the number of calls since its foundation in 1984 have been very high (127,454 by 30 June 1992).

As far as the social welfare services proper are concerned, the small number of public organizations providing them may be misleading. In reality, the Family Counselling Units provide counselling services for patients' families and HIV-positive persons, for example, but not on a systematic basis. This is done when the opportunity arises, or at the request of the clients. What the public facilities have so far overlooked is the organization of shelters, safe houses, or home care services, leaving these to the private non-profit sector.

Finally, it seems that the for-profit sector has not yet considered social welfare and health care assistance for AIDS patients, HIV-infected persons and their families as possible clients. The only examples are a home nursing service and three other services for drug addicts which are commercially operated. Since the disease frequently affects persons with high incomes, one may wonder why this service is not being provided more often. One answer may be that the families cover the costs of treatment themselves, resorting to assistance from outside the organized institutions. When the patient is alone, however wealthy, or the family does not want to help the patient, self-help groups often assist.

The self-help groups' comparatively large number among the AIDS organizations in Italy suggests that they are meeting a need which is being increasingly felt. They particularly cater for needs that are not strictly medical in character, but relate to the provision of support, comfort, reassurance and hope which a purely medical approach is not always able to give.

2.1.5 Organizational Responsiveness of Exclusive and Inclusive Organizations

At first sight, a comparison of the organizational response between the two groups of organizations would have little meaning given the great disproportion in number between them (1,298 to 36). Yet, as will be noticed in section 2.2, a relative concentration of activities of the exclusive organizations in the field of interest representation is also evident. This is the logical consequence of the fact that most of them were set up just for that purpose, whereas this seems to be of secondary importance to the inclusive organizations.

However, the exclusive ones keep offering most of the activities mentioned in the different subsectors. To explain their scarce incidence in the general picture of the Italian organizations responding to HIV/AIDS, several factors should be considered. These are: the need for specialized personnel, the high cost of the facilities, the level of public finance which is still inadequate.

Drug service organizations are inclusive organizations since their policy is to accept and integrate everybody in the social life of their community. Only when persons get ill are they sent to hospital.

Beside the 27 social services mentioned in Table 7.3, the other 9 exclusive organizations can be found under the term "interest and self-help groups". The other

11 out of 20 in this latter group stated that their field of interest is not limited to promoting policies for people with HIV/AIDS alone, but embraces activities present in other categories available to the general population, as is the case with the services for drug users, homosexuals, blood transfusion patients, etc.

Another reason for why there are so few exclusive organizations in Italy might be that in Italy, as in many other Western countries, AIDS brings fear and intolerance into the population. The typical perception of this disease is coloured by its mysterious nature, its incurability and the fear of contagion. Those who have contracted this very serious and incurable disease share little of the relief that comes from the solidarity and support often shown by healthy people (relatives, friends, colleagues) for patients suffering from other equally serious diseases. This is precisely because of public indifference and hostility towards AIDS patients and HIV-positive persons.

It is assumed that it is therefore more difficult to create exclusive organizations which are not offshoots of other existing inclusive organizations – known to and accepted by the public (such as Caritas, to quote one example) – precisely because of their rejection in the local environment. This is compounded by the fear of many patients of being isolated and discriminated against because they are clients of such organizations.

It might be argued, however, that this climate should be in fact the opposite, i.e. an additional motivation for promoting exclusive organizations. This would have been true for a category that is suffering from double discrimination, like homosexuals affected by HIV/AIDS. Yet even their organizations, with very few exceptions, have emphasized the fact that the orientation of their activities is of a general nature.

2.1.6 Organizational Responsiveness by those Groups most Affected

Both the census of all the organizations and the in-depth interviews have revealed that not one of the organizations analysed was established by the groups most affected themselves. Even the self-help groups mentioned were promoted and still function on the initiative of and under the management of their respective organizations, e.g. LILA (with the exception of very few services in Northern Italy sponsored by the families of PWAs).

These organizations are both exclusive and inclusive, and almost all of them private non-profits. These were set up by people whose interest in the problem was motivated by humanitarian or social reasons, not by personal involvement, and they are still run by people not affected by the virus, even though a number of HIV-infected persons participate in the activities.

This is why it is not possible to state that there is a defined organizational response to AIDS by the "groups at risk" at present.

However, it can be said that some of them play a more active role in the field of interest representation – Forum AIDS Italia, the coordinating body mentioned in section 1.1, being the most outstanding example of this activity. The national association of haemophiliacs (Associazione emofiliaci e politrasfusi) and multiple transfusion patients recently began to participate in TV debates, urging for more adequate measures of protection for their members. As for the homosexuals, who are estimated to be around one million in Italy, it has been said that there is a kind of self-isolation of this group, probably due to the fact that the culture of the country's majority tends to marginalize them. But the decisions of the Council of Europe in matters like marriage, adoption and a possible changing mentality in our country are encouraging this group more and more to openly discuss their own problems and to better organize themselves. Their associations are still very few and far between and can be found in the northern and central parts of the country; they are almost non-existent in the South. Those functioning are able to take care of their own members (still a minority) especially through prevention and anti-AIDS educational campaigns. In most instances it is from these organizations that people already affected by the disease receive the best health and welfare provisions as well as psychological support.

However, the major group at risk, the drug users (or former drug dependants) are not organized. Their needs are represented within Forum AIDS Italia and on many other occasions by the people responsible for the therapeutic communities as well as by social and health workers. It should be said that most decisions taken by the authorities and most strategies for combating the drug problem and the related AIDS issue are determined by those working directly with drug addicts.

2.2   Volume of Subsectoral Response

2.2.1 Number of Organizations and Activities across the Different Subsectors

When one considers the number of organizations, namely 549 for the public sector, 779 for the private non-profit sector, and 5 for the for-profit sector, one can see that even though the majority of activities are performed by the private non-profit sector – both in numerical terms and in view of the variety of activities undertaken (except in the case of control and monitoring) – the ratio between the number of organizations and the number of activities performed is higher when it comes to the public sector (6.8 compared with 5.1 in the private sector).

A comparison based on the inclusive versus exclusive character of the organizations shows that the activities performed by those specializing in AIDS are mainly in the field of prevention; they are proportionally fewer in number than those offered by organizations of a more general nature. However, they are more numerous in terms of number and percentage as far as mediating interests and collecting funds are concerned, even though the ratio between exclusive and inclusive organizations is 1:37.

Table 7.10: Number and Percentage Distribution of Activities by Subsector and the Organization's Legal Status

	Public		Private Non-Profit		Private For-Profit		Total	% Total
	n	%	n	%	n	%		
Prevention	1,652	44.2	1,764	44.2	11	40.8	3,427	44.2
Care	1,387	37.1	1,947	48.8	13	48.1	3,347	43.2
Control/ Monitoring	686	18.3	143	3.6	3	11.1	832	10.7
Interest Representation	14	0.4	125	3.1	0	0	139	1.8
Fund-raising	2	0.1	8	0.2	0	0	10	0.1
Total	3,741	100	3,987	100	27	100	7,755	100

Table 7.11: Number and Percentage of Activities by the Organization's Inclusive/Exclusive Orientation

	Inclusives		Exclusives	
	n	%	n	%
Prevention	3,323	44.6	104	34.9
Care	3,254	43.7	93	31.2
Control/Monitoring	810	10.9	22	7.4
Interest Representation	68	0.9	71	23.8
Fund-raising	2	0	8	2.7
Total	7,457	100	298	100

2.2.2 Organizational Responsiveness by Legal Status across the Different Subsectors

As shown in Tables 7.11 and 7.12, by far the largest number of activities are offered by the public and non-profit organizations in the fields of both prevention and care.

The division of labour by legal status of the organizations is also fairly evident in these fields. Four information campaigns were sponsored at a national level by the Ministry of Health by 1992: two in 1990, one in 1991, and one in 1992. These campaigns basically consisted of pamphlets, videos, and TV spots, partly aimed at the general public, partly at professional groups (teachers, health workers, volunteers), and partly at high-risk groups (youth, prisoners, drafted soldiers, etc.).

While the quality of the information material was good as it was reduced to a few essential points not only directed towards the medical profession, its dissemination seems to have been less effective. Many schools, workplaces, youth centres, and, above all, prisons, were not supplied with enough material.

As for the content, there was some criticism regarding the persistently moral tone and some inconsistencies, e.g. the use of condoms was clearly explained in material aimed at teachers but not in that aimed at students. Above all, the most significant inadequacy concerns the absence of an evaluation of the impact these information campaigns are having on improving the awareness of the population and curbing risky behaviour.

Since the all-out AIDS information campaigns require considerable resources and the possibility of disseminating information on a very large scale in order to inform the largest possible number of individuals and environments, they are practically monopolized by the public sector.

Table 7.12: Number of Activities in the Area of Prevention by the Organization's Legal Status

	Public	Private Non-Profit	Private For-Profit	Total
Hotline	15	36	0	51
Production of Information Material	197	189	2	388
AIDS Information Campaigns	404	32	0	436
Educational and Information Work	365	413	4	782
Drug-related Prevention	353	391	3	747
Training of Volunteers and Health Care Professionals	318	703	2	1,023
Total	1,652	1,764	11	3,427

Table 7.13: Percentage Distribution of Activities in the Area of Prevention by the Organization's Legal Status

	Public	Private Non-Profit	Private For-Profit	% Total
Hotline	29.4	70.6	0	100
Production of Information Material	50.8	48.7	0.5	100
AIDS Information Campaigns	92.7	7.3	0	100
Educational and Information Work	46.7	52.8	0.5	100
Drug-related Prevention	47.3	52.3	0.4	100
Training of Volunteers and Health Care Professionals	31.1	0.2	68.7	100

However, other activities that are strictly related to the information campaigns, e.g. the production of information material and educational work, are shared almost equally between the public and private sector.

The private non-profit organizations are stimulated to produce and disseminate their own information material probably because of the shortcomings of the "official" material mentioned above and for the need to adapt it to their own target groups. Educational work is a logical consequence of another kind of activity where the non-profit organizations outnumber the public ones, i.e. psychological support and face-to-face counselling.

There are in fact quite a number of public organizations which provide psychological support and face-to-face counselling. The vast majority of them are represented by the services for drug addicts where psychologists must be involved by law.

The hotline activity can be seen as part of counselling and psychological support. This is particularly true if it is not limited to giving information of a practical nature and is accompanied by an expression of interest for the person calling and his/her problem. It is therefore not surprising that we find the private sector represented more than twice as much in this field in comparison to the public sector. This does not imply that public organizations are unable or unwilling to perform this activity. There is rather a problem regarding priorities of time and personnel to be assigned to these individual activities, as has also been confirmed by the in-depth interviews. This is why the vast majority of the non-profit organizations tend – or are forced – to carry out personnel training on their own initiative. About half of them carry out information and prevention work, thereby exceeding the number of public organizations doing so – particularly with regard to education, counselling and public information which appears when demand arises. This has been confirmed by the fact that more than twice as many private as public organizations have a help-line to answer questions from the public.

As far as practical help such as home care, shelters or housing are concerned, an enormous inadequacy exists. Considering that the incubation period for AIDS varies from between two to three years or less and eight to ten years or more, and that most persons lose their jobs and sometimes the support of their families as soon as they develop AIDS (even though they can still live a virtually normal life to a certain extent until the terminal phase), one must wonder how Italy intends to deal with the AIDS emergency. This will arise as a result of an increasing mass of people, mostly young, being without work and without resources, for whom virtually no provision has been made for social support or welfare. The number of persons who are being left to their own devices between hospital admissions for treatment is growing all the time. And this applies particularly to those who are not drug addicts: drug users can generally rely upon the assistance from the therapeutic communities, at least until they require specialized health services.

Table 7.14: Number and Percentage Distribution of Activities in the Area of Health Care and Social Services by Legal Status

Type of Activity	Public		Private Non-Profit		Private For-Profit		Total	Total
	n	%	n	%	n	%	n	%
AIDS Specialized Medical Care	490	97.4	11	2.2	2	0.4	503	100
Care/Psychological Support	416	35.5	752	64.2	3	0.3	1,171	100
Face-to-Face Counselling	390	48.3	414	51.3	3	0.4	807	100
Home Care Services	3	11.5	22	84.6	1	3.9	26	100
Hospices, Shelters, Housing	8	40.0	11	55.0	1	5.0	20	100
Voluntary HIV-Testing	47	90.4	4	7.7	1	1.9	52	100
Buddy System	0	0	2	100	0	0	2	100
Referral Services	33	4.3	729	95.4	2	0.3	764	100
Food Bank	0	0	2	100	0	0	2	100
Total	1,387		1,947		13		3,347	

Virtually all drug organizations are part of the public sector. In view of the nature of the AIDS disease, the high level of specialization required for treatment, as well as the costs, it is obvious that well-trained para-medical personnel are needed, which explains why the public sector predominates in this type of activity.

The same can be said for voluntary HIV-testing. However, excluding the hospitals, the number of organizations offering this kind of service is probably low when one considers that the fear of AIDS is growing and that more people are requesting an HIV antibody test.

The tables presented so far show that most types of organizations in the areas of prevention and care (for drug addicts, homosexuals, haemophiliacs, as well as for those who care for the population in general) perform nearly all kinds of activities. The differences between the public and private sector begin to appear when we consider the other areas of interest: control/intelligence, policy advocacy and support activities.

The activities regarding control and monitoring are much more frequent within the public sector (Table 7.10), with 82.8% in the public sector and only 17.3% in the private one. The reverse is true as far as interest representation is concerned: here, the proportion is 10.1% to 89.9%. In any case, these two groups of activities are offered by a much smaller number of organizations to those which provide prevention and care activities.

Again the reason can be found when one considers the national AIDS policy on the one hand, and the target groups of the organizations on the other. Control and monitoring are the responsibility of the Ministry of Health. Law no. 135/1990 (see above) aims to establish a uniform framework for the decisions of the regional governments. They are obviously mostly implemented through public organizations. In fact, it can be seen that HIV-screening, -testing and identification (contract tracing) are carried out almost exclusively by the public sector. The limited number of public organizations in charge of the monitoring of blood product safety can be explained by the fact that this is strictly centralized.

Another typical trend of the Italian AIDS policy is the emphasis which is put upon the medical aspects of the problem. This is why research is another important activity among the functions of the public organizations. However, research is much more geared towards the medical, diagnostic and epidemiological aspects than to the psychological and social ones. This explains why so many research activities are also only carried out within the non-profit sector. The non-profit organizations in charge of drug users in particular, and those for homosexuals (all non-profit), need to deepen their knowledge of the strategies best suited to meet the specific psychosocial needs of their clients through research.

As for the activities aiming to promote policies to defend the patient's interests and human and civil rights, the great disproportion in the involvement of the public versus the non-profit organizations, as well as the limited number of such

Table 7.15: Number and Percentage of Activities in the Area of Control and Monitoring by the Organization's Legal Status

	Public		Private Non-Profit		Private For-Profit		Total	Total
	n	%	n	%	n	%	n	%
Epidemiological/ Social Research	218	63	128	37.0	0	0	346	100
AIDS Policy Coordination and Implementation	11	47.8	12	52.2	0	0	23	100
Control of Blood/Plasma Product Safety	9	75	2	16.7	1	8.3	12	100
HIV-Screening, -Testing, Identification	448	99.3	1	0.2	2	0.4	451	100
Total	686		143		3		832	

activities in general, should also be understood in the light of the national AIDS policy.

Law no. 135/1990 contains a number of provisions designed to protect the interests and rights of the HIV-infected person:

> Health care personnel ... shall provide the necessary assistance taking all the measures required to guarantee patient confidentiality.

> ... statistics on HIV infection must nevertheless be compiled using methods which make it impossible to identify the individuals concerned. (§ 5[2])

> No-one may be required, without their consent, to be tested for HIV infection save for clinical needs in the individual's own interest. Tests are permitted ... under epidemiological programmes only when the samples to be analysed are anonymous, and when it is absolutely impossible to identify the individuals tested. (§ 5[3])

> The results of the tests ... may only be given to the person concerned. (§ 5[4])

> Proven infection with HIV may not be a motive for discrimination, particularly with regard to enrolment at school, practising sports, or obtaining or maintaining employment. (§ 5[5])

> Employers, public or private, are forbidden to carry out investigations to ascertain whether any of their employees or persons under consideration for future employment are HIV positive. (§ 6[1])

Italian AIDS legislation would therefore be sufficient to protect the fundamental rights of the individual: freedom from interference in one's private life and respect for personal dignity, the possibility of receiving an education, of working, and of participating in social life. However, as often occurs, the practical implementation of this law, which is to a certain extent one step ahead of the attitudes of the man on the street or might clash with strongly-felt needs, is encountering difficulties and limitations.

This is why the non-profit organizations are nevertheless active in this field. This might seem rather paradoxical, but just because the law might theoretically meet all the needs related to the individual rights of patients as citizens and human beings, the non-profit sector has to fill the gaps left by public intervention.

It is well known that bureaucracies follow patterns of behaviour that "must" be rigid, insofar as they are regulated in advance by fixed norms that can only be changed slowly and with difficulty. For instance, the public organizations analysed in this chapter are not equipped to offer legal advice or counselling on insurance and/or welfare entitlements – with a few exceptions. They would go beyond their competence by organizing self-help groups or interventions for combating discrimination (except for the few exclusive organizations quoted further down) – even more so as far as political lobbying is concerned, which is usually out of the question for a public organization.

A government decree of 8 June 1991 is meant to protect prisoners suffering from HIV/AIDS, the vast majority of whom are drug users. AIDS patients and HIV-infected persons at a more advanced stage in their illness are treated in health care organizations outside the prison system. Prisoners suffering from full-blown AIDS can also be released from prison.

Both the public and private AIDS organizations which provide social or medical services cannot work directly in the prisons themselves but can operate under contract with the prison's administration. However, Parliament has not yet adopted a draft bill which provides a special pension for AIDS patients, including those who have not paid national insurance contributions.

In practice, many hospital patients are being HIV-tested without being told. In some rare cases, mandatory testing has occurred in certain companies (clearly before the 1990 law). Naturally the workers could have refused to have been tested at that time, but that would have put him/her in a difficult situation. This resulting dismissal of HIV-positive persons (prior to the 1990 law) was dealt with by the labour tribunals which ruled that they had to be reinstated.

Some cases of discrimination against children at school have also recently emerged: but here it was not a matter of applying a new law, but one of changing the attitude of the parents of children who refuse to allow their own children to attend the same school, kindergarten or playing fields as HIV-positive children. It was also in these cases that the institutions (the school, or sometimes the munici-

Table 7.16: Number and Percentage of Activities in the Area of Interest Representation by the Organization's Legal Status

	Public		Private Non-Profit		Private For-Profit		Total	Total
	n	%	n	%	n	%	n	%
Self-help Groups	4	0.7	25	3.2	0	0	29	2.2
Counselling for Insurance/ Welfare Entitlements	3	0.6	21	2.7	0	0	24	1.8
Civil/Human Rights/ Protection against Discrimination	4	0.7	36	4.6	0	0	40	3.0
Political Lobbying	2	0.4	25	3.2	0	0	27	2.0
Legal Advice	1	0.2	18	2.3	0	0	19	1.4
Total	14	2.6	125	16.0	0	0	139	10.4

pal authorities) acted to put an end to the protest themselves – sometimes without success.

Carrying out support activities for AIDS programmes is obviously more necessary for private than for public organizations. In fact, eight non-profit organizations stated that they carried out fund-raising campaigns – only one of them actually belongs to the public sector.

The latter is an out-patient centre linked to the Higher Institute of Health (ISS). It performs virtually every type of activity included in the questionnaire, including the organization of self-help groups, but its main purpose is to screen for HIV infection. It was created in 1985 – the year in which the number of AIDS cases in Italy suddenly soared from 36 to 195, and when the public health authorities realized that it was necessary to organize an official monitoring system for the disease.

Fund-raising activities may be so limited in number because, in general, non-profit organizations receive their funding from the state. As indicated earlier, since 1990, the Government has allocated over 4,000 billion lire (approx. $ 2,500 m.) for various AIDS prevention programmes, including contributions and grants to organizations in the third sector. However, particularly because of the need for structures to organize hospices, home care, information and prevention campaigns covering a wide area, these contributions are not sufficient. The difficulties faced by the non-profit organizations, both religious and secular, are increased by the fact that there is no widespread tradition among the general public for privately contributing to these particular initiatives – as there is with other diseases or social and health problems to which public opinion is more sensitive.

2.2.3 Organizational Responsiveness of Exclusive and Inclusive Organizations across the Different Subsectors

It is useful to examine the differences between the inclusive and the exclusive organizations in relation to the different types of activities performed. On an aggregate level, it becomes clear that the activities performed by the inclusive organizations are preponderant both in absolute and relative numbers. However, it is more meaningful to analyse the specific types of activities to which the two groups give priority.

The analysis shows that inclusive organizations within the area of prevention are most active with regard to training. This might be explained by the fact that most of the inclusive organizations are drug abuse service organizations which rely on qualified and trained personnel. Drug-related prevention and information activities are the second-most offered activities.

The most interesting result as far as the exclusive organizations are concerned is the fact that their activities are equally distributed among all types of activities, except drug-related prevention. Exclusives seem to have mainly been established to provide group-specific information.

Table 7.17: Number and Percentage of Activities in the Area of Prevention by the Organization's Inclusive/Exclusive Orientation

	Inclusives		Exclusives		Total	Total
	n	%	n	%	n	%
Hotline	32	62.8	19	37.3	51	100
Production of Information Material	366	94.3	22	5.7	388	100
AIDS Information Campaigns	416	95.4	20	4.6	436	100
Educational and Information Work	763	97.6	19	2.4	782	100
Drug-related Prevention	742	99.3	5	0.7	747	100
Training of Volunteers and Health Care Professionals	1,003	98.1	20	2.0	1,023	100

The distribution of activities between inclusive and exclusive organizations in the field of care once again shows that the inclusives provide more medical care, psychological support and personal counselling. But there is one anomalous finding regarding the referral of patients to other services, i.e. the high number of this type of activity offered by the inclusive organizations. Although these are organizations which, while also occupied in other areas, nevertheless run their own programmes or units for people with HIV/AIDS – as confirmed by the fact that 98.6% of them also provide medical assistance to their clients. The most probable explanation for this is that they refer their clients to hospitals when their condition worsens or when complications arise and that, apart from medical assistance, they are more active than the exclusives in looking for other institutions better suited to meet the particular needs of their clients. Another hypothesis is that exclusive organizations work in greater isolation as far as relationships with agencies and people involved with them are concerned, which confirms what was said in section 2.1.5.

Whereas both exclusive and inclusive organizations give priority to the provision of psychological support and personal counselling, the differences begin to emerge in the availability of activities in the area of medical care, which is ranked fourth in the case of inclusive organizations and only sixth for exclusive ones. Most of the social services (hospices, home care), however, are handled by exclusive organizations, even though they are, in absolute numbers, extremely few.

Table 7.18: Number and Percentage of Activities in the Area of Care by the Organization's Inclusive/Exclusive Orientation

Type of Activity	Inclusives n	%	Exclusives n	%	Total n	Total %
AIDS Specialized Medical Care	496	98.6	7	1.4	503	100
Care/Psychological Support	1,148	98.0	23	2	1,171	100
Face-to-Face Counselling	788	97.7	19	2.4	807	100
Home Care Services	12	46.2	14	53.9	26	100
Hospices, Shelters, Housing	16	80.0	4	20.0	20	100
Voluntary HIV testing	43	82.7	9	17.3	52	100
Buddy System	1	50.0	1	50.0	2	100
Referral Services	748	97.9	16	2.1	764	100
Food Bank	2	100	0	0	2	100

It is in the field of care where the medical profession predominates. It is worth noting that the exclusive organizations, being so few and mostly non-profit organizations, seem particularly interested in policy coordination in order to strengthen their role, while the inclusive organizations where AIDS patients are small in number, are not. This might also explain why there is a constant problem of coordination in Italy.

Although some of these exclusives were instituted at the request of the government (ANLAIDS, the *National Associations to Combat AIDS*) in order to encourage the coordination of local policies, their relative isolation and limited power is perhaps due to the fact that they are always voluntary, non-profit associations. Other exclusive organizations which have spontaneously emerged and whose original primary purpose was not AIDS policy coordination, but the defence of the rights of their clients, also perform similar activities in order to be able to build up a dialogue with government agencies.

Despite what was said about the primary purpose of most exclusive organizations, especially those promoted most recently, i.e. to defend the rights of people with AIDS/HIV, there is no distinct prevalence of exclusives over inclusives, as one might have expected, either in percentage terms or in the number of activities performed. Indeed, comparison between the groups shows us that at least as far as the creation of self-help groups, the combating of discrimination and lobbying are concerned, there is certainly greater commitment on the part of the exclusive organizations. Naturally, in view of the huge numerical disproportion between the two groups (1,298 as against 36), this may not be meaningful at all, but it is revealing when one thinks that this is one of the main *raisons d'être* for the initial emergence of the exclusive organizations.

Table 7.19:　Number and Percentage of Activities in the Area of Control and Monitoring by Inclusive/Exclusive Orientation

	Inclusives n	Inclusives %	Exclusives n	Exclusives %	Total n	Total %
Epidemiological and Social Research	340	98.3	6	1.7	346	100
AIDS Policy Coordination and Implementation	15	65.2	8	34.3	23	100
Control of Blood/Plasma Product Safety	11	91.7	1	8.3	12	100
HIV-Screening, -Testing and Identification	444	98.5	7	1.6	451	100

Table 7.20: Number and Percentage of Activities in the Area of Interest Representation by Inclusive/Exclusive Orientation

| | Inclusives | | Exclusives | | Total | Total |
	n	%	n	%	n	%
Self-help Groups	15	51.7	14	48.3	29	100
Counselling for Insurance/Welfare Entitlements	10	41.7	14	58.3	24	100
Civil/Human Rights/Protection against Discrimination	21	52.5	19	47.5	40	100
Political Lobbying	15	55.6	12	44.4	27	100
Legal Advice	7	36.8	12	63.2	19	100

2.3 Analysis of Selected Single Activities

2.3.1 Number of Organizations and Distribution of Single Activities

From Tables 7.10 and 7.11, presented in section 2.2 of this chapter, it appears that the largest number of activities is concentrated on certain types of activities, namely prevention and care and social services.

It is interesting to analyse how the specific activities are distributed within these fields, keeping in mind that the data refer to the organizations analysed in depth, i.e. 50 selected organizations (see Appendix).

As far as prevention is concerned, the activities are distributed as presented in Tables 7.21 and 7.22.

Information material is produced by 34 organizations among those interviewed in the form of leaflets, pamphlets, brochures (26 organizations), posters (19 organizations), journals or magazines (12 organizations), advertisements and films, videos (9 organizations). Seven organizations publish newsletters, collect bibliographies or use stickers and badges while only five of them have also published self-help guides. It should be pointed out that amongst these latter organizations only one is a public inclusive: it is a service for mental health located in Genoa (north-west). As for the other four, they are all non-profit and exclusive, except one whose major field of interest is focused on drug users and other marginalized groups.

We know that the drug-related prevention of AIDS is a subject of major concern for the Italian social and health policy. It is therefore no wonder that 32 organizations perform this specific activity. This is mostly done through education on needle sterilization (22 organizations) and by making use of therapeutic commu-

Table 7.21: Number and Percentage of Organizations by Single Activities in the Area of Prevention (n = 50)

	Number	Percentage
Educational and information work	44	88%
Counselling the use of condoms	24	48%
Media relations	30	60%
Organizing educational events	39	78%
Safe sex educational campaigns	14	28%
Streetwork	9	18%
Press conferences, press surveys	21	42%
Publicity campaigns in printed media	15	30%
Publicity campaigns in public places	12	24%
Publicity campaigns on TV and radio	11	22%
Production of information material	34	68%
Advertisements	9	18%
Bibliographies	7	14%
Films, videos	9	18%
Journals or magazines	12	24%
Leaflets, pamphlets, brochures	8	16%
Newsletters	26	52%
Posters	15	30%
Self-help guides	5	10%
Stickers, buttons	6	12%
Hotline	20	40%
Drug-related prevention	32	64%
General drug abuse counselling	22	44%
Free distribution of one-way needles	6	12%
Methadone maintenance programmes	7	14%
Therapeutic community	5	10%
Training of volunteers and health care professionals	29	58%
Occupational therapy instructions	17	34%
Promoting safety measures for clients of dentists, beauty shops and barbers	5	10%
Training of volunteers	29	58%

Table 7.22: Number and Percentage of the Organizations by Single Activities in the Area of Care and Social Services (n = 50)

	Number	Percentage
Primary health care, medical services	20	40%
Medical care and information	19	38%
Ambulant health care services, hospital outreach services	1	2%
STD information and treatment	16	32%
Care and psychological support	32	64%
Identity house	3	6%
Organizing recreation and leisure-time activities	12	24%
Organizing residential and neighbourhood care networks	4	8%
Pediatric AIDS day care	3	6%
Spiritual and religious support services	4	8%
Suicide prevention and emergency counselling	5	10%
Support for self-help groups (Self-help groups)	14	28%
Transportation service for PWA	14	28%
General face-to-face counselling	29	58%
Counselling for mothers/parents	22	44%
Counselling for terminally-ill patients	19	38%
Family planning and therapy	19	38%
Home care services	19	38%
Hospices, shelters, housing facilities	13	26%
Hospices, shelters, housing facilities for PWAs	9	18%
Emergency housing	4	8%
Housing enrichment for people unable to obtain/ maintain adequate housing	7	14%
Voluntary HIV testing	29	58%
Buddy system	–	–
Referral services	3	6%
Centralized case management for PWAs	2	4%
Adoption and foster care for children with AIDS	2	4%
Others		
Food bank, free meals	11	22%

nities when necessary (15 organizations). Much less frequent are the methadone maintenance programmes (7 organizations) and the distribution of one-way needles (6 organizations).

In the area of care/psychological support, face-to-face counselling and training are strictly interrelated activities. To be effective, face-to-face counselling for people with HIV/AIDS needs people with preferably specialized training: not only doctors or psychologists but in particular volunteers and even social workers. This is why almost all structures that offer counselling have taken care to organize training activities; this is often based on an interprofessional approach.

The same organizations link counselling to activities of a more practical type (with few exceptions) as presented in Table 7.23.

The relative frequency of home care services might seem to contradict the general picture of the organizational responsiveness described in section 2.2. This is the result of the sample of organizations interviewed – since the most active ones have been included, i.e. among them the exclusive ones. Despite their commitment, it is clear, however, that only a small percentage of the clients' needs can be met through their efforts.

Voluntary HIV-testing and counselling are activities offered by 29 organizations. Here, it is interesting that only 8 of them are health units. Ten more are services for drug users and 1 for mentally-ill persons. The others are organizations or associations for homosexuals (most active as far as prevention is concerned), or with a statutory aim to act in favour of marginalized groups.

Among the 21 organizations which carry out epidemiological and social research, we find 10 social services for drug users, 8 health units, 2 of the best structured

Table 7.23: Number and Percentage of Organizations by Single Activities in the Area of Control/Monitoring (n = 50)

	Number	Percentage
Epidemiological/social research	21	42
AIDS policy coordination and implementation	10	20
Governance by national committees	2	4
Regulating bath houses/sex clubs, etc.	0	0
Control of blood/plasma product safety	1	2
HIV-screening, -testing, identification	13	26
Mandatory testing	3	6
Voluntary HIV-testing	11	22
Drug abuse control	13	26
Help to handle and control shooting galleries	0	0

non-profit organizations for AIDS patients and gay men respectively, and, finally, an institution promoted by Caritas.

Primary health care and medical services are provided by 20 organizations. This is provided through medical care and information except in one case. In addition, 16 organizations offer STD information and treatment. However, there is only one organization (for homosexuals, private and inclusive, located in Rome) which offers ambulant health care and hospital outreach services.

As for the activities less well represented, besides the provision of housing facilities (13 organizations, of which 4 are able to offer emergency housing and 7 permanent housing facilities) and that of free meals (11 organizations), we find them in the areas of control, i.e.:

- HIV-screening, -testing, identification (contact-tracing) are carried out by 13 organizations.
- In 6 cases we find that the same organizations which offer HIV-screening, -testing and identification have the monitoring of drug abuse among their activities, which is also carried out by 7 more organizations – a total of 13.
- AIDS policy coordination is carried out by 10 organizations, 2 of them are governed by national committees.
- The relatively frequent presence of activities like counselling for insurance/ welfare entitlements (17 organizations), legal advice (16 organizations) and civil/ human rights/protection against discrimination (14 organizations) reflects the general lack of security and little acknowledgement of the rights of PWAs and HIV-positive persons.

However, the defence of the patient's rights is probably meant in generic terms. In fact, although 5 organizations have a complaint hotline, fewer are able to offer enforceable safeguards regarding labour or the medical and health system (3 organizations), housing (2 organizations) or insurance (1 organization).

The organizations involved in political lobbying and in promoting self-help groups and the bringing together of people with HIV/AIDS are more active. These activities are carried out by 12 organizations; 6 of them offer both forms of support.

Cultural or organizational conditions may be the reason why an ombudsman exists only in one organization (i.e. LILA – the *Italian League for Combating AIDS*, a private and exclusive organization). Buddy systems and the regulation of bath houses/sex clubs are activities which were not provided by the organizations interviewed. Finally, the strict regulations of the Italian legal system and the presence of a large number of social agencies specializing in adoption makes it difficult for the organizations to promote adoption and foster care for children with AIDS, which is carried out by only 2 organizations among those in charge of PWAs.

2.3.2 Type of Organizations across Selected Activities

The activities analysed seem to be the most relevant ones within the framework of the Italian AIDS policy, not only because of the number of organizations involved, but also because they clearly indicate the trends of the general organizational response – regardless of the specific aims, organization or resources of the services considered.

Since prevention is by far the field where the efforts of the organizations have been focused from the beginning, it might be interesting to look more closely at the means by which they try to achieve this objective.

As we have seen, educational events, media relations, press conferences and publicity campaigns are widely used by most organizations. In many cases, their activities have helped to fill the gaps of the national information campaigns sponsored by the government. The kind of message addressed to the whole population is in fact anonymous because it cannot have a concrete, real interlocutor: the "human, individual case" is, however, what the organizations have most experience in. This explains why, in practice, the great majority of the organizations are involved to varying degrees in educational work and production of their own information material. Their purpose is to personalize the message for their own clients. The scarcity of resources is an obstacle to the involvement of the organizations in these activities, however.

Counselling on the use of condoms is an activity provided by about half of the 50 organizations interviewed. It is sometimes difficult to understand, in the light of their organizational nature, why some of them perform this activity and some not. In the group which is performing this activity, there are of course several health units and ambulatory services for drug users. But organizations of the same kind do not counsel on the use of condoms. One might guess that the decision to instruct clients on the use of condoms is more due to the personal initiatives of the medical and social staff than to the formal rules and structure of the organizations.

The government's prevention campaigns have been stressing the necessity to use condoms. Also, all the organizations for homosexuals now provide condoms, which might explain the drastic reduction of AIDS cases among them. None of the Catholic organizations interviewed, on the other hand, gave a positive reply to the question as to whether they promote the use of condoms. A similar discrepancy can be found as far as the coordination bodies for combating AIDS are concerned: LILA and ANLAIDS are both private and exclusive organizations, represented throughout the country. However, LILA carries out counselling on condoms, ANLAIDS does not. Note that the establishment of the latter, although non-profit, was sponsored by the Ministry of Health.

In view of the great commitment of most organizations to drug-related prevention when it comes to AIDS, one might wonder why education regarding needle sterilization is offered by a good number of them, including all the public socio-health units for drug addicts and most of the private ones. While the actual distribution of one-way needles is carried out by a much lower number of organizations and never by the public units mentioned above. It is interesting to observe how this official AIDS policy has been differently implemented at the grass-roots level. The reason here is simple enough: the SERTs (Servizi per Tossicodipendenti, i.e. public services for drug addicts) are multifunctional, have a very complex organization and perform tasks inspired by different therapeutic models. Consequently, they tend to avoid those interventions that can easily be implemented by other institutions or by the clients themselves, i.e. the free distribution of one-way needles by pharmacies if prescribed.

The same is true for methadone programmes. Here it is not the SERTs' responsibility any more and it is forbidden for non-profit organizations to develop such programmes. Methadone can, however, be prescribed by doctors working for the National Health Service according to their own professional diagnosis of the situation.

It is significant that while face-to-face counselling and psychosocial support are seen by most organizations as a major part of their activities, only a smaller number of them are able to offer services which require higher specialization. For example, some activities require a certain degree of personal involvement from the staff (suicide prevention, spiritual and religious support) or a certain expertise to set up services that might go beyond the normal organizational resources of the organizations but are useful (transportation services, recreation and leisure time activities, residential and neighbourhood care networks, etc.). This is why special attention should be given to those attempts to organize new models of training for professionals and volunteers which are beginning to appear.

A rather large part of the organizations provides counselling to mothers and families and to the terminally-ill. These organizations are of all types: from public to private, from inclusive to exclusive, from more oriented towards medical services to more oriented towards social work practice. It might be more interesting to see which ones do not take care of terminally-ill patients and which ones concentrate on them in preference to other clients. Among the former group, we find exclusive health units; this might be another sign of a somewhat more "detached" attitude of the medical profession or, rather, of some representatives of the profession when the problem of giving psychological help to people on the edge of death arises. Regarding care for the terminally-ill, there are most developed organizations for gay men, one operational structure for PWAs (dependent on a Southern university) and a service for drug users – also in the South. Again it seems that in several cases the organizational response might depend less on the purposes, status and management of the institutions than on the type of personnel available and, in a sense, on the "philosophy" (practical and ethical principles) which inspires the organizations.

The so-called "Centri di solidarità" (Solidarity centres) and other non-profit organizations particularly designed for relatives of drug users are those more active in family therapy and planning.

3   Policy Implications

3.1   The National Style of Organizational Response and the Health and Social Policies

AIDS and drug addiction are two problems that have been linked together almost since the moment AIDS first appeared in Italy. Even now, many national and regional government regulations deal with both drug users and people affected by HIV/AIDS at the same time; these regulations largely address the SERTs.

It has in fact been recognized that it has been since the middle of the 1980s (in line with the recommendations of the WHO World Programme on AIDS) that heterosexual HIV transmission first originated – mainly amongst the drug population.

As for the second-most prominent group at risk, that of homosexuals, it has been said that they are in general well organized – at least in the big cities of Northern and Central Italy. Their organizations are promoted and managed with little or no support from public funds. However, the general distrust that surrounds them, which causes a good number of homosexuals to keep their condition secret, not only makes it more difficult to help those infected with the HIV virus but it also represents a further risk factor in the spread of the disease. Although these are very approximate estimates, it is calculated that only 50% of them know whether or not they have contracted the virus. As of March 1993, 1.3% of AIDS cases reported in that year were heterosexuals who had contracted the virus from homosexual or bisexual partners.

The necessity to improve AIDS prevention is evident, despite the efforts that have been made both by the government and many organizations in the field. As has been mentioned, the distribution of information material is inadequate. For example, material was distributed in part to pharmacies, but not to general practitioners. A sharp tendency on the part of young people to ignore taking precautions has been observed. It is frightening – taken as indicating a tendency – that while in 1989 non-drug-addicted heterosexuals represented 4.7% of all cases, at the beginning of 1993 the number had already increased to 7.5%.

It does seem, however, that AIDS is changing the sexual behaviour of the population. Condom sales have increased sharply, and sexually transmitted diseases have been decreasing since 1984.

The role played by the Catholic Church should also be considered. Groups with a religious background are very active in promoting practical measures, above all in the area of social services. But they show strong resistance in the areas of education and information, even though it is well known that, alongside the rigid positions maintained by the hierarchy, independent efforts to adequately counsel young people who turn to individual pastors or priests closest to them do exist.

The growing number of women of child-bearing age who are seropositive, either because they are IV-drug users or because their partners have AIDS or HIV, has drawn the attention of the authorities to the very important role that can be played by the Family Advisory Bureaus (Consultori Familiari, i.e. family planning clinics as well as centres for health care for mothers and children, offering psychological consultation for partners, legal abortion, etc. – legally established as public entities since 1975) in giving information to seropositive pregnant women on the risks of transmitting the infection to their children and in sending them to specialized clinics. The involvement of these agencies is very new, and the results are still unknown. As one of the basic functions of the Advisory Bureaus is seen to administer sex education, it would be important to study their activities in more depth.

As for the risk of infection from transfusions, two ministerial decrees in June 1991 oblige associations of blood donors to promote health information and education and to establish the criteria and methods for importing human blood.

As has already been pointed out, AIDS cases resulting from transfusions have dramatically decreased in Italy and are now fewer than 400. Nevertheless, it seemed necessary to intensify the regulation of blood originating in areas where AIDS had become endemic.

In fact, another worrisome aspect regarding the problem of HIV/AIDS concerns the influx of immigrants from the Third World. Clandestine immigrants have had to hide themselves since the law of 1990, where regulations for controlled immigration are pronounced. They therefore often live hidden in the most broken-down parts of the cities where they are difficult to be reached for information distribution.

This is further proof of the fact that HIV and AIDS must be fought simultaneously on all fronts: what still seems to be lacking in Italy is the coordination of all social and health policies, both in the public and private sectors of organizations and institutions as well as those of the national and local policies.

This coordination, which is stated in principle in the legislation, has difficulties with being implemented. This is so even though it has been considered a political and operational instrument of the highest level by the Interministerial Committee and the Commission of Experts.

After Law 135/1990, the Minister of Health issued other important decrees aimed at protection from infection and the professional training of social and health workers in both the public and private sectors: the regulation of syringe and condom manufacturing; the prevention and treatment of AIDS in prisons; working out the terms of agreement between volunteer agencies and the Local Health Units concerning the home care of patients. Finally on 7 November 1991, a plan for coordinated action between the national and regional governments was decided to be revised periodically by the Interministerial Committee for the Fight Against AIDS.

Difficulties remain, however, in terms of the rapport with those responsible for local health policy who, at times, have viewed the regulations for implementing this law as something imposed "from above".

Furthermore, even though all the central administrations that might have an interest in the problem are represented on the Committee, the policy coordination to fight against AIDS is, in practice, monopolized by the Ministry of Health. Moreover, the doctors monopolize both the management of AIDS policies and the use of funds for research.

As specified in the "Plan for Implementing Research on AIDS", administered by the Higher Institute of Health (ISS), of the 28.5 billion lire ($ 17 m.) allocated for research, only 3.4 billion ($ 2.1 m.) are destined for financing the "organizational and psychosocial aspects of care". Another problem is that this research takes place within the universities and the results are circulated in an academic environment, so it would not be easy for the volunteer groups which are on the front lines of providing care to learn about the new research results.

3.2   The Personnel's Points of View and the Need for Training

The in-depth interviews which have been conducted for this study and many informal exchanges of ideas with those interviewed have revealed a widespread feeling of discouragement among the heads of non-profit organizations, and even among some of the more committed individuals in the public sector. They maintain that "good will is not enough", that funds are absolutely inadequate, that there is a need, not only to increase, but also to legally regulate the collaboration between organizations that take care of the various aspects of AIDS.

Even though there are strong economic and professional incentives for health workers in the hospitals that handle AIDS patients, psychological burn-out remains very high. The staff complain that they do not receive enough support, neither in the specialization courses that are given regularly by the Higher Institute of Health (ISS) – which deal with various medical aspects of the disease – nor in the daily practice of their job, to help them control and rationalize the feelings of anxiety and impotence that arise from their contact with their patients. From this point of view, the best conditions are to be found inside residential communities for drug addicts that house seropositive or AIDS patients. It seems that life in a community has a therapeutic effect both on the staff and on the people they are caring for. The terminally-ill patients are physically separated from the others who use the facility, but they are visited regularly and receive manifestations of solidarity that have a positive effect. This helps them to face the final phase of the illness, and to help the staff (doctors, psychologists, social workers, and volunteers) to overcome their own anxiety and uncertainty.

In both the treatment of the patients and in assisting those who are seropositive, some non-profit organizations have made the greatest progress. That is, they have succeeded in putting together an integrated approach to the disease, e.g. where the intertwining of biological, psychological, and social factors requires an ability to meet a demand that entails all-encompassing and complex needs, and where it is necessary to overcome professional compartmentalism.

However, along with these exemplary experiences, there are also some initiatives – though few, e.g. training programmes and operational methodology – in the public sector which follow the same criteria, with excellent results. The problem, however, is always the same: the isolation in which these agencies work. The integrated approach model created through these experiences ought to become widely known and be implemented on a much vaster scale.

The same is true for some pilot experiments in supplementary training for employees belonging to diverse professions. In this model, besides experts in medical problems linked to AIDS, the teaching staff consist of experts in organizational analysis, in psychological research, and in transactional analysis, too. The content of the training sessions and the teaching methods are aimed at exploring and overcoming the difficulties that the employees encounter in their various roles. They also aim for better communication, not only between the workers and their patients, but between them, the services they belong to, and the family context. So far they have been limited in scope but should be considered to be organized on a broader scale.

After 1991 laws have been implemented by the regional governments for organizing services to care for patients at home (D.P.R. [Decreto Presidente della Republica] 14/9/1991). One can thus conclude that this area of activity, until now so absent, has good prospects for developing in the near future; this will require the preparation of an interdisciplinary team, which is particularly difficult. It is not merely a matter of making collaboration possible between the different professions or that of helping the workers to resolve their own emotional difficulties, as in the examples already given. It is also important to prepare them to face duties that are completely new in our culture (though saturated in Catholic tradition), such as those related to helping the ill and their family members to give meaning to the period of life that remains as well as to death.

Once more, these very particular experiences should be made widely accessible and put in practice outside the limited circle in which they develop. A constant problem in Italy lies precisely in the fragmentation of such initiatives.

3.3 Concluding Remarks

On the whole, Italian policy related to the fight against AIDS has seen a swift enough response concerning diagnostic testing and health remedies on the part of the government. This was first organized within the public institutions, in particular for those that care for drug addicts. In the hospitals of the larger cities, specialized departments have been equipped for patients infected with HIV. Indeed, in Italy, as in other industrialized countries, AIDS is concentrated in the most urbanized areas; the cities of Milan, Rome, Naples, and Turin have almost one third of all Italian AIDS cases.

Nevertheless, there is still an insufficient number of hospital beds for AIDS patients, despite the funding that has been allocated by the government. Technical, organizational, and financial difficulties remain, however, especially concerning the renovation of old hospitals.

Even if the commitment of the Italian policy for the fight against AIDS is expressed primarily at the level of prevention, care, and research, from a medical point of view, attention has been given to the psychological and social aspects of the disease in the legislation. The decree of 13 September 1991 has been mentioned that determines the form and kind of agreement concerning home care and the plan to coordinate national and regional activities ("Act of Intention" of 7 November 1991), in which explicit reference has been made to "an important involvement in charitable, psychological, social, and educational activities on the part of volunteer associations ... whose contribution should be considered in the context of general coordination". But the practical implementation of these provisions is still in an initial stage.

There has been a certain delay in becoming aware of the fact that the disease does not only touch specific social groups such as IV-drug users and homosexuals, and that AIDS and HIV are not simply medical and health problems. In fact, a whole range of other aspects, from legal to economic and from political to ethical questions have been taken into account in the meantime.

If one can perceive some signs of positive change in the attitudes of the authorities and the population, this is certainly due to the efforts of non-profit organizations and many motivated persons. This is especially the case in the area of services for drug addiction, who have demonstrated that the approach must not be towards the disease but towards the ill "person". It has been precisely the non-profit organizations and volunteers that have concerned themselves with drug dependency who, since 1987, have underscored the need for care outside the hospital.

Exclusive public and non-profit organizations should be strengthened in number and given more independence. This is precisely because knowledge of the disease is becoming more widespread and thus there is better understanding of what kind and level of specialization is required of institutions and staff for various kinds of activity.

Although every area of health policy in the country openly recognizes that an integrated approach to the social and health aspects is necessary, the organizational methods of the AIDS policy remain of a "residual" type, in the sense that they concentrate on the hospitals. The professional competence within the hospitals continues to be compartmentalized, excessively specialized, and hierarchical.

It therefore seems all the more necessary to develop activities outside the hospitals. This is becoming more and more urgent, given that HIV infection is rapidly saturating hospital facilities, which are already inadequate to meet the needs of the general population, especially in the South and in the large cities. The national anti-AIDS plan calls for the creation of around 6,000 beds, but it will take another two or three years before this can be realized. The rising curve of the epidemic together with longer survival periods of the patients indicate that this could become insufficient before long.

References

AA.VV. (1987) *l'infezione da HIV e AIDS: modello per la prevenzione e l'educazione sanitaria nei tossicodipendenti e negli operatori* . Verona: CNR.

AA.VV. (1988) 'Atti della tavola rotonda su', *Aids fuori dalla paura.* Roma: Parsec.

AA.VV. (1988) *Infezione da HIV e Aids. Manuale di prevenzione e educazione sanitaria.* Verona: CNR.

AA.VV. (1988) *Aids: immagini contro. Il modo di pensare che genera il male del secolo.* Milano: Rizza.

AA.VV. (1989) 'L'Aids e l'ambiente di lavoro', *l'operatore sanitario* 12

AA.VV. (1989) 'Speciale Aids e sieropositività: i diritti civili alla prova. Percorsi di solidarietà e della prevenzione', *Prospettive sociali e sanitarie.*

AA.VV. (1989) 'Indagine sugli atteggiamenti nei riguardi dell'AIDS e delle principali categorie a rischio', *marginalità e società* 10.

AA.VV. (1990) 'Numero monografico: Aids', *Bollettino per le farmacodipendenze e l'alcolismo* 1.

AA.VV. (1990) *3a giornata mondiale contro l'abuso e il traffico illecito di droga. Legge sull'Aids e tossicodipendenze.* Roma: Ministero della Sanità.

AA.VV. (1992) 'La prevenzione dell'Aids. Aspetti preventivi nella formazione degli operatori', *Prospettive sociali e sanitarie* 16/17.

Agnoletto, V. (1990) 'Sieropositività e AIDS; prospettive per la terapia', *Prospettive sociali e sanitarie.*

Aspe (1989) Speciale: 'AIDS e diritti umani 1', *Aspe* 27.

Autonomie Locali e Servizi Sociali (1990) 'Programma di interventi urgenti per la prevenzione e la lotta contro l'AIDS (legge n. 135/1990)', *Autonomie locali e servizi sociali* 1.

Autonomie locali e servizi sociali (1992) 'Rapporto dell'Istituto di Sanità sulle attività di formazione per operatori socio-sanitari per lotta Aids', *Autonomie locali e servizi sociali* 1.

Betta, A./Cembrani, F. (1989) 'Problematiche connesse all'infezione da virus HIV nei luoghi di lavoro', *Difesa sociale* 3.

Bozzuffi, L. (1989) 'Il prima piano sanitario nazionale 1989-1991: Interventi nel settore AIDS e tossicodipendenze', *Bollettino per le farmacodipendenze e l'alcolismo* 3.

Calleri, G. (1989) 'Costo ospedaliero del malato AIDS', *Epidemiologia e prevenzione* 39.

Cattorini, P. (1989) (a cura di) *Aids e segretezza professionale*. Padova: Liviana.

Cimino, T./Gemelli, F./Bertucci, R./Sernia, S./Marino (1991) 'Rischio occupazionale da HIV e sua tutela in ambito INAIL quale infortunio lavorativo', *Difesa sociale* 4.

Clemente, A. (1990) 'Aids: Interventi di prevenzione ed educazione sanitaria', *Professione infermieristiche* 3.

Codini, G. (1989) 'Aids. All'insegna della speranza: i risultati del congresso nazionale di Napoli', *Vivere oggi* 10.

Codini, G./Corsi, L./Paterson, M. (1989) 'La famiglia nell'occhio del ciclone Aids', *Vivere oggi* 7.

Corradini, L. (1989) 'Educare alla salute: tra famiglia e scuola', *Famiglia oggi* 41.

Del Colle, B. (1990) 'Quali rimedi contro l'AIDS', *Famiglia oggi* 47.

De Simone, C. (1987) (a cura di) *Affrontare l'AIDS. Indicazioni per la sanità pubblica, la salute del singolo e la ricerca*. Roma: Sigma-Tau.

Dolazza, L./Commoli, F. (1992) (a cura di) *Oltre l'Aids. Malati e operatori si incontrano*. Bologna: edizione Dehoniane.

Ferri, F./Carito, M. (1988) 'Sieropositività e Aids in tossicodipendenti: osservazioni psicologiche', *Marginalità e società* 8.

Giruni, E. (1992) 'L'accertamento della sieropositività', *Salute e territorio* 78.

Greco, D./Filibeck, U./Monzali, C./Salmaso, S. (1989) 'La politica nazionale per la lotta contro l'AIDS in Italia', *Bollettino per le farmacodipendenze e l'alcolismo* 3.

Grillone, V./Davanzo, G./Fassino, S. (1991) *Aids. Prevenzione, cura, assistenza*. Torino: edizione Camilliane.

Gulia, P. (1989) 'Aids: una malattia dei poveri?', *Italia Caritas* 4.

Lampronti, V./Maciocco, G. (1989) 'L'Aids', *Salute e territorio* 6667.

Lazzari, C./Di Renzo, R./Carlozzo, B.M./De Cinque, C. (1992) 'Il supporto psicoterapeutico di soggetti con Aids', *Psicoterapia e psicoanalisi* 2.

Maggi, M. (1989) 'Il virus dell'intolleranza paura e ignoranza ostacolano le comunità di recupero', *il Delfino* 6.

Ministero Della Sanità (1984) Circolare n. 64/83 'sindrome di immunodeficienza acquisita'. Roma: Ministero della Sanità.

Ministero della Sanità (1990) 'Serie Aids' 2, *bollettino per le farmacodipendenze e l'alcolismo* 2

Ministero della Sanità (1990) 'Serie Aids' 3, *bollettino per le farmacodipendenze e l'alcolismo* 3.

Ministero Della Sanità (1991) 'Campagna di informazione sull'AIDS: informazione per gli operatori professionali dell'assistenza', *Federazione medica* 7.

Montalto, B. (1989) 'Aids e trattamenti coercitivi', *Federazione medica* 1.

Nizzoli, U./Bosi R. (a cura di) *I nuovi ultimi. Ricerca di percorsi di avvicinamento per l'ascolto e la presa in carico dei malati di AIDS*. Ed. Francisci.

Pandolfo, A. (1990) 'L'Aids: una sfida anche per il diritto del lavoro', *Tutela* 2/3.

Parnanzini, L. (1989) *Infezione da HIV e gravidanza*. Aquila: Associazione prevenzione droga.

Rotondo, A./Ranci, D. (1989) 'Aids e crisi degli approcci di cura ed assistenza', *Prospettive sociali e sanitarie* 21.

Salmaso, L. (1989) 'Etica e dignità della persona', *Famiglia oggi* 41.

Serpelloni, G. et al (1989) 'Screening e monitoraggio epidemiologico dell'infezione da HIV nei tossicodipendent', *Epidemiologia e prevenzione* 37.

Simonetti, L. (1987) *L'Aids: problema medico e sociale: informare per prevenire.* Aquila: associazione prevenzione droga.

Sulger Buel, E. (1991) *Aids. Dossier di un'epidemia. una guida per i giovani.* Teramo: Isola del Gran Sasso.

Zanni Minoia, L. (1989) 'Aids: minaccia e difesa', *Famiglia oggi* 41.

Zigrino, F. (1988) 'Il problema dell'Aids nel pubblico impiego con particolare riguardo alle USL', *Il vicino è vicino* 3.

Appendix: List of Organizations Interviewed

Public Inclusives

Centro Malattia a Trasmissione Sessuale	Turin
SERT USL 6	Turin
SERT USL 75/4	Milan
SSM USL 11	Genoa
Centro diagnostico malattie infettive	Bologna
SERT USL 29	Bologna
Centro Malattie a Trasmissione Sessuale	Florence
SERT USL 10/H	Florence
Unità operativa Allergologia e Immunologia	Florence
SERT USL 8	Rome
Unità operativa AIDS II livello	Rome
Progetto ALEPH	Naples
SERT USL 42	Naples
GOT USL 10	Bari
Centro Malattie a Trasmissione Sessuale	Catania
SERT USL 34	Catania

Public Exclusives

Gruppo C – SERT USL 25	Verona
Casa Luciana	Rome
Sezione screening HIV, Cotugno	Naples
Unità operativa AIDS, Istituto d'Igiene	Bari

Private Non-Profit Inclusives

Gruppo Ablele	Turin
Associazione A77	Milan
AISEL	Milan
Cooperativa Archimede	Milan
Centro Solidarietà	Verona
Comunità dei Giovani	Verona

Centro Solidarietà	Genoa
AFET	Genoa
ZEPHIROS	Genoa
ASAT	Bologna
ARCI GAY	Bologna
Centro Solidarietà	Florence
Centro socio-sanitario Magliana	Rome
Circolo Mario Mieli	Rome
Operatori Sanitari Associati	Rome
Associazione SAMAN	Naples
Associazione La Tenda	Naples
APRI	Bari
Amici Fondazione Emofilia	Bari
Casa Nazareth	Catania

Private Non-Profit Exclusives

Gruppo Solidarietà AIDS	Turin
Informagay	Turin
LILA, Sezione Piemonte	Turin
Centro patologie HIV correlate	Milan
Associazione Solidarietà AIDS	Milan
Cooperativa Azalea	Verona
Coordinamento ligure persone sieropositive	Genoa
ANLAIDS, sezione Emilia Romagna	Bologna
LILA, sezione Lazio	Rome
LILA, sezione Catania	Catania

Annex I: Reported AIDS Cases in Selected European Countries

**Figure A1: Cumulative Number of AIDS Cases and AIDS Ratios
(per Million Population) (1984-1994)**

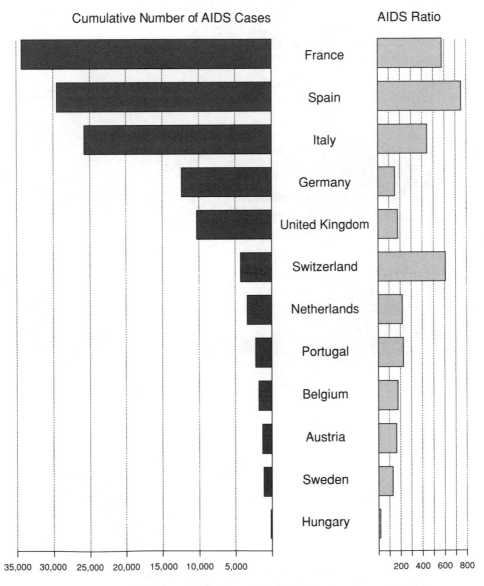

Source: European Centre for the Epidemiological Monitoring of AIDS.
   HIV/AIDS Surveillance in Europe. Quarterly Reports.

Figure A2: Development of AIDS Cases (Rates per Million Population) (1984-1994)

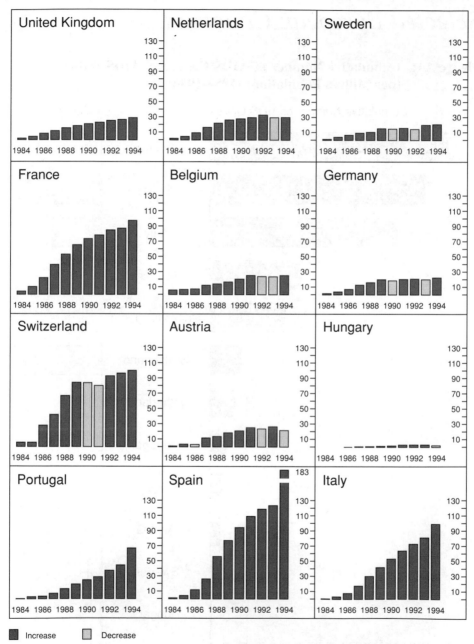

■ Increase   □ Decrease

Source: European Centre for the Epidemiological Monitoring of AIDS.
         HIV/AIDS Surveillance in Europe. Quarterly Reports.

Figure A3: Cumulative Adult/Adolescent AIDS Cases by Transmission Group in Per Cent (1989/1994)

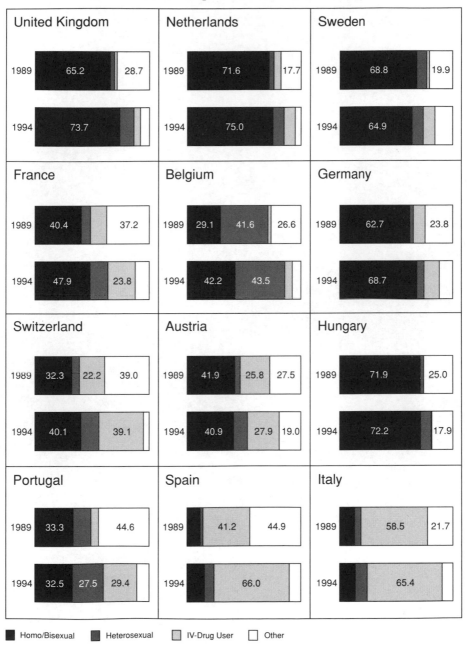

Source: European Centre for the Epidemiological Monitoring of AIDS. *HIV/AIDS Surveillance in Europe. Quarterly Reports.*

Annex II: The Original Research Design

MANAGING AIDS –
THE ROLE OF PRIVATE NONPROFIT INSTITUTIONS
IN PUBLIC HEALTH AND WELFARE POLICY

A RESEARCH PROPOSAL FOR AN
INTERNATIONAL COMPARATIVE STUDY

(Supported by WHO – Euro / RPA and WHO / GPA)

Bernd Marin / Patrick Kenis

EUROPEAN CENTRE / VIENNA

August 1989

Introduction

This is the first international, comparative study ever done on managing AIDS on an institutional, (inter-)organizational, policy-field level.

This is even more surprising, given the fact that in the absence of any medical remedy for the AIDS pandemic so far, prevention of further diffusion of the disease and adequate care for people affected, i.e. health & welfare *management* within an encompassing AIDS-policy design is *the* key – the single most crucial set of factors determining success or failure in coping with AIDS on a global level.

Consequently, the study aims at a comprehensive overview of all major institutions working in AIDS-related health & welfare, be it prevention and education, care and human services, control, policy coordination, surveillance, monitoring, research and intelligence or policy advocacy, interest organization, civil and human rights, be they public or private; and at understanding their functioning in terms of activities performed, professional services offered, clients and publics served, work organization, managerial processes, public policy functions performed, etc.

More than in other sectors of health and welfare, it seems, are AIDS-prevention and AIDS-service organizations run by voluntary associations, volunteers, charitable and philantropic organizations, community-based self-help groups, advocacy groups and other political intermediaries. Without their (largely unpaid) work and commitment, AIDS-management would most probably collapse rapidly in most countries seriously hit by the plague. AIDS-institutions are, therefore, a paradigmatic case in point to test some supposed strengths and weaknesses of voluntary, private nonprofit, non-governmental health & welfare organizations in general.

At the same time, next to nothing is known in a systematic and comparative way about the thousands of organizations "out there", be they specialized AIDS-service associations, be they institutions constituted for other purposes but performing significant (or even predominantly) AIDS-programmes; next to nothing is known about their functional capacities, their institutional properties, their inter-organizational linkages, their cooperation, division of labour etc.; and next to nothing is known about the role and integration of these mainly private nonprofit institutions into an overall public health / welfare / risk-management - policy.

This empirical study is to fill this conspicuous knowledge gap. To the extent that AIDS-institutions will start to establish a European / global network for exchange of experiences among themselves under the leadership of the World Health Organization Global Programme on AIDS (WHO / GPA), the know-how accumulated through this international comparative research might serve some brain trust functions.

Goals and Objectives

The main outcomes to be expected from the research project are:

1) An *AIDS-Institutions Directory (AIDSINST)*, providing a comprehensive mapping of all major public and all voluntary AIDS-prevention- / -service- / -policy - institutions in a given country. This *"Organizational Directory" Database* of private nonprofit non-governmental AIDS service organizations will list names, addresses, legal status, founding dates/start of AIDS programmes, specialized vs. encompassing institutions, types of organization, main AIDS-related activities, geographical scope, access to services / representation / benefits, formal affiliations to other organizations, financial and manpower resources incl. volunteers of European AIDS service organizations.

2) An *Integrated AIDS-Policy-Management Information System (MANAIDS / "Managing AIDS")*, combining a database on all major public institutions and all voluntary private nonprofit AIDS-associations, their functional capacities (including "Task Profiles", "Service Statistics" etc.), organizational properties and inter-organizational / intersectoral cooperation networks (or missing links) with functional profiles of AIDS-institutions, national AIDS-policies within the overall health & welfare system, national problem loads and epidemiological AIDS-profiles and institutional characteristics of AIDS-institutions compared to organizations in other health & welfare sectors and to AIDS-organizations in other countries.

3) A continuous *expertise-input* to ongoing WHO / GPA and WHO-Euro activities such as meetings of European AIDS-service organizations, participation in AIDS-scenarios and the World AIDS-Day as well as to efforts of CSDHA / UNOV and other UN-related agencies.

4) A comprehensive *research report* with national country reports and an international comparative analysis, focusing on managerial aspects, inter-organizational, intersectoral and public / private integration as well as international coordination in AIDS-policy.

5) A short *summary assessment* with *recommendations* for institutional design and public AIDS-policies in health and welfare.

WHO, the UN-System, and the European Centre on AIDS

The General Assembly of the United Nations in its resolutions 42/8 of October 1987, 43/L.12 of 20 October 1988 urged all appropriate organizations of the United Nations system to support the worldwide struggle on AIDS under the leadership of WHO and in conformity with its global strategy. WHO globally directs and coordinates AIDS prevention, control, research and education and national government programmes. It has established, as endorsed in the Resolution WHA40.26 of the Fortieth World Health Assembly, a special "Global Programme on AIDS" (GPA) in Geneva and "stresses its high priority"; it has, by March 1989, set up a "Global Commission on AIDS" (GCA) to review, evaluate, advise and recommend to the Director-General; it has developed inter-agency mechanisms, facilitated international information exchange and research, mobilized support from heads of state or government, the World Summit of Health Ministers and from the representatives of the European Community; it has collaborated with other organizations of the United Nations system (in particular with UNDP, UNESCO, UNICEF, UNFPA), with other intergovernmental organizations such as the World Bank and the International Labour Organisation (ILO) and with nongovernmental organizations such as the Commission of the European Communities, the League of Red Cross and Red Crescent Societies, Family Health International, the International Federation of Social Workers etc. – and with the European Centre for Social Welfare Policy and Research in Vienna, which carries out this research project on contract with WHO / GPA and in coordination with the Centre for Social Development and Humanitarian Affairs of the United Nations Office at Vienna (UNOV / CSDHA), in particular its Working Group on AIDS, its Social Development Division, its Division for the Advancement of Women, its Crime Prevention and Criminal Justice Branch and its Division on Narcotic Drugs.

There is a series of convergences between the WHO Global Programme on AIDS and the European Centre's Programme of Activities in Preparation 1990 - 1992: Surveillance, forecasting and impact assessment, scenarios, the development of databanks, family planning, children and AIDS as well as traditional and alternative care in managing health and welfare systems. In particular, UN and WHO concerns with coordination and unification of national and international efforts in AIDS-management, with "integration of initiatives", with "developing, implementing, monitoring and evaluating well-coordinated, multisectoral national AIDS plans in line with the global strategy on AIDS " (WHO / UNDP Alliance to Combat AIDS: policy framework), and with a "closer involvement of NGOs" in public health and welfare policy fully coincide with the general orientations of the European Centre and with the main focus of this research project.

In fact, the most recent report of the Global Commission on AIDS of 12 April 1989 makes the following particular recommendation on "*Closer involvement of*

NGOs: There is a crucial need at this stage of the global and national activities relevant to AIDS actively to involve in national programmes, all relevant nongovernmental organizations (NGOs), community-based organizations and the private sector. GPA should in every appropriate way take steps to increase the awareness of other relevant international organizations and national AIDS committees concerning the desirability of involving NGOs, community-based organizations and private voluntary organizations ..." And an intergovernmental authority outside the UN-system, the Council of Europe Committee of Ministers in its Recommendation No. R (87) 25 adopted on 26 November 1987, "recommends the governments of member states", among other, to "intensify co-operation within Europe in pursuing studies on specific aspects of the control of AIDS with a view to ... optimising the effectiveness of such policies by avoiding duplication of efforts through exchange of information, comparison and assessment of strategies; identifying common areas of research ...; achieving a concerted harmonised European policy in the fight against AIDS." In the Guidelines appended, it stresses, among others, the importance "of ensuring a regular flow of information and vertical and horizontal co-operation in the implementation of the policy and co-ordination of actions", of monitoring "the implementation of the policy by instituting an appropriate feedback system for permanent revision and adaptation of the policy" and of "Evaluation and research. Development of research and co-operation at European level through the designation of reference centres in all AIDS-related fields is an urgent priority to combat AIDS, would be of great benefit both in terms of effectiveness of programmes and costs, and should therefore be strongly supported ..." This research project should help to fulfil these requests.

The Overall Research Design

Some Basic Distinctions

"AIDS - (RELATED) INSTITUTIONS"

This investigation focuses on policies and institutions. While it is interested in better understanding *AIDS-prevention- / -service- / -policy-institutions*, i.e. in *AIDS-coping organizations*, it must broaden its view to *AIDS-related institutions* in general in order to include major *AIDS-affected institutions* and their interaction with AIDS-coping institutions.

With respect to AIDS-coping institutions, s*pecialized AIDS-prevention- / -service- / -policy-organizations* exclusively dedicated to the purpose of AIDS-management ("*exclusives*") are to be distinguished from *institutions performing AIDS-programmes predominantly or significantly* apart from other domains of activities ("*inclusives*"), e.g. hospitals with AIDS-units providing extramural care, STD-clinics with sexual counselling services, drug therapeutic communities, methadone clinics with health education programmes, community care centres, family planning agencies, self-help group clearinghouses, local health initiatives, social work agencies, home-nursing institutions, patients rights and human rights organizations, philantropic and charitable foundations, plasma product (organ, tissues, cells, semen) banks, blood donation associations, to name just a few.

"Inclusives" might through specialization convert themselves into "exclusives", "exclusives" might gradually broaden their domain beyond AIDS-service and -management and evolve into "inclusives". Many "exclusives", specialized AIDS-organizations will be *transformed organizations* which formerly had nothing to do with AIDS-management at all and have appropriated this task quite recently, whereas others will be *newly founded*, constitutively specialized AIDS-organizations.

Obviously, the nature and origin of AIDS-prevention- / -service- / -policy-institutions will also influence their structures and constitute important assets and liabilities for their everyday modes of functioning. Newly set-up AIDS-organizations might have the advantages of clear, even monopolistic mandates, political and financial support, regulatory authority, task specialization etc., but they might simultaneously lack the embeddedness, consistently high reputation, professional recognition, organic linkages and resource access of an old, well-established non-specialized institution performing AIDS-programmes among others, or of a transformed / converted institution.

"Inclusive" organizations, on the other hand, might incorporate AIDS-programmes within a generally advantageous institutional texture and could thereby cross-subsidize and professionally support them in an optimal way, but they might also prove to be unable or (more or less openly) unwilling to occupy themselves with a new, scientifically ill-understood, institutionally difficult to handle, risky, medically unhealable, culturally often stigmatized disease, inducing a series of serious, partly unconscious, mostly unconfessed, but hardly deniable fears, prejudices and also institutional resistances. In such cases, if an inclusion of AIDS-management cannot be avoided by an institution resistant to do it, it might be tempted to segregate it in isolated subunits, task forces, committees, etc., to marginalize AIDS-programmes or, the other way round, allow other programmes to suffer from a preoccupation with AIDS raising resentment and even hostility towards the "intruding" issue or the beneficiaries of the new care unit.

In any case, "inclusive" institutions will be well characterized by the very mode of inclusion or incorporation of AIDS-programmes / -units into their overall health and welfare management system, as are transformed organizations by the very conversion process and newly founded AIDS-prevention- / -service- / -policy-institutions by the foundation circumstances and the political will reflected in constitutive statutes, licenses and mandates, public status and authority, entitlements, endowments, etc.

But not all AIDS-related institutions, obviously, are coping (more or less effectively) with the disease and its prevention; many institutions or organizations, constitutively outside AIDS-management proper, and without any AIDS-programmes themselves, are or might become nevertheless profoundly affected by the health, social, economic, administrative, etc. impact of the AIDS-risk and pandemic – such as, for instance, the military, the police forces, prostitution, bathhouses and sex clubs, prisons, hospitals without AIDS-care facilities, social security administrations, municipal housing departments, insurance companies, homeless shelters, hospices, haemophiliac associations, sexual and ethnic minority community institutions, women and family associations, youth clubs, kindergartens, etc. Whereas these major AIDS-affected institutions as such are outside the focus of this study, their interaction with AIDS-coping organizations – of which they might often constitute main target groups or clienteles – makes them relevant environments of AIDS-prevention- / -service- / -policy-institutions.

A 4-SECTOR "WELFARE-MIX" MODEL

As other EC-projects, this study follows a 4-sector welfare-mix model, which conceptualizes overall welfare as generated in varying mixes by all sectors of society (state, markets, civil society, community / family / households); which distinguishes organizations by their functional logic and the sector within which they operate; and by the kind of activities performed, i.e. by their output, theoretically categorized as types of goods / welfare-services produced.

The following overview table outlines the correspondence between societal sectors, their constitutive organizations and the type of output-activities or welfare-services produced:

Societal Sectors Activities	Constitutive Organizations	Type of Output-Welfare-Services Produced
State	Public Agencies	Monopolistic Authoritative Public Citizenship Categoric (Private / Commercial)
Markets	(Private) Corporations, Business Firms, Enterprises, Companies	Private / Commercial
Intermediaries between Markets and Third Sector	(Consumer) Cooperatives	Private / Commercial Membership Solidaristic / Communitarian / Self-Help
Third Sector ("The World of Associations ", "Social Economy") Civil Society	Voluntary Nonprofit Associations Nongovernmental Organizations Interest/Advocacy Organizations Organized Popular Movements Membership Organizations Charitable and Philantropic Associations Churches, Religious Associations Solidaristic/Communitarian/ Foundations	Monopolistic Authoritative Public Citizenship Categoric Private / Commercial Membership Self-Help
Intermediaries between Third Sector and Unorganized Informal Sector	Self-Help Groups, Mutual Aid Networks, Social Club-like Groups without Membership, Social Movements	Solidaristic/ Communitarian/ Self-Help
Primary Community ("Primary Social Support Systems") Unorganized Informal Sector	Private Households; Family, Solidaristic/Communitarian/ Kinship, Neighbourhood "Moral Economy"	Self-Help

Whereas public agencies, private corporations and voluntary nonprofit associations partly also serve each other, they all and above all serve private households, i.e. the unorganized informal sector which itself is a major producer and *the* consumer, client or beneficiary of welfare-services.

As indicated in the table above (but without further elaborating on this theoretically), voluntary nonprofit associations play a crucial role in overall societal welfare generation: while all other sectors crystallize around the production of some specific type of good / service – public agencies around public / authoritative services, corporations around private / commercial services and private households around solidaristic / communitarian / self-help – the Third Sector is the only one which generates the whole range of goods / welfare-services – from monopolistic over public, private / commercial, membership services to solidaristic self-help.

As it was already used implicitly, let us explicitly outline an output-typology by defining types of goods / services produced as applied to AIDS-coping institutions:

Monopolistic Services: services provided only by the state or with exclusive special authorization delegated from the state or other public authorities.

Examples: Control of blood or plasma product safety done by one organization only; mandatory testing; National AIDS-Coordinating Committees as proposed by the Council of Europe.

Generally: Control, intelligence, surveillance, monitoring activities, policy coordination, regulatory (also compulsory and coercive) measures, etc. by the state only or exclusively authorized agencies on its behalf.

Authoritative Services: services provided by the state or with special authorization delegated from the state or other public authorities.

Examples: All kinds of screening or testing; official health education and promotion programmes.

Generally: Control, intelligence, surveillance, monitoring activities, policy coordination, regulatory (also compulsory and coercive) measures, etc., but also prevention and certain licensed care activities delivered by the state or authorized agencies on its behalf.

Public Good Services: services provided free of charge and with free access to everybody.

Examples: Publicity campaigns; AIDS-information hotlines; anonymous voluntary testing.

Generally: Most preventive activities and health education / promotion programmes.

Citizenship Services: services provided free of charge and with free access to all citizens, but citizens of a given nation-state only.
Examples: Ombudsman; personalized health information services; family therapy; advocacy for entitlements, counselling for eligibility for entitlements, discrimination complaint centre.
Generally: Many preventive activities, care and social services, mostly policy advocacy, interest, civil rights action.

Categoric Services: services provided free of charge for specific populations / entitled beneficiaries.
Examples: Medical care for persons with AIDS; pediatric AIDS day care and foster care for children with AIDS; occupational safety instructions for health care professionals; free distribution of one-way needles to drug addicts; emergency housing or foodbanks for terminally-ill patients; lobbying for gay interests.
Generally: Many preventive activities, mostly care and social services, some control and mostly policy advocay, interest organization and civil rights activities.

Private / Commercial Services: services provided for charge (except for minimal, purely symbolic charges) with free access for everybody.
Examples: Psychosocial support services; legal advice; commercial home nursing.
Generally: Some care and social services, practically no preventive, control and advocacy activities.

Membership Services: services provided free of charge or at reduced rates with restricted access, i.e. to subscribed members of an association only ("selective services").
Examples: Organizing assortative mating by infection status on club-basis; spiritual and religious support services; health insurance risk pools.
Generally: All programme and service activities can be organized on membership basis, few actually will.

> *Solidaristic / Communitarian / Self-Help Action:* organized self-help, mutual aid, reciprocal benefits (consumers / clients = producers = beneficiaries).
> Examples: Identity house; emotional support ("buddy system"); organizing residential and neighbourhood care networks; support for self-help groups and mutual aid networks; PWA coalition; self-governance and control of prostitution by prostitutes; benefice events and fund-raising activities.
> Generally: All activities can be organized on solidaristic / communitarian / self-help basis, several of them and most support activities actually will.

BASIC FUNCTIONAL TASK TYPES OF AIDS-INSTITUTIONS

Using this theoretical scheme in the field of AIDS-institutions, it seems that the major domains of their activities crystallize around the following task areas:

- Prevention
- Care and social services
- Control / intelligence / surveillance / monitoring
- Policy advocacy / interest organization / civil and human rights

These major tasks could in principle all be realized by almost all types of services from monopolistic to solidaristic activities, whereas in fact (as we have seen from the table illustrating the output-typology of types of goods / services produced) they strongly tend to cluster in certain preferred patterns: control activities will, as policy coordination, usually be organized through monopolistic, authoritative and some categoric devices; prevention mainly through public, citizenship or categoric services, almost never on a commercial base; care and social services in most modes including private / commercial but except for monopolistic and authoritative activities (apart from few exceptions such as e.g. child adoption); policy advocacy and interest organization, too, will be generated in many ways, including monopolistic devices such as a public ombudsman, but rarely through private / commercial activities.

Consequently, we will find very few private firms in AIDS-management (except for the blood processing, plasma product and pharmaceutical industries), state agencies and public authorities concentrating on control and policy coordination, whereas the bulk of work to be done will be in the hands of voluntary nonprofit organizations assisted by and assisting the primary communities as well as state health and welfare authorities. Thinking in ideal types, the following scheme might help to structure the universe of voluntary nonprofit or nongovernmental AIDS-prevention- / -service- / -policy-institutions by major functional tasks:

- Health Promotion, Information, Education, Instruction, Training incl. Publicity Campaign Agencies

- Service Provision Organizations in Case Work of Personal Care and Individual Advice

- Self-Help Group-Clearinghouses, Mutual Aid Networks, Community Care Centres

- AIDS Policy Coordination and Implementation Bodies

- Authoritative Regulatory and Control Bodies (incl. screening, testing, blood product safety and quality control organizations)

- Intelligence Organizations (incl. epidemiological and social research units)

- Policy Advocacy / Interest / Civil and Human Rights Organizations

THE "WELFARE-MIX" MODEL CONTINUED

Whereas the state, markets and primary community and that is public agencies, enterprises and private households are highly differentiated from each other, with clear-cut boundaries, functional autonomy but also internal operational homogeneity, the opposite holds for the Third Sector, which overlaps with all others and whose voluntary organizations are characterized just by combining elements typical of state agencies, business firms, political interest organizations and primary community

Thus, the Third Sector does not only contribute to the overall "Welfare-Mix", it is itself a broad functional mix combining highly divergent (and often considered "incompatible") tasks and organizing principles into an "improbable" new production function. This internal mix of voluntary associations as against the "pure" forms of state agencies, business companies and private households is their specific strength and weakness at the same time: it guarantees their very existence and persistence over long periods of time on the one hand and constantly threatens their dissolution into powerfully institutionalized environments such as public administration, capitalist enterprises, political parties or primary communities on the other. Consequently, we find more longevity, occasionally over centuries, as well as more ephemeral, transitional phenomena among voluntary organizations than among business firms or even public agencies and departments.

Similarly, voluntary nonprofit associations are to be expected – and actually found – on both ends of the efficiency spectre: combining either the accumulated vices of state, markets and community such as bureaucratic rigidity, social injustice, dilettantism and nepotism, or mobilizing otherwise unreached synergetics by combining their respective comparative advantages in terms of professional quality of service as well as innovative, flexible, client-oriented and equitable delivery. Comparative efficiency, as maintenance as such, depends on the functional mix of nonprofit associations and its permanent adjustments to shifts in the overall welfare-mix between state, markets, third sector and primary community.

Therefore, the functional profile or functional mix of any voluntary association in terms of output-activities or types of welfare-services produced – together with its interorganizational linkages – is itself the single most important factor to allow to predict its daily behaviour, its constitutive dilemmas, its structural choices. Thus, it is not the input of resource acquisition and allocation, but the output produced and the mixed modes of service production – making a voluntary organization resemble in varying degrees "parastate organizations", "service firms", "political interest associations", "clubs" or "self-help groups", etc. – which are the crucial determinants of its logic of operation.

The Domain Investigated and "AIDS-Institutions Directory" Entries

FOCUS

Data collection and analysis will concentrate on

- all functional types of voluntary nonprofit AIDS-prevention- / -service- / -policy - institutions
- all major public AIDS-prevention- / -service- / -policy - institutions
- specialized AIDS service associations and institutions performing AIDS programmes
- the interaction of voluntary associations with public (health and welfare) agencies, private corporations (e.g. hospital, insurance sector, blood and pharmaceutical industry) and primary social support systems
- their interaction with major AIDS-affected institutions (e.g. social security administration, homeless shelters, hospices, haemophiliac associations, minority community institutions, prisons etc.).

Thus, the AIDS-Institutions Directory (AIDSINST), will provide a comprehensive mapping of *all major public* AIDS-prevention- / -service- / -policy - institutions and *all voluntary* organizations / institutions coping with AIDS and systematically cover their main functional capacities, organizational properties and interorganizational linkages within the overall health and welfare system.

SCOPE AND DOMAIN

Not included in the associational directory AIDSINST will be exclusively residential and local initiatives, pure self-help groups and clubs, non-organized private care, commercial activities, primary medical care within hospitals (incl. nonprofit hospitals), medical and other scientific research laboratories and institutes, as well as very small organizations (e.g. associations below a certain size in employees / volunteers).

Extramural cure and therapy, prevention, health promotion, epidemiological and social research centres, instruction, training, counselling, screening, testing, etc. agencies will be included.

The selection and choice of countries covered will be done jointly with WHO and prospective country team candidates: the focus will be on about six European countries and the United States for comparative purposes.

Special Aspects

NATIONAL PROBLEM LOADS AND AIDS-PROFILES

Quite obviously, manpower and institutional capacities required from AIDS-coping organizations will vary with national problem loads and epidemiological profiles of AIDS-cases and HIV-infections. Even within what WHO in its global surveillance and forecasting programme calls "Pattern I" of HIV / AIDS, i.e. the pattern typical of industrialized countries in Europe and North America, AIDS-incidence rates and HIV seroprevalence vary tremendously between countries, as do the profiles or socio-demographic features of population groups primarily affected by the disease. It will be the task of the international research team at the European Centre to provide, on the basis of updated WHO epidemiological data, a constantly updated time series data set on "National Problem Loads and AIDS-Profiles" and to link these objective indicators and indices to the respective organizational capacities available in a country and their geographic distribution, in order to determine adequate correspondence or mismatches between objective prevention / service / policy requirements and given institutional responses.

MANAGING AIDS: THE OVERALL NATIONAL CONTEXT / SYSTEM

Similarly, an overview of overall institutional contexts and AIDS-policies within the national health and welfare system will be provided by the EC-team. This comparative mapping of divergent national contexts in which AIDS-organizations operate offers a macro (country) and a meso (sectoral or AIDS-policy field) level framework for the associational and inter-organizational data which are the focus of the research. They will be based on three types of sources: a WHO-collected overview of different national approaches to AIDS-policy; an overview by the respective national teams of the main structural features of the national health and welfare systems along some common outline; and a series of sectoral indices, constructed by the EC-team on the basis of incoming associational data, capturing emergent properties of the AIDS-policy field through its inter-associational networks. This will allow to locate AIDS-prevention / service / policy-organizations within the institutional contexts which determine their functioning.

THE UNIQUENESS OF AIDS IN TERMS OF RISK AND HEALTH CARE MANAGEMENT AND SOCIAL SERVICE ORGANIZATION

AIDS, it has often been said, is unique a disease in many ways. We will, nevertheless, not start the project by elaborating on these premises but rather leave it to the empirical investigations to come up with insights grounded in experience and international comparative findings to specify these assumptions. Thus, a deeper understanding of the special and often unique requirements of effective HIV-risk-management and AIDS health care, welfare and social service organizations is a main result to be expected from empirical and comparative, cross-national research.

Still, there is one peculiarity which permeates all working within and inquiry about the AIDS-policy field, which will have to be taken into account systematically, i.e. a lack of consensus on fundamentals, widespread but self-denying and partly even unconscious fears, popular myths, prejudices and their cristallization into institutional resistances. Operating within the comparatively "enlightened" environment of scientists, health care professionals, committed volunteers and international policy-makers makes one all too easily forget the grim everyday realities of managing AIDS within established institutions: the incapacity or (more or less open) unwillingness to occupy oneself with a new, scientifically ill-understood, risky, medically unhealable, culturally often stigmatized disease, which seems to be "hopeless" in that no vaccines and practically no cures or palliatives exist, which needs extensive and expensive care (unavoidably at the expense of other care services) over long periods without any hope to avoid a fatal outcome and that is painful dying; a disease moreover, which because of its long incubation period allows for unknown, unwitting transmission, which in popular perception is furthermore attributed to changeable or avoidable behaviour and linked to illegal or risky practices of undoubtly limited cultural tolerance; a disease finally, the prevention, control, containment, diagnosis, medical treatment, etc. of which involves a series of serious civil liberties and human rights issues and ethical dilemmas. These institutional resistances against AIDS-management seem to be a major problem of "inclusive" institutions performing AIDS-programmes apart from other activities, whereas specialized AIDS-organizations are expected to be more immune to such regressive tendencies.

AIDS - PREVENTION - / - SERVICE - / - POLICY - INSTITUTIONS WITHIN THE HEALTH AND WELFARE SYSTEMS

DATA SETS – LIST OF VARIABLES (OVERVIEW)

I.   Macro (Country) Variables

1. "National Health & Welfare Indicators / Contexts"
2. Third Sector Configurations
3. Third Sector Health & Welfare ("The Mix of the Welfare Mix")

II. Meso (Sectoral) Variables

1. "National Problem Loads and AIDS-Profiles" (Epidemiology)
2. National AIDS-Policies (within the overall Health & Welfare System)
3. Inter-Organizational Networks, Institutional Development, Functional Profiles etc. of AIDS-Service Institutions

III. Micro (Associational) Variables

1. Status, Organizational History, Development
2. Formal Organization
3. Decision-Making and Managerial Processes
4. Volunteering, Professionalism, Leadership
5. Activities: Task Profiles and Clientele Structures
6. Activities: Work Organization and Processes
7. Activities: Output / Service Statistics and Performance Indicators
8. evv. Membership Structures
9. Input and Allocation of Resources
10. Inter-organizational / Intersectoral / International Cooperation and Competition
11. Institutionalization

LIST OF MICRO (ASSOCIATIONAL) VARIABLES

1. *STATUS, ORGANIZATIONAL HISTORY, DEVELOPMENT*
   Name/Acronym
   Address
   Contact Person
   Legal Status
   Specialized AIDS Service Associations (EXCLUSIVES) /
   Institutions Performing AIDS Programmes (INCLUSIVES)
   Type of Organization
   Founding Date (Age)
   Starting Date as an AIDS-Service Institution
   Major Organizational Changes
   "Weltanschauung" / Ideological Orientation

2. *FORMAL ORGANIZATION*
   Constitutive Associational Goals and Objectives
   Scope and Domain of Associational Competences
   Organigram/Organizational Chart
   Formalization
   Internal Structure and Differentiation
   Associational Authority and Control
   Degree of Centralization, Autonomy

3. *DECISION-MAKING AND MANAGERIAL PROCESSES*
   Internal Decision-Making
   Interest Cleavages/Conflict Potentials
   The Functional Autonomy of Frontline Service Providers/Field Workers

4. *VOLUNTEERING, PROFESSIONALISM, LEADERSHIP*
   Categories and Numbers of People Running the Organization
   Staff Development
   Professionals/Laypeople/Employees/Volunteers

PEOPLE WORKING IN AIDS-SERVICE INSTITUTIONS / UNITS

Involvement/Detachment

Manpower Recruitment

Terms of Employment

Comparative Salary Levels and other Remunerations

Staff Fluctuation/Turnover

Associational Career Opportunities

5. *ACTIVITIES: TASK PROFILES AND CLIENTELE STRUCTURES*

Goals and Objectives of the Association concerning AIDS-Management

Task Profiles

Territorial Scope of Activities

Clienteles and Target Groups

Clientele Profile

6. *ACTIVITIES: WORK ORGANIZATION AND PROCESSES*

Standard Operating Procedures

Working Time Pattern/Regime

Individual and Collective Work

Service Integration / Referral

Kind of Work

Professional Methods Used

Administrative and Informational Rationality

Quality Control, Auditing, Supervision

Job Satisfaction, Stress / Burnout, Alienation

7. *ACTIVITIES: OUTPUT / SERVICE STATISTICS AND PERFORMANCE INDICATORS*

Output/Service Statistics (by major domains)

Input Allocation to Programme and Service Activities

Performance Indicators/Coverage

Performance Indicators/Image

8. *MEMBERSHIP STRUCTURES*

    Number of Members and Membership Development

    Membership Fluctuations

    Organizational Density

    Categories of Members

    Membership Dues Formula

    Membership Renewal and Mode of Dues Collection

    Terms of Membership/Crucial Membership Services

    Explaining the Organizational Form

    Multiple Memberships

    Membership Profile

    Associational Membership Policy

9. *INPUT AND ALLOCATION OF RESOURCES*

    Total Revenue of the Association (Budget 1990)

    Total Revenue of the Association in Previous Years

    Budget Allocated for AIDS-Programme(s)

    Sources of Income

    Staffing

    Intangible and "Silent" Resources

    Most Important Patrons/Donors/Sponsors

    Equipment and Facilities

    Major Spending Patterns

    Input Allocation to Associational Activities

    Problems in Public Resource Acquisition

10. *INTER-ORGANIZATIONAL / INTERSECTORAL / INTERNATIONAL*
    COOPERATION AND COMPETITION

    External, Inter-Organizational Relations

    Most Important Partners of Cooperation

    Quality of 3 Most Important Cooperative Relationships of the Association/Unit

    Plural Views/Opponents/Adversaries

    Competitive Spaces

11. *INSTITUTIONALIZATION*

Public Policy/Regulatory Authority

Old Age Association

High Public Involvement

Public Control and Intelligence Domain

State Quality Control

Monopolistic/Authoritative and Other Public Services

High Programme and Service Coverage

Consistent High Reputation

High Organizational Density

Important State Subsidies

High Access to Public Resources

Advantageous Tax Status

Delegated AIDS Authorities

Delegated AIDS Monopolies

Staff Paid by the State

Entitlement to Public Staff Secondments

Publicly Seconded Staff

High Degree of Interorganizational/Intersectoral/ International Cooperation

Number of Tasks Related to the State or Public Agencies Performed
   by the Association

Staff Mobility from and to Civil Service

Privileged Linkages with the State

Monopolized Access

Annex III: European AIDS Service Organizations Inventory Sheet

World Health Organization (WHO) Collaborative Study
European Centre for Social Welfare Policy and Research, Vienna

---

1.1 FULL NAME OF THE ORGANIZATION:

1.2 FULL NAME OF THE HIV/AIDS-SPECIALIZED UNIT, IF ANY:

1.3 ACRONYM(S):

1.4 IS THERE AN ENGLISH VERSION OF THE NAME(S)?

---

2. ADDRESS

Street, number		Telephone no.
City or town	Post Office Box no.	Cable
Postal code	Postal code of POB	Fax no.
Country		Electronic mail no.

---

3. LEGAL STATUS OF THE ORGANIZATION
   (Choose only one)

   Governmental, public agency ....
   Private firm, enterprise, company ....
   Nonprofit, voluntary organization ....

---

4. FOUNDING DATE OF THE ORGANIZATION: ....
   IN WHICH YEAR DID YOU START HIV/AIDS PROGRAMMES: ....
   FOUNDING DATE AS AN AIDS SERVICE ORGANIZATION/UNIT: ....

5.1 THE ORGANIZATION IS
    (Choose only one)

    Specialized in HIV/AIDS only ....
    General, including HIV/AIDS programmes among other activities ....

5.2 WHICH ONE OF THE LABELS FITS BEST WHAT YOU DO IN THE FIELD OF HIV/AIDS?
    (Choose only one)

    .... Local health initiative, mutual aid network
    .... Community care centre
    .... Inpatient health care centre, hospital
    .... Nursing home
    .... Family planning/sexual education centre
    .... Drug treatment/counselling centre
    .... Fund-raising organization
    .... AIDS-specialized foundation (nonprofit funding org.)
    .... Intelligence and surveillance centre (epidemiological/ social research)
    .... Blood screening, blood product safety and quality control organization
    .... PWA case management organization
    .... Biomedical research centre
    .... Health promotion, education, prevention, instruction, training organization

    .... Clearinghouse of self-help groups
    .... HIV testing centre
    .... Outpatient, ambulatory health care centre
    .... Home care service organization
    .... Social work agency
    .... Hospice, shelter
    .... Home for persons with HIV/AIDS
    .... AIDS policy coordination and implementation body
    .... Health department
    .... STD clinic
    .... Blood/Plasma product bank
    .... Policy advocacy, civil and human rights organization
    .... Self-help group/interest organization of/for people with HIV/AIDS
    .... Hotline
    .... Other
            Please specify

5.3 For General Organizations (including HIV/AIDS programmes among other activities) ONLY:
    PLEASE INDICATE BASICALLY WHAT KIND OF ORGANIZATION YOU ARE:

5.4 ARE THERE ANY OTHER LABELS WHICH ALSO APPLY?
(Please use the categories listed in Question 5.2 and choose no more than three additional labels)

5.5 WHAT ARE YOUR MAIN HIV/AIDS-RELATED ACTIVITIES?

Prevention / Education / Information
.... Hotline (telephone counselling)
.... Production of information material
.... AIDS information campaigns (national or local)
.... Educational and information work (incl. streetwork)
.... Drug-related prevention
.... Training (of volunteers, health care professionals etc.)
Health Care and Social Services
.... AIDS-specialized medical care
.... Care/psychological support of people
         with HIV/AIDS
.... Face-to-face counselling
.... Home care services
.... Hospices, shelters
.... Housing facilities
.... Voluntary HIV testing and counselling

.... Buddy system
.... Referral services
.... Foodbank
Control / Intelligence / Surveillance / Monitoring
.... Epidemiological/social research
.... AIDS policy coordination and implementation
.... Control of blood/plasma product safety
.... HIV screening, testing, identification (contact tracing)
Policy Advocacy / Interest Organization / Civil and Human Rights
.... Self-help groups of people with HIV/AIDS
.... Counselling for insurance/welfare entitlements
.... Civil and human rights/protection against discrimination
.... Political lobbying
.... Legal advice
Fund-raising for AIDS programmes, other support activities
Other (please specify) ....

6. GEOGRAPHICAL SCOPE OF THE ORGANIZATION
(multiple answers are possible; please specify which geographical area)

    Multinational ....
    National ....
    Regional ....
    Local ....

    PLEASE ATTACH A LIST OF LOCAL / REGIONAL OUTLETS SPECIALIZED IN HIV/AIDS

7. WHO HAS ACCESS TO THE ORGANIZATION´S SERVICES, REPRESENTATION OR
    BENEFITS?

    Everybody (including foreigners) ....
    Every citizen ....
    Specific group(s) only: please specify ....

8. TO WHICH OTHER ORGANIZATIONS IS THE ORGANIZATION FORMALLY AFFILIATED?
    For General Organizations (including HIV/AIDS programmes among other activities): Please mention only those
    organizations which are active with regard to HIV/AIDS.
    For Organizations Specialized in HIV/AIDS only: Please mention all your affiliations.
    (Please indicate full names using a separate sheet if necessary)

    ....

9   WHAT IS

	Total Organization	HIV/AIDS Unit
The number of employed staff?	....	....
The number of volunteers in the organization?	....	....
The number of subscribed members? (Only if membership organization)	....	....
The annual budget of your organization?	....	....
The percentage of your annual budget used for HIV/AIDS-programme(s)?	.... %	

Please notice: General Organizations (including HIV/AIDS programmes among other activities) should fill in both columns.
                Organizations exclusively specialized in HIV/AIDS should fill in only the first column.

10. WOULD YOU LIKE TO GIVE US SOME COMPLEMENTARY INFORMATION ABOUT THE
     ORGANIZATION?
     (Please use no more than five lines)

THANK YOU FOR SENDING US WHATEVER DOCUMENTS AVAILABLE ABOUT YOUR
ACTIVITIES (ANNUAL REPORTS, BROCHURES, STATUTES etc.) !

                              Date: ....
                              Name of Contact Person: ....

Annex IV: "Managing AIDS" Questionnaire

World Health Organization (WHO) Collaborative Study
"Managing AIDS"
European Centre for Social Welfare Policy and Research, Vienna

COUNTRY:	**QUESTIONNAIRE NUMBER:**	[1-3]
		[1-3]

DATE OF INTERVIEW:

BASIC INFORMATION

I. *INTERVIEWER:* *Record name(s) and position(s) of person(s) answering questions*

....

II. What is the full name of your organization?

....

III. Could you translate this name into English?   [1-30]

....

  INTERVIEWER: *If the respondent is not able to provide the translation, please do it yourself*

....

IV. If your organization has an acronym, what is it? ....

V. What is the address of your organization?

  Street, number ....
  Town/City ....
  Postal code ....
  Post Office Box # .... Postal code of POB ....
  Country ....
  Area code and telephone # ....
  Cable ....
  Fax # ....
  Electronic mail # ....

VI. Who could be contacted for further information about your organization?

....

A. STATUS, ORGANIZATIONAL HISTORY, DEVELOPMENT

1. The AIDS epidemic represents a major public health problem. In your opinion, how satisfactory has been the response to the AIDS epidemic by the following sectors and groups in your country?
   INTERVIEWER: Please, allow for only only number in the scale

	Not at all satisfactory				Very satisfactory	
The national public health and welfare authorities	1	2	3	4	5	[1-2]
The regional government	1	2	3	4	5	[1-2]
The local government	1	2	3	4	5	[1-2]
International public health and welfare authorities (e.g., WHO)	1	2	3	4	5	[1-2]
Social security bureaucracy	1	2	3	4	5	[1-2]
The National AIDS policy committee	1	2	3	4	5	[1-2]
The medical and other professions	1	2	3	4	5	[1-2]
Insurance companies	1	2	3	4	5	[1-2]
Hospitals	1	2	3	4	5	[1-2]
The pharmaceutical industry	1	2	3	4	5	[1-2]
The blood banks	1	2	3	4	5	[1-2]
Community groups / local initiatives	1	2	3	4	5	[1-2]
Clients, including self-help groups	1	2	3	4	5	[1-2]
Policy advocacy/interest/civil and human rights organizations	1	2	3	4	5	[1-2]
Funding agencies, sponsors	1	2	3	4	5	[1-2]
Gay men	1	2	3	4	5	[1-2]
Drug addicts	1	2	3	4	5	[1-2]
The population at large	1	2	3	4	5	[1-2]

Others (please specify)

Other 1

.... | 1 | 2 | 3 | 4 | 5 | [1-2]

Other 2

.... | 1 | 2 | 3 | 4 | 5 | [1-2]

Other 3

.... | 1 | 2 | 3 | 4 | 5 | [1-2]

INTERVIEWER: For QUESTIONS 2 and 4 - 7, you can use the information collected through the directory sheet

2. We are very interested in knowing more about your organization. What is its legal status?
   INTERVIEWER: Please allow for only one   [1-2]

Governmental, public agency 1
Private firm, enterprise, company... 2
Non-profit, voluntary organization 3

3. Please specify the legal status of your organization in your own words:

    ....

4. Which of the following statements describes your organization best?   [1-2]
    INTERVIEWER: Please allow for only <u>one</u>

    - Our only activity is HIV / AIDS
      ("EXCLUSIVE" organization)   1 —>*Go to 5*
    - A specialised separate unit handles all HIV / AIDS
      activities ("INCLUSIVE" organization)   2 —>*Go to 4a*
    - We also do other things than HIV / AIDS and there is no
      special unit for HIV / AIDS ("INCLUSIVE" organization) 3 —>*Go to 5*

    4a. To whom does the special unit report?   [1-2]
        INTERVIEWER: Please allow for only <u>one</u>

        Directly to top management 1
        To the director of services 2
        Other 3
                (Please specify) ....

5. Which one of the following categories describes the *main* purpose
    of your organization?   [1-2]
    INTERVIEWER: Please allow for only <u>one</u>

    AIDS specialised foundation (non-profit funding organization) 01
    AIDS policy coordinating and implementation body 02
    Biomedical research centre 03
    Blood screening, blood product safety and quality control organization 04
    Blood / plasma product bank 05
    Clearing-house of self-help groups 06
    Community care centre 07
    Drug treatment / counselling centre 08
    Family planning / sexual education centre 09
    Fund-raising organization 10
    Health department 11
    Health promotion, education, prevention, instruction, training organization 12
    HIV testing centre 13
    Home care service organization 14
    Hospice, shelter 15
    Home for persons with HIV / AIDS 16
    Hotline 17
    Inpatient health care centre, hospital 18
    Intelligence and surveillance centre
    (epidemiological & social research) 19
    Local health initiative, mutual aid network 20
    Nursing home 21
    Outpatient, ambulatory health care centre 22
    Policy advocacy, civil and human rights organization 23

PWA case management organization 24
Self-help group / interest organization of / for people with HIV/AIDS 25
Social work agency 26
STD-clinic 27
Other 28
        (Please specify) ....

6. Which other of the above categories help to describe your organization better?
    INTERVIEWER: Please use the codes in QUESTION 5 and do not
    allow for more than <u>three</u>

                                      1. .... [1-2]
                                      2. .... [1-2]
                                      3. .... [1-2]

7. When was *your* organization founded?

    Year: ....   [1-2]

    7a. What is the starting date of your organization as an HIV/AIDS
        service institution?

        Year: ....   [1-2]
        Month: ....   [1-2]

8. Is there a predecessor of your organization?[1-2]

    No .... 2 —> *Go to 9*
    Yes .... 1 —> *Go to 8a and 8b*

    8a. What is the full name of the predecessor?
        ....
    8b. When was the predecessor founded?

    Year: ....   [1-2]

9. Was there a "founding father / mother" or patron in the founding of your
    organization?   [1-2]

    No .... 2 —> *Go to 10*
    Yes .... 1 —> *Go to 9a*

    9a. What was the founder's occupational and political background?
        ....

10. What is the *formal* orientation of your organization?   [1-2]
    INTERVIEWER: Please allow for only <u>one</u>

    Religious .... 1 —> *Go to 11*
    Secular .... 2 —> *Go to 10a*

10a. Is the *major* orientation of your organization .... [1-2]
 INTERVIEWER: Please allow for only <u>one</u>

 Political 1
 Social movement (e.g., gay liberation) 2
 Unaffiliated 3

11. Describe the particular political, religious, or social movement group
 to which you belong or feel attached to:
 ....

12. Organizations sometimes change to serve clients more effectively.
 Has your organization implemented any of the following *structural*
 changes and if yes, in which year did that happen?

	No	Yes	Year	
Change the organization's name	2	1	....	[1-4]
Change the statutes	2	1	....	[1-4]
Shift the central focus of the organization	2	1	....	[1-4]
Centralised the structure	2	1	....	[1-4]
Decentralised the structure	2	1	....	[1-4]
Created a (new) division of services	2	1	....	[1-4]
Merged with another organization	2	1	....	[1-4]
Acquired another organization	2	1	....	[1-4]
Other	2	1	....	[1-4]

 (If yes, please specify) ....

B. FORMAL ORGANIZATION

13. Does your organization have formal written statutes? [1-2]

 No .... 2 —> *Go to 14*
 Yes .... 1 —> *Go to 13a and 13b*

 13a. What are the constitutive goals of your organization as they
 appear in the statutes?
 (Please specify)
 ....

 13b. Do the constitutional statutes of your organization explicitly
 refer to AIDS? [1-2]

 No 2
 Yes 1

14. What is the organization's geographical area of activity?

	No	Yes	
supranational / international	2	1	[1-2]
multinational (more than one country)	2	1	[1-2]
national	2	1	[1-2]
state or regional ("provinces", "Länder")	2	1	[1-2]
subregional (county, metropolitan area, "department","Kreis")	2	1	[1-2]
local	2	1	[1-2]

15. Is there a ready-made chart of your organization?　　　　　　　　　　　[1-2]

　　No .... 2 —> *Go to 15a*
　　Yes .... 1 —> *Ask for a copy*

15a. Could you please draw on paper an approximate chart
　　　of your organization?　　　　　　　　　　　　　　　　　　　　[1-2]

　　　　Yes 1
　　　　No 2

16. Which of the following activities or areas apply to your organization
　　and for which of those does your organization keep written records ?

	apply to our organization		written records		
	No	Yes	No	Yes	
Policy and strategic planning	2	1	2	1	[1-4]
Services offered	2	1	2	1	[1-4]
Service delivery performance	2	1	2	1	[1-4]
AIDS programmes	2	1	2	1	[1-4]
Organization and mode of service delivery	2	1	2	1	[1-4]
Major organizational changes	2	1	2	1	[1-4]
External relations	2	1	2	1	[1-4]
Clients	2	1	2	1	[1-4]
Management meetings	2	1	2	1	[1-4]
Professionals meetings	2	1	2	1	[1-4]
Member meetings	2	1	2	1	[1-4]
Budget proposals	2	1	2	1	[1-4]
Budget approvals	2	1	2	1	[1-4]
Statement of accounts (balance sheet)	2	1	2	1	[1-4]
Major investment decisions	2	1	2	1	[1-4]
Daily financial transactions	2	1	2	1	[1-4]
Paid personnel	2	1	2	1	[1-4]
Volunteers	2	1	2	1	[1-4]

Job profiles	2	1	2	1	[1-4]
Internal norms and sanctions	2	1	2	1	[1-4]
Research	2	1	2	1	[1-4]

17. Does your organization have outlets or branches, that is, separate units
in other physical locations? [1-2]

No .... 2 —> *Go to 18*
Yes .... 1 —> *Go to 17a and 17b*

17a. Please list the *number* of outlets and indicate how many
are specialised in HIV/AIDS

Outlets:

	number	specialised in HIV/AIDS	
Total:	....	....	[1-6]
Regional:	....	....	[1-6]
Local:	....	....	[1-6]
Task specialised:	....	....	[1-3]
Succursale (duplicate, branch):	....	....	[1-6]

17b. Please indicate types and numbers for each formal organizational
component or subunit of your organization, such as e.g., "units",
"divisions", "departments", "internal agencies", "committees",
"working groups", "task forces", "external outreach units",
"street level operative units", etc.

Name	Number of subunits	of which specialised in HIV/AIDS	
....			[1-5]
....			[1-5]
....			[1-5]
....			[1-5]
....			[1-5]
....			[1-5]

18. Does your organization have a major policy-making body or bodies? [1-2]

No .... 2 —> *Go to 19*
Yes .... 1 —> *Go to 18a*

18a. Please specify: ....

C. DECISION-MAKING AND MANAGERIAL PROCESSES

19. Please specify which body takes the ultimate responsibility with respect
    to the following areas .....
    INTERVIEWER: Please ask only for those categories which apply
    (see QUESTION 16), show CARD 1, use the categories ([X] - [T])
    specified and allow for only <u>one</u> *actor*

		does not apply	
Policy and strategic planning	....	-8	[1-2]
Services offered	....	-8	[1-2]
Service delivery performance	....	-8	[1-2]
AIDS programmes	....	-8	[1-2]
Organization and mode of service delivery	....	-8	[1-2]
Major organizational changes	....	-8	[1-2]
External relations	....	-8	[1-2]
Clients	....	-8	[1-2]
Management meetings	....	-8	[1-2]
Professionals meetings	....	-8	[1-2]
Member meetings	....	-8	[1-2]
Budget proposals	....	-8	[1-2]
Budget approvals	....	-8	[1-2]
Statement of accounts (balance sheet)	....	-8	[1-2]
Major investment decisions	....	-8	[1-2]
Daily financial transactions	....	-8	[1-2]
Paid personnel	....	-8	[1-2]
Volunteers	....	-8	[1-2]
Job profiles	....	-8	[1-2]
Internal norms and sanctions	....	-8	[1-2]
Research	....	-8	[1-2]

20. According to the statutes, are there areas of decision-making with respect
    to clients where the professionals within the organization have full
    discretion *vis-à-vis* the administrators regarding

	No	Yes	does not apply	
the range of services offered and programmes performed 2		1	-8	[1-2]
the AIDS programme(s) 2		1	-8	[1-2]
the organization and mode of service delivery 2		1	-8	[1-2]
the type of clients served 2		1	-8	[1-2]
Other 2		1	-8	[1-2]
(if yes, please specify)				
Other 1				[1-2]
Other 2				[1-2]

21. Who does actually participate with the decisive influence ("final say") on long-term and day-to-day actions of your organization in the following areas? *INTERVIEWER: Please ask only for those categories which apply (see QUESTION 16), show CARD 1 and allow for up to three of the most important categories of __internal__ actors ([X]- [H]) and up to three of the most important categories of __external__ actors ([I]- [T])*

	Internal ([X] - [H])	External ([I] - [T])	does not apply	
Policy and strategic planning	....	....	-8	[1-12]
Services offered	....	....	-8	[1-12]
Service delivery performance	....	....	-8	[1-12]
AIDS programmes	....	....	-8	[1-12]
Organization and mode of service delivery	....	....	-8	[1-12]
Major organizational changes	....	....	-8	[1-12]
External relations	....	....	-8	[1-12]
Clients	....	....	-8	[1-12]
Management meetings	....	....	-8	[1-12]
Professionals meetings	....	....	-8	[1-12]
Member meetings	....	....	-8	[1-12]
Budget proposals	....	....	-8	[1-12]
Budget approvals	....	....	-8	[1-12]
Statement of accounts (balance sheet)	....	....	-8	[1-12]
Major investment decisions	....	....	-8	[1-12]
Daily financial transactions	....	....	-8	[1-12]
Paid personnel	....	....	-8	[1-12]
Volunteers	....	....	-8	[1-12]
Job profiles	....	....	-8	[1-12]
Internal norms and sanctions	....	....	-8	[1-12]
Research	....	....	-8	[1-12]

22. Could you identify the groups that are involved in conflicts with each other in your organization, and who intermediates in those conflicts?
   ....

23. And do you identify any conflicts between your organization as a whole and other organizations, agencies, or groups in your relevant environment?
   ....

INTERVIEWER: PLEASE TRY TO TRANSLATE THE STORIES YOU HAVE
               HEARD IN THE FOLLOWING STANDARDISED FORM

Within the association (internal [(X) - (H)]):

between....   concerning....   mediated by

.... |...|....................
.... |...|....................

Between the organization as a whole and relevant environments
(external [(I) - (T)]):

between your   concerning....   mediated
organization and....   by

.... |...|....................
.... |...|....................

24. Are there areas of decision-making with respect to clients where the professionals
    and volunteers within the organization have *de facto* (regardless of formal statutes)
    full discretion *vis-à-vis* the administrators regarding:

	No	Yes	does not apply	
the range of services offered and programmes performed	2	1	-8	[1-2]
the AIDS programme(s)	2	1	-8	[1-2]
the organization and mode of service delivery	2	1	-8	[1-2]
the type of clients served	2	1	-8	[1-2]
Other	2	1	-8	[1-2]
(if yes, please specify)				
Other 1				[1-2]
Other 2				[1-2]

D. VOLUNTEERING, PROFESSIONALISM, LEADERSHIP

25. How many persons in each of the following categories are in your organization?
    *INTERVIEWER: When there are no persons in a specific category, please mark
    a Zero*

	male	female	
Executives and managers	....	....	[1-6]
Board members, elected functionaries and other officials	....	....	[1-6]
Employees	....	....	[1-6]
Volunteers	....	....	[1-6]
Professionals	....	....	[1-6]

26. How many persons in each of the following categories are in your organization?
INTERVIEWER: *When there are no persons in a specific category, please mark a Zero*

	Professionals*	Lay persons	
Paid Staff	....	....	[1-6]
Volunteers	....	....	[1-6]

*   Professionals = persons with an academic degree or a professional license (e.g nurses, social workers, etc.)

27. How many persons in each of the following categories are in your organization?
INTERVIEWER: When there are no persons in a specific category, please mark a Zero

	male	female	
as full-time paid employees	....	....	[1-6]
as part-time paid employees	....	....	[1-6]
as full-time volunteers	....	....	[1-6]
as part-time volunteers	....	....	[1-6]
as regular consultants on contracts	....	....	[1-6]

28. What was the total number of paid staff and volunteers, and the percentage related to HIV/AIDS units / services in the years listed below?
INTERVIEWER: Please record full-time equivalent paid staff and volunteers

	Paid Staff		Volunteers		does not apply	
	Full-time equivalent total number		Full-time equivalent total number			
1945	....		....		-8	[1-6]
1950	....		....		-8	[1-6]
1960	....		....		-8	[1-6]
1965	....		....		-8	[1-6]
1970	....		....		-8	[1-6]
1975	....		....		-8	[1-6]
1980	....	% HIV/AIDS	....	% HIV/AIDS	-8	[1-6]
1981	....	....	....	....	-8	[1-12]
1982	....	....	....	....	-8	[1-12]
1983	....	....	....	....	-8	[1-12]
1984	....	....	....	....	-8	[1-12]
1985	....	....	....	....	-8	[1-12]
1986	....	....	....	....	-8	[1-12]
1987	....	....	....	....	-8	[1-12]
1988	....	....	....	....	-8	[1-12]
1989	....	....	....	....	-8	[1-12]
1990	....	....	....	....	-8	[1-12]
1991	....	....	....	....	-8	[1-12]
1992	....	....	....	....	-8	[1-12]

29. Please fill in enclosed TABLE 1 on people working
    in AIDS service institutions/units

30. Are people working in the organization *personally* involved with the clients
    or issues at stake ?   [1-2]
    INTERVIEWER: Please allow for only <u>one</u>

almost nobody 1
a few 2
many 3
the majority 4
almost everybody 5
does not apply .... -8

31. Persons with AIDS/HIV sometimes organize themselves around self-help groups.
    Do these self-help groups play a significant role in your organization?   [1-2]

    No 2
    Yes 1

32. Please explain what kind of skills, backgrounds and orientations you look for when
    recruiting people for your organizations:
    ....

33. Are people working in the AIDS programmes / services / units generally recruited
    from within the overall organization or from outside?
    INTERVIEWER: *Please allow for only* <u>one</u>   [1-2]

    from within 1
    from outside 2
    does not apply .... -8

34. Is your organization unionized and/or covered by collective bargaining agreements
    between trade unions and employers organizations or other interlocutors?   [1-2]

    No 2
    Yes 1

35. Is there an elected staff representative (works counsellor or union representative)
    in your organization ?   [1-2]

    No 2
    Yes 1

36. How do average salary levels in your organization compare to those in the health and welfare system in your country in general ? [1-2]
    INTERVIEWER: Please allow for only one

    more than 30% above 7
    up to 30% above 6
    up to 15% above 5
    grosso modo comparable 4
    up to 15% below 3
    up to 30% below 2
    more than 30% below 1
    does not apply .... -8

37. What percentage of your volunteers receives some modest remuneration for the work done in your organization / unit (i.e. "paid unpaid")? [1-3]

    .... %
    does not apply .... -8

38. How many people in the *paid* staff left the organization in the past year? [1-3]

    ....employees
    does not apply .... -8

39. How many *volunteers* left the organization in the past year? [1-3]

    .... volunteers
    does not apply .... -8

40. Over the last three years, have there been changes or upgrading of occupational positions? [1-2]
    INTERVIEWER: Please allow for only one

    virtually none 1
    single 2
    several 3
    many 4
    the majority 5
    does not apply .... -8

E. ACTIVITIES: TASKS PROFILES AND CLIENTELE STRUCTURES

41. What are the goals and objectives of your organization concerning AIDS-management?
    ....
    ....

42. Are you active in the following domains regarding your HIV/AIDS programmes / services?
    INTERVIEWER: See CARD 2 for more specific descriptions of the types of services/activities

	No	Yes	
Prevention	2	1	[1-2]
Care and social services	2	1	[1-2]
Control/intelligence/surveillance/monitoring	2	1	[1-2]
Policy advocacy/interest organization/civil and human rights	2	1	[1-2]
Support activities	2	1	[1-2]

F. ACTIVITIES: WORK ORGANIZATION AND PROCESSES

43. Do those who carry out the core programme and service activities of your organization usually .....   [1-2]
    INTERVIEWER: Please allow for only one

    work in a team 1
    work individually 2
    work individually or alternating in a team 3

44. Are there specific professional methods or "techniques" used in your core programme and service activities?
    If yes, please specify which methods:

	No	Yes	does not apply	
Medical	2	1	-8	[1-2]
Psychological/psychotherapeutical	2	1	-8	[1-2]
Legal	2	1	-8	[1-2]
Social work	2	1	-8	[1-2]
Nursing	2	1	-8	[1-2]
Research	2	1	-8	[1-2]
Educational, didactic, pedagogic	2	1	-8	[1-2]
Public Relations	2	1	-8	[1-2]
Other	2	1	-8	[1-2]
If yes, please specify				

45. Is the organization as a whole accountable to outside institutions?   [1-2]

    No .... 2 —> *Go to 46*
    Yes .... 1 —> *Go to 45a*

    45a. Please specify which one(s) and in which way: ....
        ....

46. What are your daily *open (office) hours* during any given week, i.e., when can clients get in touch with you?
    INTERVIEWER: Please specify from what time to what time; when there are no open hours on a specific day, please mark a Zero

    Monday .... [1-24]
    Tuesday .... [1-24]
    Wednesday .... [1-24]
    Thursday .... [1-24]
    Friday .... [1-24]
    Saturday... [1-24]
    Sunday .... [1-24]

47. Is any work regulated by means of legal, contractual or collective bargaining in your organization?   [1-2]

    No .... 2 —> *Go to 60*
    Yes .... 1 —> *Go to 48*

48. When describing the core programme and service activities of your organization, which of the following statements characterises the every day working procedures?   [1-2]
    INTERVIEWER: Please allow for only <u>one</u>

    Most people do the same work every day in the same way 1
    Everybody has a precisely defined task to perform 2
    Most of the tasks generate new challenges 3
    Every day there are other things to do 4
    Nobody ever knows what her/his task will be the next day 5
    It is generally well known how a task has to be performed
    and single problem cases are to be resolved 6

49. What are your daily *hours of operation* during any given week?
    INTERVIEWER: Please specify from what time to what time; when there are no hours of operation on a specific day, please mark a Zero

    Monday .... [1-16]
    Tuesday .... [1-16]
    Wednesday .... [1-16]
    Thursday .... [1-16]
    Friday .... [1-16]
    Saturday... [1-16]
    Sunday .... [1-16]

50. Is overtime a regular occurrence in your organization/unit?   [1-2]

    No 2
    Yes 1

51. Is overtime normally foreseen or not?   [1-2]

    No 2
    Yes 1

52. Is there regular night or shift work?   [1-2]

    No 2
    Yes 1

53. Are there frequent emergencies?   [1-2]

    No .... 2 —> *Go to 54*
    Yes .... 1 —> *Go to 53a*

    53a. What categories of people working in the organization are most affected?
    ....

54. Are there other working time-related specificities (such as seasonal cycles)
    in your organization?   [1-2]

    No .... 2 —> *Go to 55*
    Yes .... 1 —> *Go to 54a*

    54a. Please specify which one(s): ....

55. Do those who carry out the core programme and service activities of your
    organization deal primarily .....
    INTERVIEWER: Please allow for only <u>*one*</u>   [1-2]

    with information, data, documents, files etc. ("paper work")............................... 1
    with persons ("communication")
        who are clients 2
        who are other professionals 3
        who are from other institutions and who are not professionals 4

56. What do you think is the level of burnout among the following groups of people
    in your organization?
    INTERVIEWER: Please allow for only <u>*one*</u> *number in the scale*

	Very low				Very high	Does not apply	
Employees	1	2	3	4	5	-8	[1-2]
Volunteers	1	2	3	4	5	-8	[1-2]
Professionals	1	2	3	4	5	-8	[1-2]

57. AIDS is a disease normally associated with stigmatized groups in society. How important do you think this factor is for the level of burnout among your organization's workers?   [1-2]
INTERVIEWER: Please allow for only <u>one</u> number in the scale

Not at all important		Sometimes		Very important
1	2	3	4	5

58. Does it occur that *paid staff* does not show up for work?   [1-2]
INTERVIEWER: Please allow for only <u>one</u> number in the scale

Not at all				Very frequently	does not apply
1	2	3	4	5	-8

58a. If it is frequent (4 or 5), how would you explain this?
....

59. Does it occur that *volunteers* do not show up for work?   [1-2]
INTERVIEWER: Please allow for only <u>one</u> number in the scale

Not at all				Very frequently	does not apply
1	2	3	4	5	-8

59a. If it is frequent (4 or 5), how would you explain this?
....

60. Does your organization carry out personal services?   [1-2]

No .... 2 —> *Go to 65*
Yes .... 1 —> *Go to 61*

61. Do clients have to face waiting periods for services?   [1-2]
INTERVIEWER: Please allow for only <u>one</u>

Yes, always .... 3 —> *Go to 61a*
Yes, sometimes, occasionally .... 2 —> *Go to 61a*
No, never .... 1 —> *Go to 62*

61a. For what services do they have to wait longest and how long on average?
INTERVIEWER: See list of services on CARD 2, use the codes specified in CARD 2 and do not allow for more than <u>three</u> services

type of service	average waiting time in days	
1.	....	[1-6]
2.	....	[1-6]
3.	....	[1-6]

62. Are clients served by single task forces usually passed on to other task forces ?

	Yes	No	
not at all passed on	1 (—> 63)	2 (—> 62)	[1-2]
within your organization/unit	1	2	[1-2]
to other AIDS-service institutions	1	2	[1-2]

    (if yes, please specify to which one(s))

    ....

| to hospitals | 1 | 2 | [1-2] |
| to other institutions | 1 | 2 | [1-2] |

    (if yes, please specify to which one(s))

    ....

| to the family | 1 | 2 | [1-2] |

63. Are there mechanisms to monitor and assess the quality of professional work
    and services?   [1-2]

No .... 2 —> *Go to 64*
Yes .... 1 —> *Go to 63a*

63a. Please specify which one(s):

	No	Yes	
Internal quality control circles	2	1	[1-2]
Monitoring by external professional experts	2	1	[1-2]
Other external monitoring and quality control bodies	2	1	[1-2]

64. Are there any institutional devices to support and supervise professionals
    in their daily work and service delivery?

	No	Yes	
internal psychological / psychotherapeutical supervision	2	1	[1-2]
external psychological / psychotherapeutical supervision	2	1	[1-2]
instruction and occupational training	2	1	[1-2]

G. ACTIVITIES: OUTPUT / SERVICE STATISTICS AND PERFORMANCE INDICATORS

65. Which of the following programme and service activities does your organization /
    unit provide regarding HIV/AIDS?
    INTERVIEWER: Please hand out CARD 2 to your contact person and ask him/her
    whether the organization provides any of the following services at all.
    For follow-up questions on services actually provided, please use the following
    TABLE 2 and CARD 3 for coding.

66. How is the organizational effort (i.e., time, money, staff) apportioned to the following types of HIV/AIDS activities?
INTERVIEWER: See CARD 2 for more specific descriptions of the types of services/activities. If one or more of the following types of services/activities are not existent, please mark a Zero.

Prevention .... %	[1-3]
Care and social services .... %	[1-3]
Control/intelligence/surveillance/monitoring .... %	[1-3]
Policy advocacy/interest organization/civil and human rights .... %	[1-3]
Support activities .... %	[1-3]
100%	

67. How is the organizational effort (i.e., time, money, staff) apportioned to the following types of services?
INTERVIEWER: See CARD 3 for more specific descriptions of the types of services. If one or more of the following types of services are not existent, please mark a Zero.

Monopolistic and authoritative services .... %	[1-3]
Public and citizenship services .... %	[1-3]
Categoric services .... %	[1-3]
Membership services .... %	[1-3]
Private services .... %	[1-3]
Solidaristic/communitarian/self-help action .... %	[1-3]
100%	

68. With regard to the geographical area in which you are active, how large do you estimate your target groups to be?
When applicable, what is the percentage of persons in the categories listed below, who do you think you serve or reach with your programmes and/or services?
(E.g., if in the given geographical scope of an organization there are 2000 hemophiliacs (=100%) and the organization reaches 200 of them, then "10%" should be filled in.)
INTERVIEWER: If one or more of the following groups are not covered at all, please mark a Zero. If the interviewed person is not able to estimate the size of the target group and/or does not know the percentage of people covered within a specific target group, please mark a -7 (minus 7).

	Estimated size of target groups (absolute numbers)	Percentage of persons served/reached	
Bisexual men	....	....	[1-10]
Blood donors and recipients	....	....	[1-10]
Blood processing industry / institutions	....	....	[1-10]
Children with AIDS	....	....	[1-10]
Children with parents who have AIDS or are in a high-risk AIDS group	....	....	[1-10]
Ethnic/racial minorities	....	....	[1-10]

Families of HIV-infected persons and
    of persons with AIDS   ....   [1-10]
Gay men   ....   [1-10]
Health care professionals   ....   [1-10]
Hemophiliacs   ....   [1-10]
HIV-infected persons   ....   [1-10]
Travellers   ....   [1-10]
Intravenous (IV) drug users   ....   [1-10]
Military   ....   [1-10]
Persons with AIDS   ....   [1-10]
Prisoners   ....   [1-10]
Male prostitutes and their clients ....   [1-10]
Female prostitutes and their clients ....   [1-10]
Public in general   ....   [1-10]
Sex tourists   ....   [1-10]
Street children and runaway youth ....   [1-10]
Terminally-ill persons with AIDS   ....   [1-10]
Women in general   ....   [1-10]
Young people in general   ....   [1-10]
Other   ....   [1-10]
      Please specify ....

69. If ethnic/racial minorities were mentioned, please specify which ones:
    ....

70. How do you think is the image of the overall performance of your organization/unit ?

	"excellent" "first-rate"	"good" "solid" "convincing"	"adequate" "satisfying"	"problematic" "to be improved"	"deficient" "useless"	
as seen by yourself	5	4	3	2	1	[1-2]
by your clients/target groups	5	4	3	2	1	[1-2]
by the public at large	5	4	3	2	1	[1-2]
by the political environment	5	4	3	2	1	[1-2]
by the media	5	4	3	2	1	[1-2]

H. MEMBERSHIP STRUCTURES

71. Is your organization a *membership* organization?   [1-2]

No .... 2 —> *Go to 86*
Yes.. 1 —> *Go to 72*

72. How many members does your organization have (1992)? ....   [1-4]

73. How many members did your organization have at the end of the years listed below?

does not apply

Members 1991 .... -8	[1-4]
Members 1990 .... -8	[1-4]
Members 1989 .... -8	[1-4]
Members 1988 .... -8	[1-4]
Members 1987 .... -8	[1-4]
Members 1986 .... -8	[1-4]
Members 1985 .... -8	[1-4]
Members 1984 .... -8	[1-4]
Members 1983 .... -8	[1-4]
Members 1982 .... -8	[1-4]
Members 1981 .... -8	[1-4]
Members 1980 .... -8	[1-4]
Members 1975 .... -8	[1-4]
Members 1970 .... -8	[1-4]
Members 1965 .... -8	[1-4]
Members 1960 .... -8	[1-4]
Members 1950 .... -8	[1-4]
Members 1945 .... -8	[1-4]

74. How many members left the organization in 1991?

Number .... [1-4]

75. How many new members entered the organization in 1991?

Number .... [1-4]

76. What is the number of theoretical possible members (i.e. people who could
profit from the activities your organization provides)   [1-9]

.... potential members
.... no information

77. What percentage of your members in 1992 is constituted by

clients .... %   [1-3]
volunteers/activists .... %   [1-3]
other individual members .... %   [1-3]
other organizations as members .... %   [1-3]
100%

78. What formal membership categories do your statutes or constitution contain?
Please specify: ....
....

79. How are member's dues formally assessed?
    INTERVIEWER: Please allow for only <u>one</u>   [1-2]

    as a fixed flat rate 1
    according to membership categories 2
    by member's income (sliding scales) 3
    on a voluntary basis of the members 4
    by other criteria 5
         (please specify) ....
    there is no membership fee 6

80. What is the maximum, average, and minimum fee actually paid?
    INTERVIEWER: Please specify currency

                                                                    does not apply

    minimum fee .... -8   [1-9]
    average fee .... -8   [1-9]
    maximum fee .... -8   [1-9]

81. Has membership to be renewed at all?   [1-2]

    No .... 2 —> *Go to 82*
·   Yes.. 1 —> *Go to 81a*

    81a. What percentage of your members is covered by an automatised routine dues
         collection system (through the employer, the banking system, the state, etc.)
         which relieves the single member from the re-subscription initiative ?

                                                  .... %   [1-3]

82. Are there any services you deliver to members exclusively or any policies pursued
    which are of crucial importance to your member's interest?   [1-2]

    No .... 2 —> *Go to 83*
    Yes.. 1 —> *Go to 82a and 82b*

    82a. Please specify which one(s)
         *INTERVIEWER: Please use CARD 2, use the codes (1-100) and do not allow
         for more than <u>five</u> types of services/policy advocacy*

                                          1. ....   [1-3]
                                          2. ....   [1-3]
                                          3. ....   [1-3]
                                          4. ....   [1-3]
                                          5. ....   [1-3]

    82b. Why are you providing these services/policy advocacy to members only?
         Please specify the reasons: ....
         ....

83. More general, could you try to explain why you are organized as a membership organization?

Are the reasons mainly .....

	Yes	No	
traditional/historical	1	2	[1-2]
legal obligations	1	2	[1-2]
the service commitment to your members	1	2	[1-2]
the special confidentiality required in the relationship with your members	1	2	[1-2]
membership dues as a main and stable source of organizational income	1	2	[1-2]
the political, ideological, spiritual, community, etc. affinity with your members	1	2	[1-2]
the chances for volunteer/activist recruitment to gain public recognition, status and legitimating as an interest representative	1	2	[1-2]
the capacity for political mobilization	1	2	[1-2]
the availability of financial and other public resources	1	2	[1-2]
the non-availability of financial and other public resources	1	2	[1-2]
other..	1	2	[1-2]

    (if yes, please specify)

....

84. Please name up to three of the most important other voluntary organizations of which many or most of your own members are also members:

1. .... [1-6]
2. .... [1-6]
3. .... [1-6]

85. We would like to know whether your organization is, generally speaking, rather open or restrictive with respect to new members?

	Yes	No	
Do you actively seek for new members? 1		2	[1-2]
Do you wait for new members to join? 1		2	[1-2]
Do you accept all applicants as new members?........... 1 (—> 86)		2 (—> 85a)	[1-2]

  85a. If *you do not accept all applicants as new members*, whom do you exclude and why?

....

I. INPUT AND ALLOCATION OF RESOURCES

86. What is the organization's budget (in thousands) for 1992?   [1-12]

                                        .... in national currency

(please write out the amount:)

87. What was the organization's budget (in thousands) in the years listed below,
    along with the percentage devoted to AIDS programmes?
    INTERVIEWER: Please specify currency

	Total	does not apply	% HIV/AIDS (for exclusives = 100%)	does not apply	
1991	....	-8	....	-8	[1-15]
1990	....	-8	....	-8	[1-15]
1989	....	-8	....	-8	[1-15]
1988	....	-8	....	-8	[1-15]
1987	....	-8	....	-8	[1-15]
1986	....	-8	....	-8	[1-15]
1985	....	-8	....	-8	[1-15]
1984	....	-8	....	-8	[1-15]
1983	....	-8	....	-8	[1-15]
1982	....	-8	....	-8	[1-15]
1981	....	-8	....	-8	[1-15]
1980	....	-8		-8	[1-12]
1975	....	-8		-8	[1-12]
1970	....	-8		-8	[1-12]
1965	....	-8		-8	[1-12]
1960	....	-8		-8	[1-12]
1950	....	-8		-8	[1-12]
1945	....	-8		-8	[1-12]

88. Does your organization have a certified annual financial statement?   [1-2]

   No ....2 —> *Go to 89*
   Yes ....1 —> *Ask for a copy of the annual
                                                             financial statement for each of the
                                                             years checked in QUESTION 87.*

89. What percentage of your organization's funds devoted to HIV/AIDS comes from each of the following sources?
    INTERVIEWER: "EXCLUSIVES" will continue to complete the revenue for the organization as a whole; "INCLUSIVES" will start to refer to HIV/AIDS programmes / services / units only and not any longer to the organization as a whole. If there is any source(s) of funds which does not apply, please mark a Zero.

A)	Public/governmental/international payments	.... %	[1-3]
B)	Voluntary sector contributions	.... %	[1-3]
C)	Corporate funding and income	.... %	[1-3]
D)	Household (individual and family) payments	.... %	[1-3]
E)	Service fees, commercial sales and royalties	.... %	[1-3]
		.... 100%	

A) Public/governmental/international payments   .... %
   (e.g., lump sum grants, matching grants, subsidies, etc.)

   from central (federal, national) government   .... %   [1-3]
   from regional governments   .... %   [1-3]
   from local (municipal) authorities, communes   .... %   [1-3]
   from para-state social security administration   .... %   [1-3]
   from international, intergovernmental institutions
       e.g., UN, UNDP, UNFPA, UNICEF, UNESCO,
       WHO, WHO-Euro, European Community   .... %   [1-3]
                                                        .... 100%

B) Voluntary sector contributions   .... %
   (e.g., transfers, philanthropic donations,
   membership fees, sponsorship, grants, etc.)

   from parent and affiliated organizations   .... %   [1-3]
   from other voluntary organizations including
   international non-governmental bodies   .... %   [1-3]
   from foundations and charitable trusts   .... %   [1-3]
   from churches and religious organizations   .... %   [1-3]
   from political and interest organizations   .... %   [1-3]
   from pooled funds from joint fund raising   .... %   [1-3]
   other   .... %   [1-3]
       (please specify) 100%

C) Corporate funding and income   .... %

   from corporate donations   .... %   [1-3]
   from membership fees   .... %   [1-3]
   from returns on investments and rents, interests etc. .... %   [1-3]
                                                        .... 100%

D) Household (individual and family) payments .... %

    membership fees and subscriptions .... % [1-3]
    personal donations, bequests and legacies .... % [1-3]
    .... 100%

E) Service fees, commercial sales and royalties .... %

    from individuals, families, private households .... % [1-3]
        (without public insurance coverage, including
        private insurance reimbursements)
    from corporations .... % [1-3]
    from voluntary organizations .... % [1-3]
    from public institutions .... % [1-3]
        (reimbursements for case related payments)
    .... 100%

90. Which *three* of the preceding five possible sources of funds (inside the frame in QUESTION 89) do you think are becoming increasingly important for the organization?
INTERVIEWER: Please use the codes A - E.

        1. .... [1-2]
        2. .... [1-2]
        3. .... [1-2]

91. Does your organization have regular free access to resources from other institutions for its HIV/AIDS services (e.g. access to premises, services from other organizations, exemptions from charges, transfers in kind, etc.)? [1-2]

    No .... 2 —> *Go to 92*
    Yes .... 1 —> *Go to 91a and 91b*

    91a. Please specify of which kind: ....
    ....

    91b. Please estimate its/their value in thousands (in national currency): .... [1-12]
    ....

92. Does the tax status of your organization differ from that of other voluntary organizations in your country? [1-2]

    No .... 2 —> *Go to 93*
    Yes .... 1 —> *Go to 92a*

    92a. Is your tax status generally higher or lower? [1-2]

        Higher 2
        Lower 1

93. Are there any overall savings through tax privileges and other fiscal benefits: such as tax exemptions, reduced (e.g., postal) charges, special loans and guarantees, import privileges, etc. [1-2]

    No .... 2 —> *Go to 94*
    Yes .... 1 —> *Go to 93a and 93b*

    93a. Please specify: ....

    93b. Estimate, if possible, the value of savings in per cent:
    .... % [1-3]

94. As an HIV/AIDS service institution, does your organization have special authorization delegated from the state or other public authorities (e.g. to screen, test, diagnose, control, monitor, coordinate, etc.)? [1-2]

    No .... 2 —> *Go to 95*
    Yes .... 1 —> *Go to 94a and 94b*

    94a. Please specify of which kind: ....

    94b. Is any of these delegated authorizations exclusively granted to your organization? [1-2]

    No .... 2 —> *Go to 95*
    Yes .... 1 —> *Go to 94c*

    94c. Please specify which one(s): ....

95. How many persons working in your organization are seconded by (on the payrolls of) other institutions ?

    .... seconded persons [1-2]

    95a. If any, from which institutions?

	Yes	No	
Governmental, public agency	1	2	[1-2]
Private firm, enterprise, company	1	2	[1-2]
Non-profit, voluntary organization	1	2	[1-2]

96. Is your organization entitled to special public secondments – e.g., through civil service or unemployment insurance schemes ("*Zivildiener*" / "substitutory social service", "employed unemployed", "stage" / "internship" / "*Praktikum*", "workfare", etc.)? [1-2]

    No .... 2 —> *Go to 97*
    Yes .... 1 —> *Go to 96a*

96a. How many persons working in your organization does it concern?

.... seconded persons   [1-2]

97. In general, what are your three most important public or private patrons / donors / sponsors / funders?

For EXCLUSIVES and INCLUSIVES: for the organization as a whole

1. ....   [1-6]
2. ....   [1-6]
3. ....   [1-6]

For INCLUSIVES: HIV/AIDS programmes / services / units only
1. ....   [1-6]
2. ....   [1-6]
3. ....   [1-6]

98. How many square metres does your organization have available for administration and service provision related to HIV/AIDS?

.... square metres   [1-4]

99. How many rooms does your organization have available for administration and service provision related to HIV/AIDS?

.... rooms   [1-2]

99a. Of which are rooms for administrative purposes   .... rooms   [1-2]

99b. Of which are rooms for service provision purposes   .... rooms   [1-2]

100. Does your organization have any of the following equipments in use in the HIV/AIDS area?

	Yes	No	
Library and/or documentation room	1	2	[1-2]
Facsimile machine (TELEFAX)	1	2	[1-2]
Telex	1	2	[1-2]
Photocopying machine	1	2	[1-2]
Audiovisual equipment	1	2	[1-2]
Special medical equipment	1	2	[1-2]
Car or transport facilities	1	2	[1-2]

101. Do you have computers?   [1-2]

No .... 2 —> *Go to 102*
Yes .... 1 —> *Go to 101a - 101f*

101a. Are computer facilities used in the following areas relating
to HIV/AIDS activities?

	Yes	No	
Administration and organization.......................... 1		2	[1-2]
Individual client records 1		2	[1-2]
Access to external data banks 1		2	[1-2]
Counselling by information system support 1		2	[1-2]
Other 1		2	[1-2]
(if yes, please specify)			

101b. Do you have or are you linked up to a main-frame computer?   [1-2]

No 2
Yes 1

101c. How many PCs do you have?   [1-2]

.... PCs

101d. Are your PCs linked up in a network?   [1-2]

No 2
Yes 1

101e. Do you have regular access to specialised Data Banks?   [1-2]

No 2
Yes 1
If yes, to which one(s)? ....

101f. Do you use electronic mail (e.g., BITNET, DATEX-P)?   [1-2]

No 2
Yes 1

102. Do you have hospice facilities for HIV/AIDS-related services?   [1-2]

No .... 2 —> *Go to 103*
Yes .... 1 —> *Go to 102a and 102b*

102a. How many residential housing units do you have?

.... residential housing units   [1-3]

102b. What is your occupancy rate in general?

.... %   [1-3]

103. Do you have beds for HIV/AIDS-related services?   [1-2]

    No .... 2 —> *Go to 104*
    Yes .... 1 —> *Go to 103a and 103b*

    103a. How many beds do you have?

                                            .... beds   [1-3]

    103b. What is your occupancy rate in general?

                                           .... %   [1-3]

104. In your organization, what percentage of total expenses for the *HIV/AIDS-related activities* was devoted to following categories?

		does not apply	
Personnel Costs .... %		-8	[1-3]
= Staff Expenses for Employees .... %		-8	[1-3]
= Non-Staff Expenses (Regular Consultants on Contracts, Free-Lancers, Remuneration for Officials and Volunteers, Fees for Professional Services etc.) .... %		-8	[1-3]
100%			
Overhead (Office and Operating Expenses) .... %		-8	[1-3]
Direct Programme and Service Delivery Costs .... %		-8	[1-3]
100%			

105. How is the organizational effort (i.e., time, money, staff) apportioned to the following activities?

		does not apply	
Professional Programme and Service Activities .... %		-8	[1-3]
(Internal) Organization and Administration .... %		-8	[1-3]
(External) Relations to secure Associational Existence and Maintenance .... %		-8	[1-3]
Membership Recruitment (for membership organizations only !) .... %		-8	[1-3]
100%			

106. Which of the following statements describes best the experience of your organization with grant applications for HIV/AIDS services? *INTERVIEWER: Please allow for only <u>one</u> statement!*   [1-2]

    Writing a grant proposal in order to get money for our HIV/AIDS services

        is impossible for us because we lack the expertise 1
        is far too much effort for the money we could possibly obtain 2
        distracts our scarce resources from actual service provision 3
        is just one additional administrative burden for us 4
        represents no major problem for our organization 5
        we never apply for grants 6

107. Would you refuse taking support from any source or of any kind?   [1-2]

    No .... 2 —> *Go to 108*
    Yes .... 1 —> *Go to 107a*

    107a. Please specify which ones and why:
        ....

J.   **INTERORGANIZATIONAL/INTERSECTORAL/INTERNATIONAL COOPERATION AND COMPETITION**

108. To which of the following types of organizations does your organization/unit keep regular contacts of some importance?
Please name up to three of the most important ones for each of them.
INTERVIEWER: If there is no contact to a specific type of organization, please mark a Zero

                                                            Number of
                                                         organizations

    Churches and religious organizations   ....   [1-2]
    - ....
    - ....

    Educational institutions   ....   [1-2]
    - ....
    - ....

    Funding organizations   ....   [1-2]
    - ....
    - ....

    Hospitals   ....   [1-2]
    - ....
    - ....

Interest organizations and professional organizations   .... [1-2]
- ....
- ....

International/Intergovernmental organizations (e.g., WHO)   .... [1-2]
- ....
- ....

Non-state social security administration   .... [1-2]
- ....
- ....

Other HIV/AIDS service institutions/units   .... [1-2]
- ....
- ....

(Other) civic, social action, advocacy and
popular-movement-related organizations   .... [1-2]
- ....
- ....

Other voluntary non-profit organizations   .... [1-2]
- ....
- ....

Peak organizations   .... [1-2]
- ....
- ....

Political parties   .... [1-2]
- ....
- ....

(Private) corporations (including private insurances)   .... [1-2]
- ....
- ....

Research and scientific organizations   .... [1-2]
- ....
- ....

Self-help groups and other primary social support systems   .... [1-2]
- ....
- ....

State/public agencies   .... [1-2]
- ....
- ....

Others   .... [1-2]

\-   ....

\-   ....

109. Of the aforementioned relationships with other organizations, please name the
      three most important partners of cooperation:

      1) ....

      2) ....

      3) ....

110. Please indicate the form, content and frequency of the three most important
      cooperative relationships just named in QUESTION 109
      *INTERVIEWER: Please indicate up to three categories concerning form
      and content of cooperation*

Organizations	Form of Cooperation	Content of Cooperation	Frequency of Cooperation
	1. Vertical integration	1. Exchange of experiences on programme and service activities	1. Several times a week
	2. Formal inclusion (= membership)	2. Control of programme and service activities	2. Once a week
	3. Interlocking executives= sharing of officials	3. Establishing joint task forces	3. Several times a month
	4. Staff sharing	4. Sharing/passing on clients	4. Once a month
	5. Sharing of financial resources in joint ventures	5. Exchange of information	5. Several times a year
	6. Strictly economic transactions	6. Buying and selling	6. Once a year
	7. Other (please specify)	7. Other (please specify)	7. Other (please specify)
1.	....	....	.... [1-7]
2.	....	....	.... [1-7]
3.	....	....	.... [1-7]

111. Could you please name the three most important institutions with which you
      disagree most profoundly regarding managing AIDS and HIV/AIDS policies?

      1). ....

      2). ....

      3). ....

112. Could you please name the three most important HIV/AIDS service institutions with which you share overlapping domains (regarding tasks, clients, territorial scope) and/or you candidate for the same funds:

   1). ....

   2). ....

   3). ....

K.   INSTITUTIONALISATION

INTERVIEWER: If the interviewed organization is a governmental, public agency (see QUESTION 2), please skip questions 113-116a and go to question 117.

113. Does your organization/unit provide statistical data or other documented information on clients (and/or members) to government bodies upon their request?   [1-2]

   No 2
   Yes 1
   does not apply .... -8

114. Does your organization/unit administer state grants, subsidies, HIV/AIDS policy programmes etc. on behalf of public authorities?   [1-2]

   No .... 2 —> *Go to 115*
   Yes .... 1 —> *Go to 114a*

   114a. Please specify which ones and why
   ....

115. How often a year does the organization maintain contacts of the following type with government bodies?

   Informal contacts with civil servants   .... times   [1-2]
   Formal consultation in drafting legislation and representation
         before Parliament and Parliamentary committees   .... times   [1-2]
   Contacts with Cabinet Ministers or groups of Cabinet Ministers   .... times   [1-2]
   Legally guaranteed consultations by public bodies
         on HIV/AIDS-related health and welfare policies   .... times   [1-2]
   Represented on public/semi-public bodies   .... times   [1-2]

116. Is there any state agency to which the organization monopolises certain contacts?   [1-2]

   No .... 2 —> *Go to 117*
   Yes .... 1 —> *Go to 116a*

   116a. Please specify which one(s)
   ....

117. How often do civil servants join the organization's/unit's staff or vice versa? [1-2]

    never 1
    rarely 2
    frequently 3

118. Do you have any systematic information about the demographic and
    socio-economic characteristics (gender, age, education, occupation, etc.)
    of your clientele? [1-2]

    No .... 2 —> *Go to 119*
    Yes .... 1 —> *Go to 118a*
    does not apply .... -8 —> *Go to 119*

    118a. Within this context, could you please provide us with any aggregate
        and structural (collective and strictly anonymous!!) data at your disposal?

119. Do you have any systematic information about the demographic and
    socio-economic characteristics (gender, age, education, occupation etc.)
    of your members? [1-2]

    No .... 2 —> *END*
    Yes .... 1 —> *Go to 119a*
    does not apply .... -8 —> *END*

    119a. Within this context, could you please provide us with any aggregate
        and structural (collective and strictly anonymous !!) data at your disposal?

* * * * *

List of Contributors

Danielle Bütschi, Researcher at the Department of Political Science of the University of Geneva

Sandro Cattacin, Researcher at the Department of Political Science of the University of Geneva

Hilde Degezelle, Researcher at the Department of Sociology of the Catholic University of Leuven

Emma Fasolo, Consultant for International Activities at LABOS, Foundation for Social Policy Studies, Rome

Patrick Kenis, Assistant Professor at the Department of Politics and Public Administration of the University of Constance, and Research Associate at the European Centre for Social Welfare Policy and Research, Vienna

Ineke Kester, Researcher at the Leyden Institute for Law & Public Policy, Leyden

Bernd Marin, Executive Director of the European Centre for Social Welfare Policy and Research, Vienna

Koen Matthijs, Professor at the Department of Sociology of the Catholic University of Leuven

Christiana Nöstlinger, Research Associate at the European Centre for Social Welfare Policy and Research, Vienna

Christine Panchaud, Researcher at the Department of Political Science of the University of Geneva

Victor A. Pestoff, Professor at the Department of Business Administration of the University of Stockholm, and engaged in The Modern Society Programme, Södertörns högskola, Huddinge, Sweden

Bert de Vroom, Researcher at the "Fakulteit der Bestuurskunde" (Faculty of Policy Research) of the University of Twente, The Netherlands

Dagmar von Walden Laing, Freelance Researcher in Täby, Sweden

Armand van Wolferen, Researcher at the Leyden Institute for Law & Public Policy, Leyden